# African Indigenous Medical Knowledge and Human Health

# African Indigenous Medical Knowledge and Human Health

Edited by
## Charles Wambebe
**Department of Pharmaceutical Sciences**
**Tshwane University of Technology**
**Pretoria, South Africa**

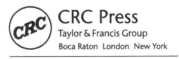

CRC Press
Taylor & Francis Group
Boca Raton London New York

CRC Press is an imprint of the
Taylor & Francis Group, an **informa** business

CRC Press
Taylor & Francis Group
6000 Broken Sound Parkway NW, Suite 300
Boca Raton, FL 33487-2742

First issued in paperback 2021

© 2018 by Taylor & Francis Group, LLC
CRC Press is an imprint of Taylor & Francis Group, an Informa business

No claim to original U.S. Government works

ISBN-13: 978-1-03-209580-6 (pbk)
ISBN-13: 978-1-138-03810-3 (hbk)

---

**Library of Congress Cataloging-in-Publication Data**

---

Names: Wambebe, Charles, author.
Title: African indigenous medical knowledge and human health / Charles Wambebe.
Description: Boca Raton : Taylor & Francis, 2018. | "A CRC title, part of the Taylor & Francis imprint, a member of the Taylor & Francis Group, the academic division of T&F Informa plc." | Includes bibliographical references.
Identifiers: LCCN 2017042029 | ISBN 9781138038103 (hardback : alk. paper)
Subjects: LCSH: Traditional medicine--Research--Africa. | Alternative medicine--Research--Africa.
Classification: LCC R651 .W36 2018 | DDC 610.7206--dc23
LC record available at https://lccn.loc.gov/2017042029

---

Visit the Taylor & Francis Web site at
http://www.taylorandfrancis.com

and the CRC Press Web site at
http://www.crcpress.com

# Contents

# Preface

A cardinal goal of health research is the development of new medicines, vaccines, and medical devices that when used properly are indispensable tools for both preventive and curative purposes. Another important goal of health research is the generation of credible data that can enhance quality of life through improved health systems and effective delivery of services. Furthermore, research data can be appropriately shared among relevant stakeholders and judiciously utilized to enlighten the public. Cumulative knowledge can become a valuable tool to guide policy makers *vis-à-vis* development of policies, regulations, strategies, and practices that will impact positively on the whole health system with multiplier effects on the socioeconomic status of the nation.

Interestingly, Africa is a continent that is richly endowed with abundant biodiversity. Sub-Saharan Africa and the Indian Ocean Islands have over 60,000 plant species (about one-quarter of the world's total). For many centuries until the advent of Western Medicine, African traditional medicine (ATM) was the only available source of health care. The preventive and curative secrets of African medicinal plants have been transferred orally from family to family and community to community.

According to the World Health Organization (WHO, 2002), approximately 80% of people living in developing countries use ATM. Undoubtedly, collaboration between traditional health practitioners and biomedical health practitioners may lead to improved primary health-care delivery both qualitatively and quantitatively. Chapter 1 provides a succinct overview of traditional medicine in Africa, including the significant development of traditional medicine in various countries in Africa.

Chapters 2 and 3 discuss the critical issues of intellectual property rights and access to genetic resources. In sub-Saharan Africa, these two issues constitute serious challenges to both traditional and biomedical health practitioners. The recommendations contained in these chapters aptly address these issues.

In spite of the relevance and empirical evidence of ATM, research and development of new phytomedicines is slow. Only 83 of the world's 1,100 leading commercial medicinal plants are African in origin. Africa is only a minor player in the global natural products market. This situation may be attributed to poverty and lack of political will. Furthermore, the disease-endemic countries lack the capacity to invest adequately in the research and development of new medical interventions. In addition, there is the gap on appropriate technologies that can be used when research funds are highly limited. Chapter 4 addresses this gap. Thus, poverty-related diseases continue to ravage Africans with devastating impact on the quality of life and socioeconomic development of African countries. It is a vicious cycle of poverty and diseases.

This gloomy situation notwithstanding, in the health sector, investing in the development of ATM may yield lifesaving new medicines of global public health impact. Chapters 4–7 provide evidence of medical products developed through African indigenous medical knowledge. A viable approach for successful research and development of medicines from African medicinal plants based on ATM is "reverse pharmacology" or "clinical observational study." When this approach is utilized, it leads to 100% corroboration between the claims of traditional health practitioners and biomedical evidence. This text deals with the principles and practical examples of a reverse pharmacology approach in the research and development of phytomedicines.

Due to limited financial resources to support research and infrastructure resulting from lack of private sector investment, value addition is generally limited while quality of products cannot be guaranteed. Human resources who can participate at all levels of research and development of medical interventions are usually not located at a single institution. Unfortunately, intra-institutional collaborations are few. The WHO Regional Office for Africa has developed many technical documents to guide member states on the research and development of herbal medicines. The West African Health Organization has developed an *Herbal Pharmacopoeia* for the subregion.

Chapter 8 provides key elements regarding the way forward and provision of an enabling environment for ATM. The concluding sentences encapsulate the key recommendation: "The upsurge of herbal medicines in Africa has bright prospects, but the pace of its development can be accelerated with promotional plans and government funding for research and development, continuous education of the practitioners, support for the local production of herbal medicines of proven efficacy and establishment of enforceable regulatory framework—the key decisions to drive the sector will have to come from the countries."

Globally, the development of new interventions for diagnosis, prevention, and treatment has witnessed an upsurge due to recent advances in science, technology, and innovation. However, Africa has not been able to participate as a functional partner in generating new knowledge and does not have the capacity and political commitment to capitalize on this exciting development. Due to disparities in economic strength, political will, and scientific resources and capabilities, Africa has lagged behind in innovations and discoveries. Indeed, it has been suggested that health investments yield the highest rates of return compared to other public investments. The benefits of health research are apparent *vis-à-vis* development and subsequent availability of more accurate diagnostic tools and new, more effective, and safer medicines and vaccines. Such new products and devices are indispensable against prevailing diseases and specific interventions leading to more comprehensive preventive measures. Subsequently, the resultant improvements in health will translate into substantial benefits for the economy including an increase in productivity, a better trained labor force, a more competitive economy, more solid enterprises, lower unemployment, among others. This text intends to serve as a catalyst for health innovations based on African biodiversity and Africa indigenous medical knowledge. Furthermore, it serves as a reference for pharmacognosists, ethnobiologists, botanists, phytochemists, pharmacologists, and all medical scientists and industries interested in the research and development of medical interventions based on African indigenous medical knowledge.

**Charles Wambebe**
*Professor of Pharmacology*
*TWAS Laureate in Medical Sciences*

# Acknowledgments

My sincere appreciation to Dr. Edith Madela-Mntia, who was the Director, International Council for Science, Regional Office for Africa until 2016, for initiating this book project. My colleague, Professor Philippe Rasoanaivo worked with me initially to agree on the chapters and potential authors. Unfortunately, he died unexpectedly. He was very humble, a highly accomplished scientist, and totally committed to science. He contributed to two chapters in this text. Although he has left us, his scientific contributions and personality will continue to speak for him. May his soul rest in perfect peace with the Lord. Furthermore, I acknowledge the ICSU Regional Office for Africa, especially Drs. Richard Glover and Daniel Nyanganyura, for their support and understanding throughout the preparation of this book.

# Editor

**Professor Charles Wambebe** obtained his PhD in Neuropharmacology from Ahmadu Bello University in 1979. He served briefly at Georgetown University Medical Center as Visiting Professor of Pharmacology and worked with the World Health Organization. He was a consultant in traditional medicine to the United Nations Development Programme, the United Nations Industrial Development Organization, the African Union, the Economic Community for Africa, and the African Development Bank. Professor Wambebe was the Pioneer Pro-Chancellor and Chairman of Council, Bingham University. His initial research focus was on the physiological roles of dopamine in the brain. He also published research articles on the neuropharmacological effects of plant extracts. Upon his appointment as Pioneer Director-General/CEO of the National Institute for Pharmaceutical Research and Development (NIPRD), Abuja, Nigeria, he switched his research interest to development of phytomedicines based on African indigenous medical knowledge. During his tenure at NIPRD, he initiated and directed the research and development of Niprisan; a standardized phytomedicine for the prophylactic management of sickle cell disorder. It was groundbreaking research that earned Wambebe the World Academy of Science Award in Medical Sciences (TWAS). Niprisan is generally regarded as clinically safe and effective. In recognition of his academic achievements, Wambebe was elected Fellow of TWAS, African Academy of Sciences, and Nigerian Academy of Science. Professor Wambebe has published over 150 peer-reviewed articles in international journals and contributed chapters to books. His current research interests involve development of phytomedicines from African indigenous medical knowledge using African food plants. Professor Wambebe is currently serving as Professor Extra-Ordinary (Pharmacology) at Tswane University of Technology, Pretoria, and Witwatersrand University, Johannesburg, South Africa.

# Contributors

**Lucile Allorge-Boiteau**
Institut Malgache de Recherches
　　Appliquées
Antananarivo, Madagascar

**Gerard Bodeker**
Department of Primary Care Health
　　Sciences
University of Oxford
Oxford, United Kingdom

and

Department of Epidemiology
Columbia University
New York, New York

**Kofi Busia**
Primary Health Care
West African Health Organization
Bobo-Dioulasso, Burkina Faso

**Robert Byamukama**
Department of Chemistry
Makerere University
Kampala, Uganda

**Abayneh Desta**
World Health Organization
African Regional Office
Brazzaville, Republic of Congo

**Drissa Diallo**
Department of Traditional Medicine
Bamako, Mali

**Sunita Facknath**
University of Mauritius
Moka, Mauritius

**Bertrand Graz**
Fondation Antennan
Geneva, Switzerland

**Fei Jiao**
Traditional Knowledge Division
World Intellectual Property Organization
Geneva, Switzerland

**Ossy MJ Kasilo**
World Health Organization
African Regional Office
Brazzaville, Republic of Congo

**David R. Katerere**
Tshwane University of Technology
Pretoria, South Africa

**Vinany Loharanombato**
Laboratoire de Phanérogamie
Muséum National d'Histoire Naturelle
Paris, France

**Alain Loiseau**
Institut Malgache de Recherches
　　Appliquées
Antananarivo, Madagascar

**André Lona**
World Health Organization
African Regional Office
Brazzaville, Republic of Congo

**Jean-Baptiste Nikiema**
World Health Organization
African Regional Office
Brazzaville, Republic of Congo

**Philippe Rasoanaivo**
Institut Malgache de Recherches
　　Appliquées
Antananarivo, Madagascar

**Yahaya Sekagya**
PROMETRA
Kampala, Uganda

**Charlotte I.E.A. van't Klooster**
Amsterdam Institute for Social Science
  Research
University of Amsterdam
Amsterdam, The Netherlands

**Emma Weisbord**
Department of Primary Care Health
  Sciences
University of Oxford
Oxford, United Kingdom

**Wend Wendland**
Traditional Knowledge Division
World Intellectual Property
  Organization
Geneva, Switzerland

**Merlin Wilcox**
Department of Primary Care Health
  Sciences
University of Oxford
Oxford, United Kingdom

# CHAPTER 1

# Traditional Medicine Situation in Africa
## *Where Are We?*

Ossy MJ Kasilo, Jean-Baptiste Nikiema, Abayneh Desta, and André Lona

## CONTENTS

## 1.1 INTRODUCTION

The World Health Organization (WHO) defines *traditional medicine* as the sum total of the knowledge, skills, and practices based on the theories, beliefs, and experiences indigenous to different cultures, whether explicable or not, used in the maintenance of health as well as in the prevention, diagnosis, improvement, or treatment of physical and mental illness (http://www.who.int/medicines/areas/traditional/definitionsen/index.html; WHO, 2002:7). It is composed of therapeutic practices in existence for hundreds of years, before the development of modern medicine.

Many products based on traditional medical knowledge (TMK) are important sources of income, food, and health care for many inhabitants of developing countries. Traditional medicine plays an important role in health care in both developed and developing countries. In fact, due to their availability and affordability, the traditional medicines and therapy systems of the developing countries provide health care to the vast majority of these countries' populations. Before the establishment of conventional medicine (also referred to as modern, Western, and/or orthodox medicine), traditional medicine was the dominant health system for millions of people in Africa, but the arrival of the Europeans led to a noticeable turning point in the history of this ancient tradition and culture (Abdullahi, 2011:116).

Herbal medicine and essential oils are the most popularly used forms of traditional, complementary, and alternative medication therapy worldwide. However, in some countries, other natural products such as animal, mineral, or other materials may also be used. Therefore, in all cases, regulations should be specifically articulated to address each country's unique situation (WHO, 2004). By definition, the "traditional" use of herbal medicines implies substantial historical use, and this is certainly true for many products that are available as "traditional herbal medicines."

In many low- and middle-income countries, a large proportion of the population relies on traditional health practitioners and their armamentarium of medicinal plants for their primary health-care needs. Although modern medicine is becoming more accessible, traditional medicines have often maintained their popularity for historical, cultural, and financial reasons. It is accepted that "traditional medicine," including indigenous, complementary, alternative, or integrative medicine, is a complex concept that includes a range of long-standing and still evolving practices based on diverse beliefs and theories. For instance, Bodeker and Burford (2008) pointed out the dichotomous situation of particular forms of traditional medicine being practiced in their countries of origin and also in countries to which they have been "imported." They suggested that the term *traditional medicine/complementary and alternative medicine* (TM/CAM) is more appropriate to describe such traditional therapies globally.

In this chapter, the term *traditional medicine* will be used as defined by WHO and will cover the role of traditional medicine in health care. In addition, some examples of trade in medicinal plants and products as well as strategies, declarations, and resolutions adopted by health and African leaders at global, continental, and regional levels are included. Furthermore, progress in the implementation of priority interventions of both of the regional strategies on promoting and enhancing the role of traditional medicine in health systems (Documents AFR/RC50/9 and AFR/RC63/6, respectively) is highlighted for the period 2001–2014. Furthermore, the implementation of plans of action on the first (2001–2010) and second (2011–2020) decades of African traditional medicine are discussed for the same period. Finally, the World Health Organization Regional Office for Africa's (WHO/AFRO) support to countries is mentioned *vis-à-vis* the implementation of the regional strategy.

Whenever possible, information on East Mediterranean countries has been included. The current progress of each country is compared to the WHO baseline survey of 1999/2000. In describing the work done by countries, WHO's Regional Office for Africa's support to countries for effective implementation of the priority interventions of these strategies is mentioned. Finally, highlighted are examples of partnerships established and challenges faced in the course of the implementation of the strategies as well as the way forward.

## 1.2 THE ROLE OF TRADITIONAL MEDICINE IN HEALTH CARE

Modern science has, in the past, considered methods of traditional knowledge as primitive and backward. Under colonial rule, traditional diviner-healers also referred to as *traditional health practitioners* (THPs) or *traditional medicine practitioners* (hereafter referred to as THPs) were outlawed. This action was based on the assumption by the colonialists that the THPs were practitioners of witchcraft. Subsequently, THPs were declared illegal by the colonial authorities, creating a war against witchcraft and magic. During that era, attempts were also made to control the sale of herbal medicines (Abdullahi, 2011) and to shun traditional practitioners despite their contribution to meeting the basic health needs of the population (Antwi-Baffour et al., 2014).

Traditional medicine has demonstrated the great potential of therapeutic benefits in its contribution to modern medicine. It is estimated that more than 25%–30% of modern medicines are derived directly or indirectly from medicinal plants, primarily through the application of modern technology to traditional knowledge (Gurib-Fakim and Kasilo, 2010; Kumari et al., 2011). In the case of certain classes of pharmaceuticals, such as active pharmaceutical ingredients for antitumor and antimicrobial medicines, this percentage may be as high as 60%. Examples of modern medicines derived from medicinal plants include anticancer medicines (vincristine and vinblastine), antihypertensive agents (reserpine), antimalarials (quinine and artemisinin), and decongestants (ephedrine).

In addition to the contribution of traditional medicine to therapeutic agents, THPs in the African region contribute to health-care coverage as they generally far outnumber Western-trained medical doctors. In Ghana and Swaziland, for example, there are 25,000 and 10,000 people for every one Western-trained medical practitioner compared to 200 and 100 people, respectively, for every THP. Similarly, in Benin and Uganda there are 8,411 and 10,000 people for every one Western-trained medical practitioner compared to 800 and only 290 people, respectively, in the urban areas and 50,000 people in the rural areas in Uganda (World Bank, 2003).

The twentieth and twenty-first centuries witnessed a revolution in human health care. The dramatic decline in mortality, the increase in life expectancy, and the eradication of smallpox are highlights of this success. Scientific innovation, leading to the development of new medicines, has played a major role in this achievement (Zhang, 2004). However, despite these successes, it is estimated that over one-third of the world's population lacks regular access to affordable essential medicines. In contrast, traditional medicine is widely available even in remote areas. Due to its local availability and low cost, it is accessible to the vast majority of people living in developing countries. Consequently, it is commonly used in large parts of Africa, Asia, and Latin America. In Africa, up to 80% of the population use traditional medicine for their primary health-care needs. This may appear an outdated data; however, even recent surveys have maintained this figure (WHO, 2013). However, this percentage may vary from country to country as indicated in Figure 1.1. In Africa, the range extends from 80% in Benin to 90% in Burundi and Ethiopia (WHO, 2013).

Traditional medicine not only maintains its function in primary health care (PHC) in developing countries, but also its use has expanded widely in many developed countries where it is referred to as TM/CAM. The most widely used TM/CAM

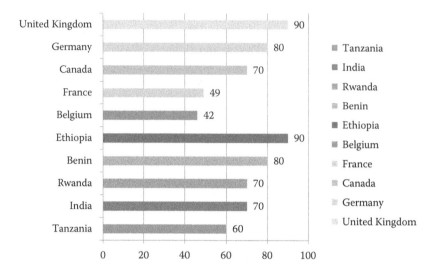

**Figure 1.1**    Percentage of populations using TM/CAM in some low-, middle-, and high-income countries. (Adapted from government reports submitted to WHO 2. Information from the document on Enhancing the role of traditional medicine in health systems: A strategy for the African Region, 60th session of WHO Regional Committee [Document, AFR/RC63/6].)

therapies are herbal medicines and acupuncture. According to various government and nongovernment reports from the countries in question, the percentages of the respective populations who used CAM at least once are as follows: 42% of the population in Belgium, 49% in France, 70% in Canada, 80% in Germany, and 90% in the United Kingdom have used traditional medicine. In these countries as well as in Australia and North America, herbal medicines are used as TM/CAM to complement standard health care (Management Sciences for Health, 2012). In the United States, in 2007, about 38% of adults and 12% of children were using some form of traditional medicine (Wachtel-Galor et al., 2011). Figure 1.1 shows the populations that use traditional medicine in some low- and middle-income countries and have used TM/CAM at least once in high-income countries.

Although traditional medicine has been used for thousands of years and has made great contributions to human health, the Alma-Ata Declaration by the International Conference on Primary Health Care (PHC) at Alma Ata, former Soviet Union, was the first official recognition of the role of traditional medicine and its practitioners in PHC by the WHO and its member states. This was the landmark declaration on the role of THPs in PHC.

The policy was an appropriate response to expressed community health needs. Consequently, African countries could not afford the high costs of modern healthcare systems and the technologies that are required. Therefore, they continued to depend on traditional medicine, which is readily available and affordable. Low- and middle-income countries, therefore, have appreciated the need to promote and integrate traditional medicine into Africa's national health-care systems.

Since the early 1960s, the Organization of African Unity (now the African Union), the WHO, Office de la recherché outré Mer (ORSTOM), and the African and Malagasy Council of Higher Education (*Conseil African et Malgache pour l'Enseignment Superieur* [CAMES]) have been leading the development of traditional medicine in the African continent and the African region, respectively. In 1976, the WHO/AFRO organized a meeting of experts in order to promote the development of traditional medicine. During the meeting, traditional medicine was first defined as "the sum total of all knowledge and practices, whether explicable or not, used in diagnosing, preventing, and eliminating physical, mental, spiritual, or societal imbalances. It relies exclusively on practical experience and observation handed down from generation to generation verbally, in writing, or otherwise" (WHO, 1978).

## 1.3 TRADE IN TRADITIONAL MEDICINAL PLANTS AND PRODUCTS: SOME EXAMPLES

The market for traditional medicine products has expanded significantly, and continues to grow. According to the report, the global dietary supplements market was valued at US$132.8 billion in 2016, is expected to reach US$220.3 billion in 2022, and is anticipated to grow at a compound annual growth rate (CAGR) of 8.8% between 2017 and 2022 (Zion Market Research, 2017). In 2002, the Secretariat of the Convention on Biological Diversity reported that the global sales of herbal products totaled US$60 billion (WHO, 2003a, b, c). Total sales of herbal medicines in Europe in 2003 reached US$5 billion, while annual revenue in Western Europe was US$5 billion in 2003–2004. In China, the total value of herbal medicines manufactured in 1995 reached 17.6 billion cedis (approximately US$2.5 billion). In China sales of herbal products totaled US$14 billion in 2005 (a 23.8% increase over the previous year) and increased to US$62.9 billion in 2011. Herbal medicines revenue in Brazil was US$160 million in 2007.

The amount of sales in the African continent is unknown for most countries (WHO, 2013). However, in 2008, it was estimated that trade in traditional medicinal plants and products in South Africa was worth ZAR 2.9 billion (US$29 million) per year (Mander et al., 2007:1). Recorded sales in Burkina Faso increased from US$2.68 million in 1998 to US$5.37 million in 2000. In Madagascar, sales increased from US$2 million in 1999 to US$3.5 million in 2000 (WHO, 2013:2). In Sudan in 2001, total sales were 7.404 million Sudanese dinars (US$28,000) and 2002 sales were worth 8.123 million dinars (US$31,000). In 2003, sales totaled 8.861 million dinars (US$34,000). Crude senna, gum Arabic, gum acacia, and hibiscus are marketed locally and internationally in commercial quantities. Digoxin and diosmin are registered as imported items. Similarly, annual market sales data including local and export sales in Egypt in 2000 were 34 million Egyptian pounds (US$5.54 million); in 2001, 38 million Egyptian pounds (US$6.2 million); and in 2002, 44 million Egyptian pounds (US$7.2 million) (WHO, 2005). Examples of herbal medicines trade in some countries in Africa as well as Brazil, China, Europe, and Western Europe are summarized in Table 1.1.

**Table 1.1    Some Examples of Trade in Traditional Medicinal Plants and Products in Some Countries in Africa, Brazil, China, Europe, and Western Europe**

| Year | Country | Estimated Market/Country | Amount in USD (US$) | References |
|---|---|---|---|---|
| 1998 | Burkina Faso | Traditional medicine sales | US$2.68 million | WHO, 2005a, b, c:58 |
| 1999 | Madagascar | Traditional medicine sales | US$2 million | WHO, 2005a, b, c:65 |
| 2000 | Burkina Faso | Traditional medicine sales | US$5.37 million | WHO, 2005a, b, c:58 |
| 2000 | Madagascar | Traditional medicine sales | US$3.5 million | WHO, 2005a, b, c:65 |
| 2000 | Egypt | Annual market herbal medicine sales data including local and export sales | US$5.54 million | WHO, 2005a, b, c:87 |
| 2001 | Egypt | Annual market herbal medicine sales data including local and export sales | US$6.2 million | WHO, 2005a, b, c:87 |
| 2001 | Sudan | Total herbal medicine sales | US$28,000 | WHO, 2005a, b, c:92 |
| 2002 | Egypt | Annual market herbal medicine sales data including local and export sales | US$7.2 million | WHO, 2005a, b, c:87 |
| 2002 | Sudan | Total herbal medicine sales | US$31,000 | WHO, 2005a, b, c:92 |
| 2002 | Global | Estimated global sales of herbal products | US$60 million | Tilburt and Kaptchuk, 2008:1 |
| 2003 | Sudan | Total herbal medicine sales | US$34,000 | WHO, 2005a, b, c:92 |
| 2003 and 2005 | Europe | Market sales of herbal medicines | US$7.1 billion | https://www.otciq.com/otciq/ajax/showFinancialReportByld.pdf?id=27951 (Accessed on April 15, 2017) |
| 2003–2004 | Western Europe | Annual revenues of herbal medicines | US$5 billion | De Smet, 2005:1 |
| 2005 | China | Sales of herbal products | US$14 billion | WHO, 2005:1 |
| 2007 | Brazil | Herbal medicines revenue | US$160 million | WHO, http://www.who.int/topics/traditional_ medicine/en/ (Accessed on April 15, 2017) |
| 2008 | South Africa | Trade in traditional medicinal plants and products | US$29 million | Mander et al., 2007:1 |
| 2011 | China | Sales of herbal medicine products | US$62.9 billion | Wachtel-Galor and Benzie, 2011:1 |
| 2012 | China | Sales of herbal medicine products | US$83 billion | Rinaldi and Shetty, 2015:1 |
| 2016 | Global | Estimated global sales for herbal medicine products | US$132.8 billion | Zion Market Research, 2017:1 |

## 1.4 STRATEGIES, DECLARATIONS, AND RESOLUTIONS ADOPTED BY HEALTH LEADERS FOR DEVELOPMENT OF TRADITIONAL MEDICINE BETWEEN 1999 AND 2014

It is over 35 years since the Declaration of Alma Ata on PHC. It is significant that member states have adopted policy decisions through resolutions and declarations on traditional medicine at global, continental, and regional levels during the World Health Assembly, African Summit of Heads of States, and Government and Regional Committee for Africa. The strategies, declarations, and resolutions adopted by health leaders for development of traditional medicine during 1999–2014 are highlighted and listed according to global, continental, and regional levels.

## 1.5 STRATEGIES AND RESOLUTIONS ADOPTED BY HEALTH LEADERS FOR DEVELOPMENT OF TRADITIONAL MEDICINE AT GLOBAL LEVEL

Upon the WHO Regional Director for Africa's recommendation, in 2002, the WHO Director General approved the institution of African Traditional Medicine Day on August 31 of each year. In May 2002, the World Health Assembly (WHA) launched the global WHO Strategy on Traditional Medicine 2002–2005 (WHO, 2002); it was adopted at the 66th Session of the WHA by its *Resolution WHA56.13 on Traditional Medicine* in 2003. In 2008, the 61st WHA adopted *Resolution WHA61.21 on WHO global strategy and plan of action on public health, innovation and intellectual property.* The resolution set a research priority agenda in traditional medicine whose effective implementation will go a long way to improving access to medicines for the people of the African region.

In addition, the WHO convened the first WHO Congress on Traditional Medicine that took place from November 7 to 9, 2008, in Beijing, China, and adopted the Beijing Declaration on Traditional Medicine. The declaration recognized the role of traditional medicine in the improvement of public health and supported its integration into national health systems where appropriate. The declaration encourages governments to create or improve national policies on traditional medicine. It also promotes improved education, research, and clinical inquiry into traditional medicine, as well as improved communication between health-care providers.

In 2009, the 62nd World Health Assembly adopted *Resolution WHA62.13 on Traditional Medicine.* The resolution noted that progress in the field of traditional medicine has been achieved by a number of member states through implementation of WHO's traditional medicine strategy 2002–2005. It further noted that African Traditional Medicine Day is commemorated annually on August 31 in order to raise awareness of the profile of traditional medicine in the African region, as well as to promote its integration into national health systems. The resolution requested the WHO to update the global WHO Traditional Medicine Strategy 2002–2005 as well as to continue providing policy guidance to countries on how to integrate traditional medicine into health systems.

In October 2013, the WHO Director General launched the updated WHO Traditional Medicine strategy: 2014–2023 at a WHO high-level meeting held at the Macao Special Administrative Region of China. Participants in Macao including national health authorities from the African Region recognized that the WHO Traditional Medicine Strategy: 2014–2023 provides useful guidance to countries in the formulation and implementation of their respective national policies and regulations and called for the adoption and adaptation of the strategy by member states. The traditional medicine strategy has three strategic objectives: (1) building the knowledge base through national policies; (2) strengthening safety, quality, and effectiveness through regulation; and (3) promoting universal health coverage by integrating services and self-health care into the national health system (WHO, 2014a, b).

In May 2014, the 67th World Health Assembly adopted *Resolution WHA67.18 on Traditional Medicine*. The resolution took note of the updated regional strategy on *Enhancing the role of traditional medicine in health systems* (Document AFR/RC63/6). Resolution WHA67.18 urged member states to integrate traditional medicine in national health systems.

## 1.6 STRATEGIES AND DECLARATIONS ADOPTED BY HEALTH AFRICAN LEADERS FOR DEVELOPMENT OF TRADITIONAL MEDICINE AT CONTINENTAL LEVEL

The Africa Summit of Heads of States and Government on HIV/AIDS, Tuberculosis (TB) and Other Related Infectious Diseases (ORID) declared traditional medicine research as a priority in April 2001 in Abuja, Nigeria. The regional strategy on *Promoting the role of traditional medicine in health systems* (Document AFR/RC50/9) (WHO, 2001) paved the way for the declaration of the first *Decade for African Traditional Medicine* (2001–2010) in Lusaka, Zambia, in July 2001 (Organization of the African Unity (OAU) 2001:1) and the adoption of a plan of action for its implementation by the African ministers of health held in Tripoli, Libya, in 2003. The adoption of this declaration by African health leaders was a landmark political commitment and recognition of African traditional medicine that has heightened the profile of traditional medicine on the African continent. It has served as a critical element in the rational development, improvement, and integration into the public health-care system on the African continent.

In July 2003, the Africa Summit of Heads of States and Government endorsed the institution of the African Traditional Medicine Day with effect from 2003 in Maputo. The summit also endorsed the plan of action for implementation of the Decade of African Traditional Medicine. Furthermore, the summit in its Maputo declaration on HIV/AIDS, TB, malaria, and ORID resolved to continue to support the implementation of the Plan of Action for the Decade for African Traditional Medicine (2000–2010), especially research in the area of treatment for HIV/AIDS, TB, malaria, and ORID (African Union, 2003).

As part of an African common position for the UN General Assembly Special Session (UNGASS) on AIDS, New York, in 2006, the Africa summit recalled the outcomes of Abuja (April 2001) in which research and development (R&D) on HIV/ AIDS, TB, and ORID, including vaccines, traditional medicines, and indigenous knowledge were identified as priority areas (UNGASS, 2006). In addition, the summit stated the "fundamental role of intensified R&D efforts in all areas particularly Traditional Medicine and microbicides as opportunities and driving forces for intensified actions" (UNGASS, 2006). Consequently, the Africa summit undertook "to increase support for research, including developing vaccines, new medicines and other tools including traditional herbal medicines, improving existing technologies to combat the diseases, undertaking operational research such as testing delivery strategies and monitoring drug resistance and drug adverse reactions" (UNGASS, 2006).

The fifth ordinary session of the African Union Conference of African Ministers of Health held in Windhoek, Namibia, on April 17–21, 2011, on the theme "the impact of climate change on health and development in Africa," discussed the End-of-Decade Review report on African Traditional Medicine (2001–2010). The implementation of the plan of action in the first decade succeeded in promoting the development of African traditional medicine in member states. This success encouraged the AU Conference of Ministers of Health to declare the Second Decade of African Traditional Medicine from 2011 to 2020 (African Union, 2011). The plan of action for implementation of AU's Second Decade of African Traditional Medicine was adopted by a special conference of African ministers of health in Geneva, Switzerland, in May 2012. The African Summit of Heads of State and Government then endorsed the Second Decade of African Traditional Medicine and its implementation plan in June 2012 in Malabo, Equatorial Guinea.

## 1.7 STRATEGIES, DECLARATIONS, AND RESOLUTIONS ADOPTED BY LEADERS FOR DEVELOPMENT OF TRADITIONAL MEDICINE AT REGIONAL LEVEL

In 1999, the 49th session of the WHO Regional Committee for Africa held in Namibia adopted a technical document and its *Resolution on essential drugs in the WHO African region: Situation and trend analysis* (AFR/RC49/R5). The Regional Committee requested the WHO to support member states to carry out research on medicinal plants and to promote their use in health-care delivery systems. The Regional Committee also called on the WHO to develop a comprehensive strategy on African traditional medicine.

In implementing the aforementioned resolution, WHO/AFRO carried out a baseline survey in 1999/2000 in which 30 of the 46 countries participated. The survey found that most countries did not have national traditional medicine policies, legal frameworks, and codes of ethics and practice. Some countries had developed training programs for THPs and conventional health practitioners (CHPs). The findings of the WHO survey were used to develop the first Regional Traditional Medicine Strategy which was reviewed by the African Forum on the Role of Traditional Medicine in Health Systems convened by WHO/AFRO in Harare, Zimbabwe, on

February 15–18, 2000. The outcomes of the forum were used to finalize the draft strategy by the WHO/AFRO Secretariat.

The 50th session of the WHO Regional Committee for Africa, held in Ouagadougou, Burkina Faso, in 2000, adopted this regional strategy document (AFR/RC50/9) by its resolution AFR/RC50/R3 on *Promoting the role of traditional medicine in health systems: A strategy for the African region,* the first ever strategy on traditional medicine developed by the WHO. The aim of the regional strategy is to contribute to the achievement of health for all by optimizing the use of traditional medicine. The regional strategy promotes the integration into health systems of traditional medicine practices and medicines for which evidence on the safety, efficacy, and quality is available, and the generation of such evidence when it is lacking.

In 2005, the WHO Regional Committee for Africa, held in Maputo, Mozambique, adopted a document on *Local production of essential medicines, including antiretrovirals,* which called on governments to promote pharmaceutical research and development, especially using locally available medicinal plants and other raw materials, in order to generate data on safety, efficacy, and quality needed for large-scale production (WHO, 2005a, b, c:6). In 2007, the 57th Regional Committee for Africa declared traditional medicine research as a priority on the occasion of the Fifth African Traditional Medicine Day held in Brazzaville, Republic of the Congo (WHO, 2007:3). The ministers of health pledged to foster strong regional, subregional, and international collaboration for information exchange, mobilization, and allocation of adequate resources, among others.

The year 2008 marked WHO's 60th anniversary and also the 30th anniversary of the Alma-Ata Declaration, adopted by WHO and UNICEF in 1978. To celebrate these anniversaries, WHO convened three high-level conferences in 2008, which resulted in three declarations related to traditional medicine: The first was the *Ouagadougou Declaration on Primary Health Care and Health Systems in Africa* in April 2008 which reiterated the Alma Ata Declaration by calling on countries "to set up sustainable mechanisms for increasing the availability, affordability and accessibility of essential medicines and the use of community-directed approaches and African traditional medicines," among others. The second was the *Algiers Declaration on Research for Health* in June 2008, which recognized the need to promote research in traditional medicine and strengthen health systems, taking into account the sociocultural and environmental situation of the people. The third was the *Beijing Declaration* in September 2008, as indicated above.

A Special Conference of Ministers of Health reviewed the Mid-Term Report on the Decade of African Traditional Medicine in conjunction with the 58th Session of the WHO Regional Committee for Africa held in Yaoundé, Cameroon, in August 2008. The conference recommended that the African Union should undertake the End-of-Decade Review on African Traditional Medicine in collaboration with the WHO and present its findings. The year 2010 marked a decade since the adoption of this regional strategy and the declaration of the African Traditional Medicine Decade. To mark the end of the Decade of African Traditional Medicine, WHO published a special issue dedicated to traditional medicine with contribution of articles from experts in member states including an overview of traditional medicine in the

African region (Kasilo et al., 2010:7) and in Economic Community of West African States (ECOWAS) member states (Busia and Kasilo 2010:17), among other articles.

The WHO/AFRO supported the development of the plan of action for implementation of AU's Second Decade of African Traditional Medicine (2011–2020), which was adopted by a special conference of African ministers of health in Geneva, Switzerland, in May 2012, and endorsed by the African Summit of Heads of State and Government in June 2012 Equatorial Guinea.

The 61st session of the Regional Committee for Africa in 2011 held in Yamoussoukro, Cote d'Ivoire, in September 2011, reviewed an information document that reported on the progress made in the implementation of both the Regional Strategy and the Decade's Plan of Action during 2001–2010. The Regional Committee recommended that the Regional Strategy for the African Region on Promoting the Role of Traditional Medicine in Health Systems should be updated. It also recommended that countries: (1) increase the allocation and mobilize additional resources to effectively implement the regional strategy, particularly to conduct research in order to generate scientific evidence of the safety and efficacy of traditional herbal medicines; and (2) strengthen the regulation of traditional medicine products, practitioners, and practices, taking into consideration the Algiers Declaration on Research for Health and the renewed Decade of African Traditional Medicine (2011–2020) (WHO, 2011a, b:4). The committee also proposed "Traditional medicine: Practices, practitioners and products in the African Region," as a topic for panel discussion at its 62nd Session of the WHO Regional Committee for Africa that was held in Luanda in 2012.

The 60th session of the Regional Committee for Africa held in Brazzaville, Republic of the Congo, in September 2013, adopted the updated regional strategy by its resolution AFR/RC63/R3 on *Enhancing the role of traditional medicine in health systems: A strategy for the African region.* The aim of the updated regional strategy is to contribute to better health outcomes by optimizing and consolidating the role of traditional medicine in national health systems. Two novel features of the updated regional strategy are (1) an emphasis on enhancing the role of traditional medicine in health systems and (2) the setting of targets to be reached in the African region over a 10-year period (2013–2023).

## 1.8 PROGRESS IN THE IMPLEMENTATION OF THE REGIONAL STRATEGY AND PLANS OF ACTION ON THE TWO DECADES OF AFRICAN TRADITIONAL MEDICINE

The following sections report on progress in the implementation of priority interventions of the updated regional strategy as well as plans of action on the first (2001–2010) and second decades of African traditional medicine (2011–2020). The priority interventions covered are summarized as follows:

- Policy formulation and implementation of strategies and plans
- Research and development

- Development of local production
- Promotion and organization of large-scale cultivation and conservation of medicinal plants
- Promotion of protection of intellectual property rights and traditional medicine knowledge
- Strengthening of human resources capacity of countries
- Development of frameworks for integrating traditional medicine in health systems
- Enhancing collaboration among multisectoral stakeholders

## 1.9  COUNTRY OWNERSHIP OF GLOBAL AND REGIONAL COMMITMENTS

Countries in the African region were engaged in the development, implementation, and monitoring of strategies and plans.

### 1.9.1  Formulation and Implementation of Policies and Regulatory Frameworks

Since the adoption of the regional strategy in 2000 (updated in 2013), more than half of the countries in the African region have adapted the WHO *Tools for institutionalizing Traditional Medicine in health systems in the African Region,* to their unique situations. The tools contain (1) *Guidelines on the formulation, implementation and monitoring of national policies on traditional medicine*; (2) *Model Legal Framework for the practice of traditional medicine: A Traditional Health Practitioners Bill*; (3) *Model Codes of Ethics and Practice for Traditional Health Practitioners*; and (4) *Guidelines for the formulation of a master plan for development of Traditional Medicine.*

By 2013, 32 countries formulated national policies, making a total of 40 out of 46 countries (by May 2013, 47 with the addition of South Sudan) in the African region with such policies as compared to only 8 in 1999/2000. In an effort to regulate, promote, develop, and standardize the practice of African traditional medicine, by 2013, a total of 29 countries had developed legal frameworks for traditional medicine practice. That was an increase of 28 from only 1 country (Zimbabwe) in 2000; while 19 countries developed *National Codes of Ethics and Practice for THPs* to enhance the safety, efficacy, and quality of services provided to patients and 21 developed *National strategic plans* for implementation of their policies from 0 in 2000, respectively. In addition, in 2011, the Ministry of Health of Uganda developed a bill entitled the *Indigenous and Complementary Medicine Bill,* which was passed by the Cabinet in 2013 and is currently awaiting discussion in Parliament. The bill seeks to establish a National Indigenous and Complementary Medicine Council with the mandate to register, license, discipline, and develop and enforce a code of ethics for TM/CAM practitioners. Thirteen countries had national policies on the conservation of medicinal plants; and 10 countries adopted national legislation for the protection of intellectual property rights and traditional medicine knowledge.

### 1.9.2 Establishment of Institutional Structures, Committees, and Facilities for Provision of Health Services for Development of Traditional Medicine

National traditional medicine offices have been established in 39 of the 46 countries, and 24 countries have traditional medicine programs in their Ministries of Health. Evidently, 12 traditional medicine offices and 14 traditional medicine programs were established during the First Decade of African Traditional Medicine (hereafter referred to as First Decade). A total of 24 countries have established national expert committees as multidisciplinary and multisectoral mechanisms to support the development and implementation of policies, strategies, and plans related to traditional medicine. Eight of these committees were established during 2001–2010.

Although traditional medicine facilities for provision of health services are required for enhancing collaboration and complementarity between the practitioners of the two systems of medicine, by 2013, few countries such as Benin, Côte d'Ivoire, and Mali have attempted to establish at least one clinic in hospitals. The Tanga regional hospital in the United Republic of Tanzania has allocated a floor to the Tanga AIDS Working Group (TAWG) to enable the testing, treating, and counseling of patients for HIV. Only Ghana has succeeded in establishing meaningful traditional medicine clinics in nine regional hospital settings. And Mali's main hospitals have departments carrying out research into traditional cures.

Although 40 countries have developed national policies, only 21 of them have developed national strategic plans for implementation of these policies. Some of the national policies have not yet been adopted by governments. Therefore, only six countries (Ethiopia, Ghana, Mali, South Africa, the United Republic of Tanzania, and Zimbabwe) have established Traditional Health Practitioners Councils as National Boards or Commissions on Traditional Medicine with legal authority to regulate the practice of traditional medicine. Countries need to enhance efforts in this regard. Other countries did not translate the policies into the national law.

### 1.9.3 The African Traditional Medicine Day

Since 2003, all countries have been celebrating the African Traditional Medicine Day. The inaugural African Traditional Medicine Day was commemorated in South Africa on August 31, 2003, in conjunction with the 53rd Session of the WHO Regional Committee for Africa with the theme, *African TM, Our Culture, Our Future*. At that occasion, WHO published a special issue in the *African Health Monitor* that covered topics such as the integration of traditional medicine into national health systems (Sambo, 2003); enhancing traditional medicine research and development in Africa (Kasilo, 2003); accelerating local production of traditional medicines in Africa (Wambebe, 2003); and building a regional initiative for traditional medicine and HIV/AIDS for Eastern and Southern Africa (Homsy et al., 2003). Ever since, these events have been celebrated annually in member states with different themes, such as *Conservation of medicinal plants: Africa's heritage* in 2011 (WHO, 2011a, b). These celebrations have drawn attention to various issues in the development of African traditional medicine.

The eighth African Traditional Medicine Day coincided with the Decade of African Traditional Medicine (2001–2010) and was commemorated with the theme, *A Decade of African Traditional Medicine: Progress so far.* A number of articles were published summarizing the achievements made and providing an overview of activities that countries have undertaken in implementing the priority interventions of the regional strategy in the past 10 years. The articles ranged from policies (Kasilo and Trapsida, 2010), practices (Mhame et al., 2010), and research (Nikiema et al., 2010; Diallo et.al., 2010) to local production (Kasilo et al., 2010) and intellectual property rights (Sackey and Kasilo, 2010).

Some countries, such as Benin, Burkina Faso, The Gambia, Ghana, Mali, Senegal, and Uganda, have instituted a National Traditional Medicine Week (Kasilo et al., 2010). These events are called different names depending on the geographical area where they are held. For instance, in Burkina Faso it is the International Exhibition of African Traditional Medicines (Kasilo, 2010; IRIN, 2004) and in Mali it is the International Week of African Traditional Medicine (Aid to the Development of Traditional Medicine) (AIDEMET, 2007). These events have created enabling environments for training, collaboration between practitioners of traditional medicine and conventional medicine, networking, and information exchange.

## 1.10 PROMOTION OF RESEARCH AND DEVELOPMENT

### 1.10.1 Research to Produce Scientific Evidence on Safety, Efficacy, and Quality of Traditional Herbal Medicines

The baseline WHO survey carried out in 1999/2000 revealed that 11 countries (Benin, Burkina Faso, Côte d'Ivoire, Ghana, Kenya, Madagascar, Mali, Nigeria, South Africa, Tanzania, and Zimbabwe) that responded were conducting research including ethnomedical surveys on traditional medicines used for the treatment of malaria, opportunistic infections related to HIV/AIDS, and sickle cell disease. Mali had issued marketing authorizations for seven traditional medicines and included them in its *National Essential Medicines List* (NEML).

The number of National Traditional Medicine Research Institutes increased from 18 in 2000 to 28 in 2013. These institutes researched the use of traditional medicine products for priority diseases using WHO guidelines (WHO, 2004a, b, c, d, e). These diseases are malaria, HIV/AIDS, sickle cell disease, diabetes, and hypertension. These are the diseases that WHO/AFRO had selected to focus on in the first decade of implementation of the regional strategy on traditional medicine and for whose treatment, research, and development must be accelerated. It is for this reason that other research activities are not covered in this section. Some of the research institutes have reported promising results.

For example, the National Institute for Health Sciences in Burkina Faso (Nikiema et al., 2010) and the National Institute for Pharmaceutical Research and Development

(NIPRD) in Nigeria (Gamaniel, 2003) have reported to have developed traditional medicinal products used for the treatment of sickle cell disease from medicinal plants and medicinal and food plants (Wambebe et al., 2001), respectively. Published data indicate significant clinical efficacy in that a majority of patients were protected from crises, while the frequency and severity of crises were significantly reduced resulting in reduction of hospital visits and increased school and work attendance. Research conducted in Burkina Faso by Simpore et al. (2003) and country reports from Zimbabwe (Mashava, 2005) and Tanzania (Kajuna, 2009; Malebo, 2014) on tests carried out after administration of the traditional herbal medicines in people living with HIV/AIDS for the management of opportunistic infections, showed a decrease in viral load, increase in CD4 and CD8 counts, weight gain, a regain in energy and appetite, and improvement of overall clinical conditions and quality of life. In addition, other studies from Burkina Faso showed evidence of the risk of drug interactions between traditional herbal medicines and antiretrovirals (ARVs) (Nikiema et al., 2009).

By 2013, a total of 13 countries (Burkina Faso, Cameroon, Côte d'Ivoire, Democratic Republic of the Congo, Ghana, Madagascar, Mozambique, Niger, Nigeria, Republic of the Congo, Tanzania, Zambia, and Zimbabwe) used research results to authorize the marketing of certain traditional medicine products after evaluation of their safety, efficacy, and quality for registration purposes using WHO guidelines (WHO, 2004a, b, c, d, e:1), in addition to Mali. The number of countries that included traditional medicine products in their NEMLs has increased to eight (Burkina Faso, Cameroon, Democratic Republic of the Congo, Ghana, Madagascar, Mali, Mozambique, and Niger) as compared with only Mali as of 1999/2000. Examples of traditional herbal medicines in the NEMLs include "N'dribala" (Benoit-Vical et al., 2003) and "Saye" (Traoré et al., 2008) used for malaria treatment and "Faca" for sickle cell disease (Nikiema et al., 2010) in Burkina Faso. "Malarial" (Diallo et al., 2004) used for malaria in Mali, and "Madeglucyl" (Ratsimamanga, 2006) for uncomplicated diabetes treatment in Madagascar. The compositions of these medicines are listed in Table 1.3. Some countries increased research efforts, used WHO documents on R&D of traditional herbal medicines, conducted ethnomedical surveys, and documented available recipes.

## 1.10.2 Development of Monographs on Medicinal Plants and Herbal Pharmacopoeias

The work on development of monographs and herbal pharmacopoeias is very important, particularly in the African continent, because most countries lack suitable technical specifications and quality control standards for African medicinal plants and herbal medicines. This is a major constraint and a significant barrier to regional and international trade as well as an important barrier to integrating traditional medicine into African public health services. Despite this importance, only a limited number of countries and regional economic communities have undertaken these activities on a regular basis due to limited resources.

The WHO baseline survey of 1999/2000 revealed that some countries and partners such as Equatorial Guinea, Ghana, Guinea, Mozambique, and Uganda had developed monographs on medicinal and aromatic plants and herbal pharmacopoeias in order to set standards on safety, efficacy, and quality of traditional herbal medicines. The OAU had published the *African Pharmacopoeia* in 1982. In Mozambique the national monographs are contained in the series *Plantas Medicinais e seu uso tradicional em Mocambique* (1983, 1991, five volumes) (WHO, 2005a, b, c). The *Ghana Herbal Pharmacopoeia* was published in 1992 (WHO, 2005a, b, c: 63), and the national pharmacopoeia also contains monographs on herbal medicines. Uganda had the national pharmacopoeia entitled, *A Contribution of the Traditional Medicine Pharmacopoeia of Uganda* (1993) (WHO, 2005a, b, c). Equatorial Guinea had national monographs contained in the *Recetario plantas medicinales de Equatorial Guinea* (1996), which contains 18 monographs (WHO, 2005a, b, c), whereas national monographs in Guinea exist in the *Plantes médecinales guinéennes* (1997) (WHO, 2005a, b, c).

The *Egyptian Pharmacopoeia* (1972, 1980) is the national pharmacopoeia that contains monographs on herbal medicines, and it is legally binding (WHO, 2005a, b, c). In lieu of a national pharmacopoeia, Sudan uses the *British Herbal Pharmacopoeia,* and it is considered to be legally binding, and in place of national monographs, the *WHO Monographs* are used (WHO, 2005a, b, c). Ghana published the second edition of its *National Herbal Pharmacopoeia* (The Government of Ghana, 2007), whereas Nigeria (The Government of Nigeria, 2008) and the Democratic Republic of the Congo (Ministry of Health, 2009: 1) printed the first editions of their national herbal pharmacopoeias in 2008 and 2009, respectively. Benin developed 418 monographs of medicinal plants used for the treatment of uncomplicated malaria during 2009–2014. The country also developed 304 monographs of medicinal plants used for the treatment of opportunistic infections of HIV/AIDS with support from the African Development Bank (ADB) (WHO, 2015). Similarly, experts of the Association for African Medicinal Plants Standards (AAMPS), founded in 2005 to support the African herbal industry and regulatory authorities by developing quality control and quality assurance standards for African medicinal plants and herbal medicines, published the *African Herbal Pharmacopoeia* (AAMPS, 2010: 1). This pharmacopoeia has monographs on 51 selected African medicinal plants, including well-known examples such as *Catharanthus roseus, Prunus africana, Harpagophytum procumbens, Pelargonium sidoides,* and the South African cancer bush, *Sutherlandia frutescens.*

On its part, in 2013, the West African Health Organization (WAHO) published the herbal pharmacopeia for the Economic Community of West African States (ECOWAS) subregion (WAHO, 2013:1). The WAHO herbal pharmacopoeia contains 52 commonly used and geographically distributed medicinal plants in West Africa, which are used for the priority diseases selected by the WHO Regional Office (together with tuberculosis and hepatitis) and for which some information exist in the *African Pharmacopoeia*, the Ghanaian, and Nigerian herbal pharmacopoeias, as well as in WHO monographs. By 2013, 20 countries (Benin, Burkina Faso, Cameroon, Chad, Côte d'Ivoire, Equatorial Guinea, Ethiopia, Gambia, Ghana, Guinea, Madagascar, Mali, Mauritius, Mozambique, Niger, Rwanda, Senegal, Seychelles, South Africa, and Uganda) have developed monographs on medicinal and aromatic plants, an increase of 18 countries compared to the baseline survey mentioned above.

Although some countries established standardization protocols and promoted clinical studies in collaboration with the National Medicines Regulatory Authorities and

WHO, Phase III clinical trials are still a challenge because of the substantial financial resources required. There are also a limited number of operational research studies that analyze factors related to the role of traditional medicine practices in different health systems. There is still limited scientific research data to ensure the safety, efficacy, and quality of herbal medicines. Where this information is available, research results are not used for policy making and are not widely disseminated, and most institutions are far from measuring consistency in the quality of different batches of traditional herbal medicines or warrant an interrupted small-scale local production of medicines.

## 1.11 PROMOTION AND ORGANIZATION OF LARGE-SCALE CULTIVATION AND CONSERVATION OF MEDICINAL PLANTS

### 1.11.1 Cultivation and Conservation of Medicinal Plants

The WHO survey of 1999/2000 revealed that Botswana (1990), Burkina Faso, Ghana (2000), and Lesotho (1997) had established policies related to the conservation of medicinal plants. Furthermore, Mali had a code on forests and legislation for the collection and conservation of medicinal plants (1999). In 2007 Cameroon and Mali developed guidelines related to the collection and conservation of medicinal plants. By 2013, 17 countries (Benin, Botswana, Burkina Faso, Burundi, Cameroon, Democratic Republic of the Congo, Ethiopia, Equatorial Guinea, Ghana, Guinea, Madagascar, Namibia, Mali, Mauritania, Republic of the Congo, Swaziland, and Zimbabwe) had small-scale cultivation of medicinal plants and aromatic plants as raw materials used for preparing, researching, and producing traditional medicine products.

Thirteen countries (Benin, Burkina Faso, Cameroon, Chad, Democratic Republic of the Congo, Ethiopia, Ghana, Nigeria, Republic of the Congo, Rwanda, South Africa, Sierra Leone, and Tanzania) had adopted the *WHO Guidelines on Good Agricultural and Collection Practices*. Fourteen countries (Benin, Burkina Faso, Ethiopia, Ghana, Guinea, Madagascar, Mali, Mauritania, Republic of the Congo, Rwanda, Senegal, South Africa, Swaziland, and Zimbabwe) had adopted national policies on the conservation of medicinal plants, while six countries had developed new medicinal plant varieties. Twelve countries (Cameroon, Ethiopia, Ghana, Kenya, Malawi, Mali, Mozambique, Senegal, United Republic of Tanzania, Uganda, Zambia, and Zimbabwe) are involved in the cultivation of *Artemisia annua* for malaria treatment.

### 1.11.2 Development of Botanical Gardens

Countries such as Benin, Côte d'Ivoire, and Mali have made good progress in this area, and this can be considered best practice that can be emulated by other countries. For instance, in 2011 the traditional medicine program of Côte d'Ivoire established a botanical garden of medicinal plants in extinction. There is also a botanical garden of medicinal plants of the Association of Traditional Health Practitioners for development of African traditional medicine (GIDMA) in Côte d'Ivoire. Between 2001 and 2007, Benin established 42 botanical gardens among which 7 were established by a research institute, a national laboratory, and a nongovernmental organization, and the other 35 by the national program of traditional medicine and pharmacopoeia of the ministry of health (Akpona et al., 2008:7). These gardens were established and managed through strategies adopted by the model of Benin that established such gardens during 2001–2007. The activities and challenges encountered by Benin in the establishment and management of botanical gardens are provided in Table 1.2.

Cultivation and conservation of medicinal plants are generally inadequate, and the application of good agricultural and collection practices (GACPs) are still limited. Most of the raw materials are collected from forests, while large-scale and mechanized cultivation and conservation of medicinal plants are still a challenge for many countries. There is still a need for additional efforts in promoting home and botanical gardens as well as selective use of modern biotechnology to develop improved medicinal and aromatic plant varieties with higher yields. There is also a need to promote practices that will guarantee consistent quality of the plant raw materials, to train stakeholders including THPs, and to translate WHO guidelines on GACPs into local languages. Also needed are intersectoral collaboration and adequate information on well-researched and nonresearched medicinal plants required for commercial cultivation. In addition, given that the pharmaceutical potentials of African medicinal plants are immense, in order to improve the situation of medicinal plants in Africa, urgent action is needed for research that focuses on the generation of baseline information on medicinal and aromatic plants and for promoting value-added processing of herbal medicines from local materials for local industries with simple dosage forms being standardized and packaged at low cost using appropriate technology. Governments should establish the necessary institutional and financial support to promote the potential role of the herbal industry in socio-economic development (Rukangira, 1996).

## 1.12 DEVELOPMENT OF LOCAL PRODUCTION FOR TRADITIONAL MEDICINE PRODUCTS

The weak cultivation and conservation of medicinal plants limits development of local production. The WHO baseline survey of 1999/2000 revealed that 15 countries had small-scale manufacturing facilities for the production of traditional medicine products. As far back as 1989, the Laboratory Galefomy of Côte d'Ivoire obtained approval for the industrial production of "Dartran" (antifungal) and "Dimitana" and "Baume Alafia" (both anti-inflammatory) herbal medicines. By 2013, the three herbal medicines had been approved by the National Commission of Côte d'Ivoire for marketing authorization.

## 1.13 FEASIBILITY STUDIES AND NEEDS ASSESSMENT ON LOCAL PRODUCTION

Between 2001 and 2005, six countries (Benin, Burkina Faso, Democratic Republic of the Congo, Mali, Nigeria, and United Republic of Tanzania) carried out feasibility

Table 1.2 Strategies Used by Benin to Establish and Manage 42 Botanical Gardens during 2001–2007 and Challenges Encountered

| Strategies | Activities Related to the Establishment and Management of 42 Botanical Gardens | Challenges for Sustainable Development of Botanical Gardens (Not Related to Strategies) |
|---|---|---|
| 1. Identification of garden sites | Involved participatory prospection, identification, and validation of sites with local communities and district authorities. | • *Agriculture*: Some farmers plot at the edge of the gardens, and this can especially facilitate the propagation of late fires to the gardens.<br>• *Cattle breeding*: Gardens shelter permanent water sources, which attract cattle.<br>• *Fire management*: Some gardens have been destroyed annually by fire. |
| 2. Creation of village botanical gardens committees | Organization of a meeting in each selected village and establishment of the committee with all stakeholders (president, secretary, accountant, two wise persons of each ethnic group and two guards), and the gender issue was considered in selecting members of the committee. | *Social considerations*<br>• Integration of all local stakeholder groups in the garden planning, especially the different ethnic groups present in the region and all those who may eventually be affected by the protection measures, in order to avoid local conflicts.<br>• Integration of traditional (e.g., Council of the elders) and modern authorities.<br>• Sensitization, by means of workshops, excursions, etc., of all villagers affected directly by exploitation restrictions.<br>• Community-elaborated code of conduct, the protection measures being agreed by all members of the local community. |
| 3. Identification of priority plants | Through participatory listing of main species people want to promote according to extinction risks and needs for traditional medicine considering national list of threatened plants. Estimation of needs in seedlings according to the garden area. | *Creation of synergy and functional network*<br>Ministry of Health, NGOs, universities, research projects, Ministry of Environment and Protection of Nature |

*(Continued)*

**Table 1.2 (Continued)  Strategies Used by Benin to Establish and Manage 42 Botanical Gardens during 2001–2007 and Challenges Encountered**

| Strategies | Activities Related to the Establishment and Management of 42 Botanical Gardens | Challenges for Sustainable Development of Botanical Gardens (Not Related to Strategies) |
|---|---|---|
| 4. Production of plants, reforestation and enrichment | Through training and creation of local nurseries, tree nursery: multiplying threatened local species, but also selling highly demanded exotic fruit trees like cashew nut and mango trees. This is an important source of additional income for the population, and delimitation of the edge of each garden with fast-growing species such as *Gmelinaarborea*, *Eucalyptus camaldulensis*. In the gardens, threatened medicinal species were planted: *Khayasenegalensis*, *Kigelia africana*, *Afzelia africana*, *Afrae glepaniculata*, *Vitex doniana*, *Strophantus sarmentosus*, and *Moringa oleifera*. | *Integrate genetic aspects into botanical gardens development* Botanical gardens development has to consider the preservation of the existing genetic diversity *Create a link between botanical gardens development and policymaking process* Taking into account that knowledge on botanical gardens has to be efficient and easily transformable into usable information for decision making. |
| 5. Awareness and promotion of gardens | Including protection of gardens against late bush fires by establishing 2–3 meters firebreak; realization of boards for identification of gardens, for orientation, and public awareness about "no fires, no pasture"; and publication and promotion of leaflets on the new concept of botanical gardens. | Integrate genetic aspects into botanical gardens development Botanical gardens development has to consider the preservation of the existing genetic diversity *Create a link between botanical gardens development and policymaking process* Taking into account that knowledge on botanical gardens has to be efficient and easily transformable into usable information for decision making. |
| 6. Additional garden activities | Beekeeping in the garden core zone for honey production; creation of a traditional pharmacy, and the foundation of a women's group for market-orientated vegetable gardening; and eco-tourism was planned to be integrated in the garden program in the future. | Sustainable development of botanical gardens in Benin. Pay attention to three major principles: i. *Have a close look:* In many places, people already preserve their environment: Look for sites such as holy groves, sacred forest, etc., as well as for starting point for such activities. They may be especially well suited as starting points for local botanical gardens. ii. *Go to the roots:* Ask the local populations about their perceptions of environmental changes and discuss with them their ideas of remedies and measures to be taken: you will admire their creativity and energy and realize that you are preaching to the already converted. iii. *Think small:* In countries like Benin, small projects often reveal to be more efficient than big ones; with little money, a lot can be done. |

*Note:* THETA-Uganda, a not-for-profit Ugandan Non-Governmental Organization (NGO) promoting collaboration between the traditional and modern health practitioners together against AIDS and other diseases.

studies with WHO support. Similarly, between 2004 and 2006 11 countries (Benin, Burkina Faso, Côte d'Ivoire, Democratic Republic of the Congo, Ghana, Kenya, Madagascar, Nigeria, South Africa, United Republic of Tanzania, and Egypt) undertook needs assessment on the local production of traditional medicines with WHO support in collaboration with the African Union's Scientific and Technical Research Commission. The feasibility studies and needs assessments contributed to the strategic plan for strengthening capacities for local production of traditional herbal medicines, including which countries adapted to their specific situations. These efforts resulted in more countries conducting R&D for ensuring safety, efficacy, and quality of traditional medicines for local production, establishment of registration systems, and issuing marketing authorizations for commercialization of traditional medicine products.

### 1.13.1 Small-Scale Manufacturing Facilities for the Production of Traditional Medicine Products

In 2009, Rwanda reported to have produced some pharmaceutical products from medicinal plants and other botanical products for patenting and commercialization, such as "Batankor" (a syrup derived from *Plantago lanceolata* used as an expectorant, anti-inflammatory, and antipruritic) and "Umugote" (a medicine derived from the *Syzygium parvifolium* tree which has powerful anti-amoebic and antibacterial properties and is used to treat infectious diarrhoeas and amoebic dysentery) (Nkurunziza, 2009:130). By 2013, 17 countries (Benin, Burkina Faso, Cameroon, Democratic Republic of the Congo, Ghana, Madagascar, Mali, Mauritania, Niger, Nigeria, Rwanda, Sao Tome and Principe, Senegal, Seychelles, South Africa, Togo, and Zimbabwe) had reported having small-scale manufacturing facilities for the production of traditional medicine products. Table 1.3 shows examples of traditional herbal medicines manufactured locally in some countries and included in their NEMLs.

As African TMK is mainly oral and passed down from generation to generation, additional countries need to document it to prevent the erosion of TMK with the death of the knowledge holder, to have wider applicability, to get the TMK registered/patented for the benefit of the knowledge holder and community, and for commercialization of TMK if applicable with prior informed consent.

### 1.13.2 Registration Systems and Marketing Authorizations

Countries with registration systems that provides for locally produced traditional herbal medicines increased from eight (Cameroon, Democratic Republic of the Congo, Ghana, Mali, Niger, Nigeria, Sierra Leone, and Uganda) in 1999/2000 to 15 in 2005 and to 17 (Benin, Burkina Faso, Cameroon, Central African Republic, Democratic Republic of the Congo, Ethiopia, Ghana, Madagascar, Mali, Niger, Nigeria, Sierra Leone, Togo, Uganda, Zambia, Côte d'Ivoire, and Mozambique) in 2013. For instance, in 2006, the national medicines regulatory authority (NMRA) in Burkina Faso issued marketing authorizations (MAs) for 11 locally produced traditional medicines including two for malaria which have been included in the NEML. By 2013, Burkina Faso had issued MAs for 37 traditional medicine products

**Table 1.3    Examples of Traditional Medicines Locally Produced in Five Countries and Included in Their National Essential Medicines List**

| Country | Traditional Medicine | Constituents | Indications | Reference |
|---|---|---|---|---|
| *Burkina Faso* | N'dribala | *Cochlospermum planchonii Hook.f* | Treatment of malaria | Benoit-Vical et al., 2003:111 |
| | Saye | *Cochlospermum planchonii Hook.f, Cassia alata L., and Phyllanthus amarus Schumach. et Thonn* | Treatment of malaria | Benoit-Vical et al., 2003:111 |
| | Faca | *Calotropis procera and Zanthoxylum zanthoxyloides* | Treatment of sickle cell disease | Nikiema et al., 2010:52 |
| | Anibex | *Euphorbia hirta.* | Treatment of amoeba and diarrhea | Njume and Goduka, 2012: 3915 |
| *Cameroon* | Pola Gastral AT-200 | *Emilia coccinea* | Treatment of gastrointestinal ulcers | http://congress-ise2012.agropolis.fr/ ftpheb.agropolis.fr/en/Congress_4_ components/Academic_colloquium/ Panels_files/s29_presentations.pdf (Accessed on May 8, 2017) |
| | Hepasor | *Enantia chlorantha* | Treatment of hepatic disorders in Cameroon | http://congress-ise2012.agropolis.fr/ ftpheb.agropolis.fr/en/Congress_4_ components/Academic_colloquium/ Panels_files/s29_presentations.pdf (Accessed on May 8, 2017) |
| | Gamma Syrup | *Pentadiplandra brazzeana* | Treatment of hemorrhoids in Cameroon and patented and registered in seven African countries including Democratic Republic of the Congo and Nigeria | http://congress-ise2012.agropolis.fr/ ftpheb.agropolis.fr/en/Congress_4_ components/Academic_colloquium/ Panels_files/s29_presentations.pdf (accessed on May 8, 2017) |

*(Continued)*

**Table 1.3 (*Continued*)  Examples of Traditional Medicines Locally Produced in Five Countries and Included in Their National Essential Medicines List**

| Country | Traditional Medicine | Constituents | Indications | Reference |
|---|---|---|---|---|
| Ghana | Diagelletes Elixir | *Psidium guajava* | Treatment of diarrhoea | Personal communication with DRA, Ghana |
| | Golden Malacure | *Cryptolepis sanguinolenta, Alstonia bonei, Vernonia amygdalina, Azadirachta indica, Hoslundia opposita* | Treatment of uncomplicated malaria caused by *Plasmodium falciparum* | Personal communication with DRA, Ghana |
| Madagascar | Madeglucyl | Eugenia Jambolana | Treatment of diabetes | Ratsimamanga, 2006:1 |
| Mali | Balembo | *Crossopteryx febrifuga* | Dry coughs | Diallo et al., 2004:117 |
| | Dysentéral | *Euphorbia hirta* | Amoebic dysentery | Diallo et al., 2004:117 |
| | Gastrosédal | *Vernonia kotschyana* | Gastritis, peptic ulcer | Diallo et al., 2004:117 |
| | Hépatisane | *Combretum micranthum* | Indigestion (especially of fats), nausea, poor appetite, constipation | Diallo et al., 2004:117 |
| | Laxa cassia | *Cassia italica* | Constipation | Diallo et al., 2004:117 |
| | Malarial | *Senna occidentalis Caesalpinaceae: 62%, Lippia chevalieri (Verbenaceae): 32%, Acmella oleracea (Asteraceae): 6%, and* | Treatment of malaria, fever | Diallo et al., 2004:117 |
| | Psorospermine | *Psorospermum guineense* | Eczema | Diallo et al., 2004:117 |

of which two were for malaria, one for sickle cell disease, and two for the treatment of opportunistic diseases in people living with HIV/AIDS (PMG151 and FMG131).

Ghana and Nigeria reported they had issued over 1,000 MAs for locally produced traditional herbal medicines, respectively, used for the treatment of various diseases including malaria, HIV/AIDS, diabetes, hypertension, and sickle cell disease (WHO, 2011a, b:3). In 2005 MAs were renewed in Madagascar for some medicines including diabetes. Other efforts include those by Ethiopia and Uganda, which adapted WHO guidelines on registration of traditional medicines to their specific situations to develop national documents for registration of traditional medicine products and the Southern African Development Community (SADC) developed for countries of its subregion.

Despite these efforts, governments need to play a key role in scaling up the creation of an enabling policy and economic and regulatory environments for local production of traditional herbal medicines and for the development of national regulations. The countries in the African region are still unable to fully translate TMK into viable medicines due to barriers such as limited knowledge sharing between scientists and THPs; insufficient manufacturing capacity; limited investment by the pharmaceutical industry; weak private-public partnerships; regulatory hurdles; lack of national standards regarding quality specification, quality assurance, and control of traditional medicine products; and limited national capacity and financial resources required for regulation, quality assurance, and control of traditional medicine products. In addition, traditional medicine products included in NEMLs are still not widely prescribed in health facilities even within the countries where they are commercialized.

There is therefore the need to create enabling environments for the establishment and scaling up of postmarket pharmacovigilance studies; the production of regular supplies of plant raw materials; and local production of, use, and especially marketing of African traditional herbal medicines. This would contribute to the utilization of uninterrupted production capacity and registration of additional medicines from medicinal plants.

## 1.14  PROTECTION OF INTELLECTUAL PROPERTY RIGHTS AND TRADITIONAL MEDICAL KNOWLEDGE

Intellectual property rights (IPRs) and TMK is a relatively new subject area in Africa. As a result, only a few countries have made progress. In 1999/2000 no country had developed a national policy or framework on IPRs for the protection of TMK. However, in 2000 the Council of Ministers of the Organization of the African Unity (OAU) adopted the OAU Model Legislation for the Protection of Local Communities, Farmers, Breeders and Access to Biological Resources (Organization of African Unity, 2000).

### 1.14.1  Documentation of Traditional Medical Knowledge

For traditional knowledge to be protected, it needs to be documented in various forms such as inventories, monographs, herbal pharmacopeias, and databases. In this regard, the WHO/AFRO country survey of 1999/2000 found that some countries such as Equatorial Guinea, Ghana, Guinea, Mozambique, and Uganda as well as the OAU had documented TMK in the form of monographs and pharmacopeias.

In 2004, a nongovernmental organization, THETA (Traditional and Modern Health Practitioners Together against AIDS and other diseases) based in Uganda, documented and published a booklet indicated in Figure 1.2 on *Herbs commonly used for the treatment of HIV/AIDS, related infections and other common illnesses.* The booklet includes the indications for treatment, the methods of preparation, and the dosing schedules. This booklet is a key resource of traditional medicine practitioners and members of the public who wish to know more about medicinal herbs for the treatment of HIV/AIDS in Uganda. It has already been mentioned in the section on development of monographs and pharmacopoeias that the Democratic Republic of the Congo (2009), Ghana (2007), Nigeria (2008), the Association for African Medicinal Plants Standards (AAMPS) (2010), and WAHO (2013) have developed herbal pharmacopoeias.

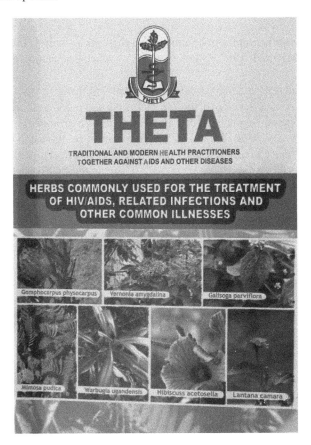

**Figure 1.2**  Booklet listing herbs commonly used for the treatment of HIV/AIDS, related opportunistic infections, and other common illnesses in Uganda.

By 2013, 10 countries (Benin, Cameroon, Chad, Côte d'Ivoire, Ethiopia, Gabon, Ghana, Mali, Rwanda, and United Republic of Tanzania) compiled inventories of medicinal plants and documented traditional remedies used for the treatment of malaria and hypertension, opportunistic infections for people living with HIV/AIDS, sickle cell diseases, diabetes, and hypertension. In addition, by 2013, 21 countries (Angola, Benin, Burkina Faso, Cameroon, Republic of the Congo, Democratic Republic of the Congo, Equatorial Guinea, Ethiopia, Gabon, Ghana, Kenya, Madagascar, Mali, Mozambique, Niger, Nigeria, Senegal, Seychelles, South Africa, Uganda, and United Republic of Tanzania) had documented traditional medicine in the form of experiences. Eight countries (Benin, Cameroon, Democratic Republic of the Congo, Ghana, Guinea, Mali, Senegal, and South Africa) had established databases on medicinal plants, THPs, and TMK.

## 1.14.2 Progress in Development of Frameworks and Institutional Structures for the Protection of IPRs and TMK during 2002–2014

Table 1.4 shows examples of countries and institutions with frameworks for the protection of TMK and IPRs. Some examples of misappropriation are highlighted in this section.

In 2002, Chad reported to have developed a national framework for the protection of IPRs. South Africa developed the *Indigenous Knowledge Systems (IKS) Policy* adopted by Cabinet in November 2004 and a *National Environmental Management: A Biodiversity Act in 2004* (No. 10 of 2004), followed by the establishment of the *National IKS Office* (NIKSO) in 2006. South Africa also developed *Draft national policy for intellectual property rights in 2013* (Government of South Africa, 2013:1).

In 2006 the Regional Intellectual Property Organization (ARIPO) and the Organisation africaine de propriete intellectuelle (OAPI [African Organization for Intellectual Property]) produced jointly a draft framework for an African instrument on the protection of traditional knowledge: *ARIPO/OAPI Draft Legal Instrument for the Protection of traditional knowledge and Expressions of Folklore*. On its part, Nigeria has developed a national legislation and a Traditional Knowledge Bill in 2006 and 2007, respectively. In addition, Cameroon and Ghana have developed national frameworks for protection of IPRs 2007 and 2008, respectively. Botswana adopted an *Industrial Property Act of 2010 for the protection of traditional medical knowledge (TMK)*.

By adopting the OAU Model Law on Access to Biological Resources, 10 countries (Burkina Faso, Cameroon, Congo, Democratic Republic of the Congo, Ghana, Guinea, Madagascar, Mali, Rwanda, and South Africa) strengthened their legal frameworks related to collection and export of medicinal plants. Seven countries (Benin, Democratic Republic of the Congo, Ghana, Guinea, Mali, Mauritania, and Republic of the Congo) adopted the *regulatory framework for the protection of traditional medical knowledge*. By adopting the OAU Model Law on Access to Biological Resources (Ekpere, 2000).

In 2013 Côte d'Ivoire established the Committee (access to genetic resources and fair and equitable sharing of benefits arising from their use) (APA) and has

Table 1.4    Examples of Countries and Regional Institutions with Frameworks for the Protection of TMK and IPRs

| Country | Document Developed by the Country or Partner on Protection of Indigenous Knowledge and IPRs | Year Done |
|---|---|---|
| Chad | Developed a national framework for intellectual property rights | 2002 |
| South Africa | Developed an indigenous knowledge system policy | 2004 |
| South Africa | Promulgated the Biodiversity Act | 2006 |
| South Africa | Established the Indigenous Knowledge System Office | 2006 |
| South Africa | Developed draft national policy for intellectual property rights | 2013 |
| Nigeria | Developed a national legislation for intellectual property rights | 2006 |
| Nigeria | Developed a traditional knowledge bill | 2007 |
| Malawi | Proposed laws for traditional knowledge, trade in genetic resources | 2006 |
| Kenya | Proposed laws for traditional knowledge, trade in genetic resources | 2006 |
| Cameroon | Developed a national framework for intellectual property rights | 2007 |
| Ghana | Developed a national framework for intellectual property rights | 2008 |
| Botswana | Adopted the Industrial Property Act | 2010 |
| Cote d'Ivoire | Developed a draft framework for the protection of indigenous knowledge | 2013 |
| Gambia | Adopted a framework for the protection of indigenous knowledge and intellectual property rights | 2014 |
| African Union | OAU Model legislation for the protection of the right of local communities, farmers, and breeders, and for the regulation of access to biological resources | 2000 |
| ARIPO/OAPI | Draft Legal Instrument for the Protection of Traditional Knowledge (TK) and Expressions of Folklore | 2006 |
| ARIPO | Swakopmund Protocol on the Protection of Traditional Knowledge and Expressions of Folklore | 2010 |
| WHO | WHO Policy guidance for the protection of traditional medical knowledge (Document AFR/EDM/TRM/2016.3) | 2016 |
| WHO | WHO Regional Legislative Framework for a Sui generis system for the protection of traditional medical knowledge (Document AFR/EDM/TRM/2016.4) | 2016 |

developed draft documents for the protection of traditional knowledge and attitudes. Other countries such as Eritrea, South Africa, Uganda, and Zimbabwe have developed or reviewed their legislation to include the safeguards provided for in the Trade-Related Aspects of Intellectual Property Rights (TRIPS) Agreement. The United Republic of Tanzania held sensitization workshops on IPRs for the past few years, and the indigenous knowledge legal framework has been under development by the Ministry of Industry, Trade and Marketing since 2013.

To promote awareness on indigenous knowledge and development of ethnoveterinary medicines between 2005 and 2007 Mali held a series of training workshops on IPRs and with WHO support, published two books: on Indigenous Veterinary Medicine and on African Traditional Medical Treatment (Koumare, 2008:1) and (Koumare, 2008:1). Development of these frameworks by countries in the African continent is important to prevent biopiracy and pharmaceutical companies patenting the inventions from medicinal resources from the continent without benefit-sharing agreements.

### 1.14.3 Examples of Misappropriation of Traditional Medical Knowledge in Africa

Currently, traditional medicine/complementary and alternative medicine (TM/CAM) plays an increasingly important role in the reform of the health sector of many developing and developed nations. Consequently, there is an urgent need to protect the IPRs of traditional medicine systems. However, the available instruments—the patenting system and the arrangements for guarding trade secrets—are inadequate for this task, and new arrangements need to be formulated. There is rampant misappropriation of TMK without prior informed consent of the knowledge holders or benefit sharing of resources accrued from the TMK. For example, in 1971, laboratory experiments verified the activity of extracts of a plant *Artemisia annua* against *Plasmodium berghei*, a mouse model of malaria. This discovery has since revolutionized the treatment of malaria around the world, but with little recognition for the THPs of the African region who have used *Artemisia* spp. for centuries, but who lacked the technology or financing to prove its efficacy against malaria in a laboratory (Robinson and Zhang, 2011:2).

In 2006, McGown published a book entitled, *Out of Africa: Mysteries of Access and Benefit Sharing* which reported on the details related to biopiracy in Africa (McGown, 2006:6), and this was an eye opener. For instance, vaccines from microbes were out of Egypt; a treatment for diabetes was out of Libya (McGown, 2006:2); and *Hoodia*, the appetite suppressant, was out of Angola, Botswana, Namibia, and South Africa (McGown, 2006). Similarly, four multipurpose medicinal plants were out of Ethiopia and neighboring countries: *Millettia ferruginea, Glinus lotoides, Hagenia abyssinica,* and *Ruta chalepensis* (McGown, 2006:7). As indicated by McGown, there is currently rampant misappropriation of resources from Africa. Partly, this is due to the fact that there is a lack of detailed documentation of TMK, which is generally transferred orally. However, if TMK is documented, it will be safeguarded, promoted, and made available in a more systematized manner to a wider audience. This latter includes researchers, students, and entrepreneurs, among others and it will also be possible to transmit TMK to future generations.

There is a need for information sharing between researchers and THPs on IPRs, as well as development of national regulatory frameworks for the protection of TMK by the Ministries of Health involving all national stakeholders. There is a need for one lead Ministry to deal with issues of TMK and to coordinate the efforts of other Ministries in this regard. In developing policy and regulatory frameworks, legal considerations for *sui generis system* countries need to take into account and respond to the following questions: What does one want to protect (subject matter)? Why does one wish to do so (policy objectives)? Which acts should be prevented/subject to prior authorization (scope of protection)? Who should benefit from this protection (rights holders and beneficiaries)? How would rights be obtained and lost, managed and enforced (formalities, term, administration)?

There is a need to develop well-considered legislative instruments at the national and regional levels to protect all aspects of TMK; establish institutional structures needed for effective implementation of the legislation; and coordinate and develop partnerships among stakeholders and communities to present a united body of opinion. African leadership will be critical in providing direction to the international debates and outcomes.

### 1.14.4 Strengthening of Human Resources Capacity of Countries for Development of Traditional Medicine

In the 1999/2000 baseline survey, 17 countries reported to have initiated training programs to improve traditional health practitioners' (THPs) skills and PHC knowledge. Ten of these countries (Burkina Faso, Côte d'Ivoire, Ghana, Guinea, Mali, Mozambique, Nigeria, Swaziland, United Republic of Tanzania, and Zimbabwe) provided training in traditional medicine for pharmacists as traditional medicine modules or through botany, phytotherapy, pharmacognosy, and public health. Other countries provided training on traditional medicine for doctors (Ghana and Zimbabwe) and nurses (Ethiopia, Ghana, Mozambique, and Zimbabwe).

## 1.15 THE JOURNEY TO INTEGRATION OF TRADITIONAL MEDICINE IN CURRICULA OF TRAINING INSTITUTIONS FOR HEALTH SCIENCES STUDENTS

Countries were expected to strengthen the capacity of training institutions to integrate traditional medicine (TM) modules in the curricula of health sciences students and health professionals during the first decade of the implementation of the regional strategy on traditional medicine. This aimed at enhancing the exposure of health science students and health professionals to the role of TM in health systems. To support the process six countries (Cameroon, Democratic Republic of the Congo, Ghana, Mali, Nigeria, and United Republic of Tanzania) field-tested draft WHO training tools in traditional medicine for health sciences students for university pharmacy students. Four countries (Cameroon, Congo, Democratic Republic of the Congo, and South Africa) did so for medical students.

### 1.15.1 Examples of Training Institutions That Have Integrated Traditional Medicine in the Curricula in Economic Community of West African States (ECOWAS)

In 2001, the Kwame Nkrumah University of Science and Technology in Ghana established a bachelor of science degree in herbal medicine to train medical herbalists and as of 2009 had trained over 100 graduate medical herbalists (https://www.knust.edu.gh/admissions/prospective/ugprogrammes). In 2009 some training institutions in West Africa such as Guinea and Sierra Leone indicated that a master's degree program in traditional medicine was necessary for pharmacists, whereas in Burkina Faso a diploma course was in progress. In 2010, the ECOWAS Deans of Pharmacy and Medical Schools adopted the WAHO tools in traditional medicine. In 2011, Burkina Faso established a bachelor of science degree in herbal medicine. In Nigeria, some courses in traditional medicine in certain universities are being taught to undergraduate pharmacy students within the context of pharmacognosy, ethnopharmacology, and history of pharmacy. In addition, Nigeria has recently established a college to offer a degree in complementary and alternative medicine.

By 2013, nine countries from the ECOWAS subregion (Benin, Burkina Faso, Ghana, Guinea, Mali, Niger, Nigeria, Senegal, and Sierra Leone) reported to have developed training programs on traditional medicine. For example, the University of Ghana, Department of Pharmacognosy and Herbal Medicine offers a course for a bachelor of pharmacy (http://pharmacy.ug.edu.gh/overview), the college of integrated medicine has a training program in complementary health care at certificate level in Ghana (https://www.villagevolunters.org/village-news/ghana-college-of-integrated-medicine/), and the Endpoint homeopathic training institute in Ghana offers a diploma and degree in alternative medicine (https://www.businessghana.com/site/classifieds/other-classified-items/396424/Admission-End-Point-College-Of-Alternative-Medicines). In addition, the University of Bamako, Department of Health Sciences, and the University of Ibadan, College of Medicine, in Nigeria (http://www.wahooas.org/spip.php?article1017), and the Obafemi Awolowo University, Ile-Ife, Pharmacy Department, also in Nigeria, offer training curricula in traditional medicine for undergraduate pharmacy students. Furthermore, the University of Sierra Leone, Department of Pharmacology and Pharmacognosy, offers a master's degree program in traditional medicine as well as courses in traditional medicine for pharmacy and medical undergraduate students.

### 1.15.2 Examples of Training Institutions That Have Integrated Traditional Medicine in the Curricula of Health Sciences Students in the East African Community (EAC)

The Kenyatta University, Department of Pharmacy and Complementary/Alternative Medicine, offers courses for undergraduate and graduate pharmacy (http://medicine.ku.ac.ke/indesx.php/department/pharmacy-and-complementary medicine); the University of Nairobi, Department of Pharmacognosy and Phytochemistry, offers a master of science in pharmacognosy and complementary medicine (http://pharmacology.uonbi.ac.ke//non_degrees_details/733), whereas the Muhimbili University of Allied and Health Sciences, Institute of Traditional Medicine, offers a postgraduate (Msc. and PhD) programme in traditional medicine development (http://www.muhas.ac.tz/indexphp/academics/muhas-institutes/110-itm) and a module for undergraduate and graduate medical students (http://itm.muhas.ac.tz/index.php/training-programmes). In addition, the Sokoine University of Agriculture, Department of Veterinary Medicine, offers a master's of science in natural products technology and value addition (http://www.suanet.ac.tz/index.php/education/programmes-offered-at-sua).

### 1.15.3 Examples of Training Institutions That Have Integrated Traditional Medicine in the Curricula of Health Sciences Students in SADC

The University of KwaZulu- Natal, Department of Science and Technology, National Research and Foundation Centre in South Africa, offers indigenous knowledge research and postgraduate training in herbal medicine (http://aiks.ukzn.ac.za/aboutdst-nrf-ciks). The University of the Western Cape, South African Science and Herbal Medicine Institute offers postgraduate programs in herbal medicine and tailor-made short courses geared to develop professional skills for a specific health professionals community (e.g., courses on clinical trials in herbal medicine) (https://www.uwc.ac.za/Faculties/CHS/SoNM/Pages/Default.aspx; https://www.uwc.ac.za/Faculties/CHS/SoNM/Pages/Chinese-Medicine-and-Acupuncture.aspx; https://www.uwc.ac.za/Faculties/CHS/SoNM/Pages/Phytotherapy.as). The College of Natural Therapies offers postgraduate and co-graduate educational programs (http://www.collegenaturaleath.co.za), whereas the Blackford Center for Herbal Medicines offers diploma in medical herbalist (http://www.Studyonline.co.za/herbal/enrol.php). In 2009, the Zambia Institute for Natural Medicine and Research (ZINARE) established the Doctor of Naturopathic Medicine Curriculum.

### 1.16 CONTINUING EDUCATION AND SKILLS DEVELOPMENT PROGRAMS FOR TRADITIONAL HEALTH PRACTITIONERS (THPS) FOR PRIMARY HEALTH CARE (PHC)

To establish continuing education and skills development programs for THPs for primary health care and strengthen systems for the qualification, accreditation, or licensing of THPs, seven countries (Republic of the Congo, Ghana, Kenya, Mali, Senegal, United Republic of Tanzania, and Uganda) field-tested WHO training tools for THPs. The countries found the training tools very useful and requested WHO to modify the tools into modules, and WHO/AFRO did develop modules (see details on Section 1.20.6). By 2013, Burkina Faso, Ghana, Mali, and nongovernmental organizations where traditional and conventional health practitioners (CHPs) are working together have reported to have institutionalized training programs for THPs. These include PROMETRA International based in Senegal; THETA based in Uganda; the Tanga AIDS Working Group (TAWG) based in the United Republic of Tanzania; and Aid to the Development of Traditional Medicine (AIDEMET), a Malian nongovernmental nonprofit organization (AIDEMET: 1).

Effective implementation of the WHO module in traditional medicine and the module in PHC will go a long way toward building the capacities of health science students and of THPs, respectively. These documents will also facilitate the establishment of systems for the qualification, accreditation, or licensing of THPs as well as collaboration between practitioners of traditional and conventional medicine.

## 1.17  COLLABORATION BETWEEN PRACTITIONERS OF TRADITIONAL AND CONVENTIONAL MEDICINE

Collaboration between practitioners of traditional and conventional medicine in most countries is still limited to prevention and care of HIV/AIDS patients. The UNAIDS has published extensively on best practices, including *Collaboration with traditional healers in HIV/AIDS prevention and care in sub-Saharan Africa: A literature review* (UNAIDS, 2000) and *Collaborating with traditional healers for HIV prevention and care in sub-Saharan Africa: Suggestions for program managers and field workers* (UNAIDS, 2006). Examples of traditional health practitioners' and conventional health practitioners' collaborations in countries of the African region include in HIV and AIDS control in Botswana, Central African Republic, Malawi, Mozambique, South Africa, Tanzania, Uganda, and Zambia. Other examples include tuberculosis control in South Africa, malaria control in the United Republic of Tanzania, and management of sickle cell disorder and cancer in Nigeria. In addition, collaboration in research and training in Nigeria and in research and management of various diseases has also been reported in Ghana, Mali, and Senegal (WHO, 2016a, b, c, d, e, f).

Other examples of collaboration involve nongovernmental organizations (NGOs) like Women Fighting AIDS in Kenya or WOFAK. PROMETRA International based in Senegal, the Tanga AIDS Working Group based in Tanzania, and THETA based in Uganda. Apart from Burkina Faso, which has developed a system for referral of patients from THPs to Western-trained medical doctors and vice versa, in most countries such collaboration needs to be strengthened as outlined by Busia and Kasilo (2010:40) and in the *WHO Framework for collaboration between traditional health practitioners and conventional health practitioners* (WHO, 2016a, b, c, d, e, f:1).

## 1.18  ENHANCING COLLABORATION AMONG MULTISECTORAL STAKEHOLDERS

To date, countries have used different strategies to coordinate interventions related to traditional medicine, facilitate coordination of relevant stakeholders and partners, as well as enhance collaboration among multisectoral stakeholders. Thirty-nine countries have established national traditional medicine offices. Twenty-four countries have traditional medicine programs in their ministries of health, and some of the former and latter countries have established national expert committees as multidisciplinary and multisectoral mechanisms to support the development and implementation of policies, strategies, and plans (WHO, 2013). This arrangement may duplicate work in some countries if not well coordinated. Therefore, it will be necessary to establish an appropriate structure in the ministry of health to monitor the implementation of policies and strategies and coordinate intersectoral collaboration as well as the interface with regional economic communities and various ministries. These ministries include but are not limited to health, culture, agriculture, trade and industry, and research, and development, and have strategic partners such as the African Development Bank, World Bank, United Nations Conference on Trade and Development (UNCTAD), United Nations Industrial Development Organization (UNIDO), African Regional Intellectual Property Organization (ARIPO), OAPI, World Intellectual Property Organization (WIPO), WAHO, the African Union, and NGOs.

## 1.19 PARTNERSHIPS

Various partnerships were established in the course of implementation of the regional strategies with the scientific community, regional bodies, development agencies, and individual countries, and only some examples are provided. The first example of scientific partnership is the collaboration in the evaluation of traditional herbal medicines used for the management of malaria by joint efforts of the Department of Traditional Medicine of the Ministry of Health in Burkina Faso, the University of Marien Ngouabi in the Republic of the Congo, and the indigenous knowledge systems (IKSs) Unit of the Medical Research Council of South Africa. The second is collaborations involving research on traditional medicine, education and training, and staff exchange among the universities and research institutions in Benin, Burkina Faso, Cote d'Ivoire, Democratic Republic of the Congo, Mauritius, and Rwanda with the University of Liège, Belgium. These research partnerships among various institutions and networks are contributing to enhancing R&D of traditional medicines in the African region and the continent.

In some countries, ministries of health are collaborating and promoting partnerships with other ministries as well as with NGOs. These include Ministries of Trade and Industry, Science and Technology in Benin, Burkina Faso, The Gambia, Ghana, Kenya, Mali, Nigeria, Senegal, South Africa, Rwanda, Uganda, United Republic of Tanzania, and Zimbabwe. Examples of countries whose ministries are collaborating with NGOs are Mali, Senegal, Uganda, and Tanzania. This has facilitated collaboration between practitioners of traditional and conventional medicine. Collaboration between African countries and the People's Republic of China was enhanced following some exchange visits. A 5-year plan of action (POA) was adopted at the China-Africa Forum on Co-operation and Development of Traditional Medicine held in Beijing in October 2002. The POA covered priority interventions related to the regional strategy on promoting the role of traditional medicine in health systems. It is within this framework that many countries in the African region including the Southern African Development Community (SADC) Ministerial Committee on Traditional Medicine have carried out study tours to the People's Republic of China with WHO and country support, between 2003 and 2009.

Collaboration between WHO, the African Union (AU), and Regional Economic Communities (RECs) was also strengthened during the implementation of the regional strategy on traditional medicine. The collaboration is mainly related to the implementation of the Plan of Action (POA) developed with the WHO support, for the first Decade of African Traditional Medicine (2001–2010). WHO provided support to countries to implement priority interventions of the plan of action. The good collaboration and promising results of the first decade have resulted in the declaration of the Second Decade of African Traditional Medicine (2011–2020). WHO has also been collaborating with RECs, an example is collaboration between the WHO/AFRO and the Economic Community of West African States (ECOWAS). This collaboration was intensified with the establishment of the Traditional Medicine Program in 2007 at the West African Health Organization (WAHO). The focus of this collaboration has been on provision of technical support to ECOWAS Member States, implementation of agreed activities including the development of the WAHO Herbal Pharmacopoeia for ECOWAS sub region. A key result has been the institutionalized collaboration between the WHO/AFRO and WAHO in the area of Traditional Medicine.

## 1.20  WHO SUPPORT TO COUNTRIES FOR EFFECTIVE IMPLEMENTATION OF THE PRIORITY INTERVENTIONS OF THE REGIONAL STRATEGY ON TRADITIONAL MEDICINE

### 1.20.1  Mobilization of Resources and Establishment of the WHO Regional Expert Committee on Traditional Medicine

The WHO/AFRO mobilized financial resources from the Canadian International Development Agency (CIDA). Additional funds facilitated the WHO to provide support to countries for implementation of the regional strategy on traditional medicine with major emphasis to research institutes evaluating the safety, efficacy, and quality of traditional medicines used for the treatment of malaria and other priority diseases (WHO, 2011a, b). In 2001, WHO/AFRO established a regional expert committee on traditional medicine in order to put in place a regional mechanism for supporting countries to effectively monitor and evaluate progress made in the implementation of the traditional medicine strategy (Kasilo et al., 2013).

### 1.20.2  Guidelines and Forums to Stimulate the Formulation of National Policies on Traditional Medicine

To facilitate country development of national policies and implementation plans, regulatory frameworks for traditional medicine practice, and codes and ethics and practice of traditional health practitioners (THPs) for safety, efficacy, and quality-assured service delivery, the WHO/AFRO developed tools for institutionalizing traditional medicine in health systems. Subsequently, WHO submitted the documents to the WHO Regional Expert Committee (WHO, 2002:1) and to a regional forum held in Zimbabwe in 2001 (WHO, 2003a, b, c) for review and adoption. The document was then widely disseminated to countries for use. To facilitate exchange of country experiences, in 2004 WHO convened a regional meeting on institutionalizing traditional medicine in health systems in Benin (WHO, 2004a, b, c, d, e), which brought together national traditional medicine program managers from the ministries of health of various countries, training and research institutions, policy makers, and THPs. The outcome of these forums and the use of WHO tools was an increase in the number of countries with national policies, legal frameworks for traditional medicine practice, codes of ethics and practice for THPs, and implementation plans for national policies.

### 1.20.3 Strengthening of Capacities in Regulation of Traditional Medicine Product

The WHO made presentations on regulations of traditional medicine products in various regional and intercountry forums including African medicines regulatory authorities' conferences held biannually. The WHO/AFRO convened regional and intercountry training workshops on the regulation of traditional medicines for national medicines regulatory authorities (NMRAs) in South Africa in 2002 (WHO, 2003a, b, c) and in Spain (WHO, 2004a, b, c, d, e) in 2004 in collaboration with World Health Organization headquarters (WHO/HQ) in Geneva. In 2005 and 2006 the WHO/AFRO supported the strengthening of capacities of officials of the NMRAs and staff exchange for evaluation of the safety, efficacy, and quality of traditional medicines for registration purposes. The outcome of these forums was the adoption of the *WHO guidelines on registration of traditional medicines* (WHO, 2004a, b, c, d, e) and *WHO Regional Regulatory Framework for regulation of traditional medicine: Practitioners, practices and products* (Document AFRO/EDM/TRM/2015.5) (WHO, 2016a, b, c, d, e, f). These documents have accelerated countries' processes of the evaluation of safety, efficacy, and quality of traditional medicine products, facilitated the issuance of marketing authorizations, as well as facilitated the development of regulations in countries. For instance, Uganda developed its national guidelines for registration of traditional medicines; Ethiopia adopted a legal framework for regulating traditional medicine, and SADC developed guidelines for the registration of traditional medicine for its subregion.

### 1.20.4 Support for Evaluation of Safety, Efficacy, and Quality of Traditional Medicines and Practices

In order to enhance capacity development for research and training institutions on data on the safety, efficacy, and quality and intellectual property rights, the WHO convened a series of regional forums on evaluation of traditional medicines in Madagascar in 2000 (WHO, 2000) and on research and development and intellectual property rights in South Africa and Zimbabwe in 2003 and 2012, respectively (WHO, 2004a, b, c, d, e:1). In addition, *a Regional Consultation on African Traditional Medicine: Practices, practitioners and products* was convened in Zimbabwe in 2012. The outcome of the workshop was the adoption of the *Regional framework for collaboration between practitioners of traditional medicine and conventional medicine* (Document AFRO/EDM/TRM/2016.6) (WHO, 2016a, b, c, d, e, f:1) and *Tools for documenting traditional medicine practices* (WHO, 2012). The workshop also identified elements for updating the regional traditional medicine strategy, taking into account lessons learned during the implementation of the first strategy and suggestions from countries.

In addition, WHO convened several regional workshops on evaluation of the WHO/CIDA-supported research projects in traditional medicine and malaria in

Kenya in 2005 and in Burkina Faso in 2014, respectively (WHO, 2014a, b:1). Training workshops on preclinical safety testing of traditional medicines were convened in collaboration with the WHO Tropical Diseases Research Program of WHO/HQ, in South Africa in 2004 (WHO, 2004a, b, c, d, e:1) and Kenya in 2005 (WHO, 2005a, b, c:1). Furthermore, the WHO/AFRO assessed the Centre for Scientific Research into Plant Medicine in Ghana (2007) and the Department of Traditional Medicine of the National Institute for Research in Public Health in Mali (2008) in view of their designation as WHO collaborating centers (WCCs) for traditional medicine research. These efforts, regular exchange of experiences, and review of progress led to

- The adoption and publication of five WHO guidelines on clinical study of traditional medicines and protocols for evaluation of traditional medicines used for the treatment of malaria, HIV/AIDS, sickle cell disease, diabetes, and hypertension, which were combined into one volume (WHO, 2004a, b, c, d, e)
- Increased number of research institutes evaluating scientific evidence on the safety, efficacy, and quality of traditional medicines used for the treatment of priority diseases from 18 in 2000 to 28 in 2013
- Establishment or strengthening of research partnerships among various institutions and networks (see Section 1.19)
- Increased number of marketing authorizations for some traditional medicine products (also referred to as herbal medicines in some countries) from 1 in 1999/2000 to 13 in 2013
- Increased number of traditional medicine products included in NEMLs from one to eight countries

## 1.20.5  Support to Local Production of Traditional Herbal Medicines

In 2001 WHO in collaboration with the African Initiative and the Centre for Development of Enterprise and Industry of the European Union, carried out joint missions to Benin and Mali to provide technical support for local production of traditional medicines used for sickle cell disease and malaria. Between 2001 and 2005, WHO supported feasibility studies in Benin, Burkina Faso, Democratic Republic of the Congo, Mali, Nigeria, and the United Republic of Tanzania. In 2004 and 2006 WHO supported needs assessment on local production of traditional medicines in collaboration with the African Union's Scientific and Technical Research Commission in Benin, Burkina Faso, Côte d'Ivoire, Democratic Republic of the Congo, Ghana, Kenya, Madagascar, Nigeria, South Africa, United Republic of Tanzania, and Egypt. To enhance support to countries in these areas, WHO developed a strategic plan for strengthening capacities for local production of traditional medicines, which countries adapted to their unique situations.

## 1.20.6  Development of Training Materials to Facilitate Integration into the Curricula and Training Programs

In order to promote the acquisition of knowledge and skills and facilitate development of curricula and training programs in its member states, the WHO/AFRO developed draft Training Tools for Health Sciences in Traditional Medicine (WHO, 2015) and draft Training Tools in Primary Health Care (WHO, 2015). The WHO supported 10 countries in field-testing the draft training materials for health sciences students and five countries for THPs and convened a regional forum to exchange the countries' experiences of field-testing. The countries requested WHO to simplify the training tools into modules to facilitate gradual integration into the curricula.

In response, WHO/AFRO developed a *Module on traditional medicine for training of health sciences students and conventional medicine practitioners* (Document AFRO/EDM/TRM/2016.1) (WHO, 2016a, b, c, d, e, f:1). The module contains nine chapters: (1) "Basic concepts in traditional medicine," (2) "From medicinal plants to pharmaceutical products," (3) "Establishment of ethnomedical information," (4) "Policy and regulatory framework," (5) "Protection of intellectual property rights and traditional medical knowledge," (6) "Safety, efficacy, quality and rational use of herbal products," (7) "Herbal medicine research," (8) "Methods of administration, diagnosis and product preparation of Traditional Medicine," and (9) "Glossary of terms and definitions." Similarly, WHO/AFRO developed a *Module for training of traditional medicine practitioners in primary health care* (Document AFRO/EDM/TRM/2016.2) (WHO, 2016a, b, c, d, e, f:1.2). The document contains six modules: (1) "Basic principles," (2) "Health and the environment," (3) "Preventive medicine," (4) "Communicable diseases," (5) "Non-communicable diseases," and (6) "Traditional Medicine."

### 1.20.7 Protection of Intellectual Property Rights (IPR) and Traditional Medical Knowledge (TMK)

In order to establish mechanisms for the protection of IPRs and TMK, the WHO/AFRO convened a number of regional workshops in Zimbabwe in 2001, 2012, and 2014, in South Africa in 2003, and in Kenya in 2005, which discussed issues related to research as well as IPRs and TMK. In addition, in March 2006, the WHO/AFRO in collaboration with the African Union Technical and Scientific Research Commission jointly organized a regional workshop on regulatory framework for the protection of TMK and IPRs, which reviewed preliminary documents developed by the WHO/AFRO on IPRs. Given the complexity of this subject, it took many years to agree on a framework that could be used as a template for countries' adaptation to their unique situations. Finally, the experts and member states adopted the two following documents that were developed by the WHO/AFRO: *WHO Regional Policy guidance on national policy for the protection of indigenous knowledge in African traditional medicine* (Document AFRO/EDM/TRM/2016.3) and *Sui generis legislative framework for protection of indigenous knowledge in African traditional medicine* (Document AFRO/EDM/TRM/2016.4). Preliminary versions of these documents received contributions from ARIPO, OAPI, and WIPO. These documents complement the Organization of African Union Model Law and the ARIPO/OAPI continental legal instrument; consequently, ARIPO developed the *Swakopmund protocol on protection of Traditional Knowledge and Expression of Folklore* (ARIPO, 2010). The WHO will continue to work in close collaboration with ARIPO, OAPI, and WIPO as well as with the African Union on issues related to IPRs.

## 1.21 RESOURCE MOBILIZATION

Some countries of the African region reported that funds were allocated but only for specific activities such as celebration of African Traditional Medicine Day, sensitization and training of THPs, and distribution of training materials. Some countries have formulated project proposals or had used their national strategic plans on traditional medicine for attracting grants and collaboration agreements with partners and donors. Other countries succeeded in mobilizing financial resources from NGOs and bilateral and multilateral organizations. Major donors that provided funding to countries include the Global Fund to fight AIDS, TB and Malaria; various health system projects; Canadian International Development Agency (CIDA), World Bank (WB), African Development Bank (ADB), International Development Research Centre (IDRC), WHO, UNAIDS, WAHO, Phytica-USA, Japan-Overseas Development Agency, University of Oslo, OAPI, French and Taiwanese cooperation, and NGOs (Italian NGOs, PROMETRA International and Antenna Technology [Swiss]).

## 1.22 CHALLENGES

Progress has been made in implementing the regional strategies on promoting (Document AFR/RC50/9) and enhancing (Document AFR/RC63/6) the role of traditional medicine in health systems, as well as plans of action on the Decades of African Traditional Medicine 2001–2010 and 2011–2020, respectively. However, countries have faced some challenges that hamper the integration of traditional medicine into national health systems. These challenges include but are not limited to those in the following sections.

### 1.22.1 Inadequate Organizational Arrangements at National Level for Institutionalization of Traditional Medicine in National Health System

In most countries, the allocation of adequate financial resources from national budgets for implementation of traditional medicine activities is either nonexistent or highly limited. Most countries have not yet established mechanisms for the official recognition of THPs through enactment of laws that provide for establishment of governing bodies for THPs. Countries with national policies on traditional medicine have not yet effectively implemented them due to the lack of strategic implementation plans and scarce resources. Mechanisms of communication and collaboration between practitioners of conventional and traditional medicine have not yet been articulated.

### 1.22.2 Scanty Research Data on the Safety, Efficacy, and Quality of Traditional Medicines

This is partly due to limited resources for conduct of phase III clinical trials as golden standards for confirmation of safety, efficacy, and quality of medicines and partly due to nonrecognition of traditional medicine research as a priority for provision of quality-assured medical products to their population and prerequisite for economic development. These reasons, among others, have resulted in scanty documentation of effective traditional medicine products and practices.

## 1.22.3 Inadequate Modalities for Strengthening Capacities of Human Resources

The majority of countries have not yet integrated some aspects of traditional medicine in the curricula of health sciences students and other higher learning institutions. In addition, continuing education training programs for THPs are not structured.

## 1.22.4 National Policies and Legislation on IPRs

There are scarce country policies or legislation for protection of TMK and IPRs because less than half of the 47 countries in the African region have developed such policies or legislation. In addition, there is scanty documentation of TMK for its preservation due to the oral nature of the knowledge transmitted in various forms from past generations. This has made it largely invisible to the development of the community and to science. However, there is need for documenting and verifying TMK. This requires collaboration between western-trained practitioners and THPs, so that they can develop a framework for deciding which herbal medicines are valid and putting in place an education scheme for effective contribution of THPs to mainstream healthcare.

## 1.22.5 Favorable Investment Environment

Governments have not yet played their key roles in scaling up the creation of enabling policy to create favorable economic and regulatory environments for investment in small- and large-scale manufacturing of traditional herbal medicines with evidence-based safety, efficacy, and quality.

## 1.23 THE WAY FORWARD

In light of the progress made and challenges faced in the implementation of the regional strategy, member states should take action on the issues in the following sections.

## 1.23.1 Institutionalization of Traditional Medicine

Improve organizational arrangements at the national level for institutionalization of traditional medicine in national health systems, such as placing the traditional medicine program at the ministerial level for advocacy and visibility as well as to promote, coordinate, and monitor the implementation of multisectoral traditional medicine strategic plans. This will ensure allocation of adequate financial resources for implementations of country plans, establishment of mechanisms for the official recognition of THPs, and better communication and collaboration between practitioners of conventional and traditional medicine.

### 1.23.2 Funding Needs

Take concrete steps to assess the funding needs for traditional medicine research and allocate financial resources from national budgets while considering changes in financing options and innovative funding mechanisms. In addition, invest in traditional medicine operational and biomedical research to improve the safety, efficacy, and quality of traditional medicine practices and products.

### 1.23.3 National Traditional Medical Knowledge (TMK) Databases

Develop national databases for recording TMK and the use of traditional medicine products; document and preserve TMK in various forms, and develop national legislation for the protection of IPRs and access to biological resources and indigenous knowledge.

### 1.23.4 Adaptation of WHO Tools

Adapt WHO tools and guidelines on traditional medicine to each country's unique situations and implement the priority interventions as well as policies, strategies, and plans.

### 1.23.5 Marketing Authorization

Issue marketing authorization for medicines that meet national criteria and WHO norms and standards of quality, safety, and efficacy, and include them in NEMLs. Member states should also strengthen pharmacovigilance systems for monitoring adverse effects of traditional medicine products.

### 1.23.6 Training Programs

Strengthen the capacity of training institutions to develop training programs and revise curricula to include traditional medicine modules for exposure of health sciences students and health professionals to the role of traditional medicine in health systems.

### 1.23.7 Promotion of Public-Private Partnerships

Enhance the creation of an enabling policy, and economic and regulatory environments to promote public-private partnerships to raise interest in the investment for large-scale manufacturing of traditional medicine products with evidence-based safety, efficacy, and quality.

## ACKNOWLEDGMENTS

We gratefully acknowledge the Canadian International Development Agency (CIDA) for the financial support received through a specific project, which has facilitated implementation of the Regional Strategies on Promoting and Enhancing the Role of Traditional Medicine in health systems by countries and the Regional Office, a summary of which is reported in this chapter. We also thank the various partners for their contributions to the development of traditional medicine in member states in the African region as reflected in this chapter.

## REFERENCES

Abdullahi, A.A., 2011. Trends and challenges of traditional medicine in Africa. *African Journal of Traditional, Complementary and Alternative Medicines* 8 (5S). doi: 10.4314/ajtcam.v8i5S.5.

African Association of Medicinal Plants Standards, 2010. *African Herbal Pharmacopoeia.* https://www.aamps.org/african-herbal-pharmacopoeia (Accessed on April 15, 2017).

African Union, 2001. Decision on the declaration of the period 2001–2010 as the OAU Decade for African Traditional Medicine (Dco.CM/2227) (LXXIV). Assembly of Heads of State and Government. *Thirty-Seventh Ordinary Session of the AEC*, Lusaka, Zambia, July 9–11 (AHG/Draft/Dec.1-11) (XXXVII) Rev.1, AHG/Draft/Decl./(XXXVII), pp. 1–2.

African Union, 2003. The Maputo declaration on Malaria, HIV/AIDS, TB and ORID (Assembly/AU/Decl.6 [II]) made at the Assembly of the African Union, *Second Ordinary Session*, Maputo, Mozambique, July 10–12 (Assembly/AU/ Decl. 4-11), pp. 1–3.

African Union, 2006. Special summit of African Union on HIV/AIDS, tuberculosis and malaria (ATM), Abuja, Nigeria, May 2–4. *Theme: Universal Access to HIV/AIDS, Tuberculosis and Malaria Services by 2010 Sp/Assembly/ATM/3 (I), Rev. 2. An African Common Position for the UN General Assembly Special Session (UNGASS) on AIDS*, New York.

African Union, 2008. Mid-term review report on the implementation of the plan of action on the Decade of African Traditional Medicine. *Conference of African Ministers of Health*, Yaoundé, Cameroon, August 31. Report prepared by WHO Regional Office for Africa in collaboration with the African Union.

African Union, 2011. Windhoek declaration on the impact of climate change on health and development in Africa, CAMH/MIN/DRAFT/DECL (V), *Fifth Ordinary Session of the African Union Conference of Ministers of Health*, Windhoek, Namibia, April 17–21, pp. 1–6.

Aid to the Development of Traditional Medicine (AIDEMET), Editorial May 2007. Available at: http://www.aidemet.org/doc/edit_0507_2.pdf (Accessed on April 11, 2017).

Akpona, H.A., Sogbohossou, E., Sinsin, B., Houngnihin, R.A., 2008. Botanical gardens as a tool for preserving plant diversity, threatened relic forest and indigenous knowledge on traditional medicine in Benin, IUFRO Conference, Ghana, October 15–17. In: John A. Parrotta, Alfred Oteng-Yeboah Joseph Cobbinah (Eds.), *Traditional Forest-Related Knowledge and Sustainable Forest Management in Africa IUFRO World Series* Volume 23. Available at: https://www.acadcmia.cdu/7269595/Assessing_indigenous_knowledge_for_evaluation_propagation_and_conservation_ of_indigenous_multipurpose_fodder_trees_towards_enhancing_climate_change_ adaptation_in_northern_Ethiopia_Conference_proceeding_Page_39.

Antwi-Baffour, S.S., Bello, A.I., Adjei, D.N., Mahmood, S.A., Ayeh-Kumi, P.F., 2014. The place of traditional medicine in the African society: The science, acceptance and support. *American Journal of Health Research*, 2(2), 49–54. Available at: http://www.sciencepublishinggroup.com/j/ajhr; doi:10.11648/j.ajhr.20140202.13 (Accessed on April 11, 2017).

ARIPO, 2010. Swakopmund Protocol on the Protection of Traditional Knowledge and Expressions of Folklore, Swakopmund, Namibia. Available at: http://www.wipo.int/ edocs/lexdocs/treaties/en/ap010/trt_ap010.pdf (Accessed on November 9, 2017).

Benoit-Vical, F., Valentin, A., Da, B., Dakuyo, Z., Descamps, L., Mallie, M., 2003. N'Dribala (*Cochlospermumplanchonii*) versus chloroquine for treatment of uncomplicated *Plasmodium falciparum* malaria. *Journal of Ethnopharmacology*, 2003; 89(1):111–114. Available at: http://apps.who.int/medicinedocs/fr/m/abstract/Js21375en/ (Accessed on April 12, 2017).

Bodeker, G., and Burford, G., 2008. Traditional, complementary and alternative medicine: Policy and public health perspectives. *Bulletin of the World Health Organization*, 2008; 86(1), 77–78. doi:10.2471/BLT.07.046458; PMCID: PMC2647349.

Busia, K., and Kasilo, O.M.J., 2010. An overview of traditional medicine in ECOWAS Member States. Special Issue on Decade of African Traditional Medicine (2001–2010). *African Health Monitor*, 14:16–24. Available at: http://apps.who.int/medicinedocs/ documents/s21374en/s21374en.pdf (Accessed on April 15, 2017).

Busia, K., and Kasilo, O.M.J., 2010. Collaboration between traditional health practitioners and conventional health practitioners: Some country experiences. Special Issue on Decade of African Traditional Medicine (2001–2010). *African Health Monitor*, 14:40–46. Available at: http://apps.who.int/medicinedocs/documents/s21374en/s21374en.pdf (Accessed on April 15, 2017).

Conserve Africa Foundation, 2002. Medicinal plants and natural products. Conserve Africa. Available at: http://www.conserveafrica.org.uk/medicinal_plants.pdf (Accessed on March 24, 2017).

De Smet, P., 2005. Herbal medicine in Europe: Relaxing regulatory standards. *New England Journal of Medicine*, 352:1176–1178.

Diallo, D, Haidara, M, Tall, Kasilo, O.M.J., 2010. Recherche sur la médecine traditionnelle Africaine: Hypertension. Special Issue on the Decade of African Traditional Medicine (2001–2010). *African Health Monitor*, 14:58–63. Available at: http://apps.who.int/ medicinedocs/documents/s21374en/s21374en.pdf (Accessed on April 15, 2017).

Diallo, D., Maiga, A., Diakité, C., Willcox, M., 2004. Malarial–5: Development of an antimalarial phytomedicine in Mali. In: M. Willcox, G. Bodeker, and P. Rasoanaivo (Eds.), *Traditional Herbal Medicines for Modern Times: Traditional Medicinal Plants and Malaria*, CRC Press, London, pp. 117–130.

Ekpere, J.A., 2000. The OAU Model Law: The protection of the rights of local communities, farmers and breeders, and for the regulation of access to biological resources. *UNCTAD Expert Meeting on Systems and National Experiences for Protecting Traditional Knowledge, Innovations and Practices*. Geneva, Switzerland, October 30–November 1, pp. 1–18. Available at: r0.unctad.org/trade/...envi.oaulaw.pdf (Accessed on April 21, 2017).

Gamaniel, S., 2003. Country reports: Evaluation of traditional medicine for the management of sickle cell anaemia in Nigeria. Special Issue on traditional medicine: Our culture, our future. *African Health Monitor*, 4(1):27–28. Available at: http://apps.who.int/ medicinedocs/fr/m/abstract/Js21375en/ (Accessed on April 12, 2017).

Gurib-Fakim, and Kasilo, O.M.J., 2010. Promoting African medicinal plants through an African Herbal Pharmacopoeia. Special Issue on Decade of African Traditional Medicine (2001–2010). *African Health Monitor*, 14:64–67. Available at: http://apps.who. int/medicinedocs/documents/s21374en/s21374en.pdf (Accessed on April 15, 2017).

Homsy, J., King, R., Tenywa, J., 2003. Country reports: Building a regional initiative for traditional medicine and HIV/AIDS in Eastern and Southern Africa. Special Issue on traditional medicine: Our culture, our future. *African Health Monitor*, 4(1):24–26. Available at: http://apps.who.int/medicinedocs/fr/m/abstract/Js21375en/ (Accessed on April 12, 2017).

International Week of African Traditional Medicine (Sémaine Internationale de Médecine Traditionnelle Africains [SIMTA]). Available at: http://www.aidement.org/docs/ news/072008_2.pdf (Accessed on November 10, 2017).

Kajuna, S.L.P., 2009. A comparison of the efficacy and safety of NK2 against standard combination ARV treatment in patients with symptomatic primary human immunodeficiency virus type I (HIV-1) infection: A randomised controlled trial. *Final Project Report of Phase I clinical trial submitted to WHO Regional Office for Africa by Kairuki Hubert Memorial University*, Department of Biochemistry and Molecular Biology (Principal investigator, Professor Sylvester LP Kajuna, June 2009).

Kasilo, O.M.J., 2003. Enhancing traditional medicine research and development in the African Region. Special Issue on Traditional Medicine: Our culture, our future. *African Health Monitor*, 4(1):15–18. Available at: http://apps.who.int/medicinedocs/fr/m/ abstract/Js21375en/ (Accessed on April 12, 2017).

Kasilo, O.M.J., 2010. International Exhibition of African Traditional Medicines (Le Salon Internationale des Remèdes Naturels Africains (SIRENA), Available at: http://www. melilinkz.org/news/newsz.asp?NewsID=5728 (Accessed on May 1, 2017).

Kasilo, O.M.J., and Trapsida, J.M., 2010. Regulation of traditional medicine in the African Region. Special Issue on Decade of African Traditional Medicine (2001–2010). *African Health Monitor*, 14(1):25–31. Available at: http://apps.who.int/medicinedocs/docu-ments/s21374en/s21374en.pdf (Accessed on April 15, 2017).

Kasilo, O.M.J., Trapsida, J.M., Ngenda, M., Lusamba-Dikassa, P.S., 2010. An overview of the traditional medicine situation in the African Region. Special Issue on Decade of African Traditional Medicine (2001–2010). *African Health Monitor*, 14(1):7–15. Available at: https://www.aho.afro.who.int/en/ahm/issue/13/reports/overview-traditional-medicine-situation-african-region (Accessed on November 9, 2017).

Kasilo, O.M.J., Nikiema, J.B., Ota, M.M.O., Desta, A.B., Touré, B., 2013. Enhancing the role of traditional medicine in health systems: A strategy for the African Region. *African Health Monitor*, 18(November):40–43. Available at: https://www.aho.afro.who.int/en/ ahm/issue/18/reports/enhancing-role-traditional-medicine-health-systems-strategy-african-region (Accessed on April 26, 2017).

Koumare, M., 2008a. Quelques données sur la conception et la pratique de la Médecine et Pharmacopée vétérinaires indigènes. Achevé d'imprimer par CF-MAC, à Bamako, Mali.

Koumare, M. 2008b. Pour mieux comprendre et mieux se soigner. Par les pratiques de la médecine traditionnelle africaine. Achevé d'imprimer par CF-MAC, à Bamako, Mali.

Kumari, S., Shula, G., Rao, A.S., 2011. The present status of medicinal plants—Aspects and prospects of medicinal plants. *International Journal of Research in Pharmaceutical and Biomedical Sciences*, 2(1, January–March).

Malebo, H.M., Kasubi, M.J., Mtullu, S., Chiduo, M., Massaga, J.J., Kaganda, J., Mushi, A.K., Senkoro, K.P., Makundi, E.A., 2014. Efficacy and safety of Tashack used singly or concurrently by HIV patients on ARVs in Tanga municipality in Tanzania.

*Report of the Regional Workshop on Development of Work Plans for Implementation of the Regional Strategy on Traditional Medicine*, Harare, Zimbabwe, November 11–14.

Management sciences for health, 2012. Chapter 5.Complementary and alternative medicine policy. Policy and legal framework. In Part I: Policy and economic issues. pp. 5.2–5.17.

Mander, M., Ntuli, L., Diedericks, N., Mavundla, K., 2007. Economics of the traditional medicine trade in South Africa. Chapter 13. In: S. Harrison, R. Bhana, A. Ntuli (Eds.). *South African Health Review 2007*, pp. 189–195. Durban: Health Systems Trust. Available at: http://www.hst.orgza/publications/711.

Mashava, P., 2005. Experience of evaluation of herbal preparations used for the treatment of HIV/AIDS from Zimbabwe. University of Zimbabwe, Department of Science and Mathematics Education. Report submitted by the principal investigator (August).

McGown, J., 2006. Out of Africa: Mysteries of Access and Benefit Sharing. Published by The Edmonds Institute, USA in cooperation with the African Centre for Biosafety, South Africa. Available at: http://www.edmonds-institute.org/outofafrica.pdf (Accessed on April 14, 2017).

Mhame, P.P., Busia, K., Kasilo, O.M.J., 2010. Clinical practices of African Traditional Medicine. Special Issue on the Decade of African Traditional Medicine (2001–2010). *African Health Monitor*, 14(1):32–39. Available at: http://apps.who.int/medicinedocs/documents/s21374en/s21374en.pdf (Accessed on April 15, 2017).

Ministry of Health, 2009. *The First Edition of the Herbal Pharmacopoeia and Tradition*. A.G.B, Technoprint s.a.r.l., Kinshasa/Barumbu, Democratic Republic of the Congo.

Nikiema, J.B., Djierro, K., Simpore, J., Sia, D., Sourabié, S., Gnola, C., Guissou, I.P., 2009. Stratégie d'utilisation des substances naturelles dans la prise en charge des personnes vivant avec le VIH: Expérience du Burkina Faso. Dossier Spécial: Médecine traditionnelle en Afrique. *Ethnopharmacologie*, 43(July):47–51.

Nikiema, J.B., Ouattara, B., Sembde, R., Djierro, K., Compaore, M., Guissou, I.P., Kasilo, O.M.J. 2010. Promotion de la médecine traditionelle du Burkina Faso: Essai de développement d'un médicament antidrépanocytaire, le FACA. Special Issue on the Decade of African Traditional Medicine (2001–2010). *African Health Monitor*, 14(1):52–57. Available at: http://apps.who.int/medicinedocs/documents/s21374en/s21374en.pdf (Accessed on April 15, 2017).

Njume, C., and Goduka, N.I., 2012. Treatment of diarrhoea in Rural African Communities: An overview of measures to maximise the medicinal potentials of indigenous plants. *International Journal of Environmental Research and Public Health*, 9(11):3911–3933. [Published online 2012 October 26]. doi:10.3390/ijerph9113911.

Nkurunziza, J.P., 2009. Centre for Research in Phytomedicines and Life Sciences, Institute of Scientific and Technological Research (IRST). Validating traditional knowledge: Rwanda. In: *Volume 10: Examples of the Development of Pharmaceutical Products from Medicinal Plants*, pp. 127–134. Available at: http://apps.who.int/medicinedocs/fr/m/abstract/Js21375en/ (Accessed on April 12, 2017).

Organization of the African Unity (OAU), 2001. Decision on the Declaration of the period 2001–2010 as the OAU Decade for African Traditional Medicine (Dco. CM/2227 (LXXIV). Assembly of Heads of State and Government. Thirty-Seventh Ordinary Session of the AEC, 9–11 July, Lusaka, Zambia (AHG/Draft/Dec.1-11 (XXXVII) Rev.1, AHG/Draft/Decl./ (XXXVII), pp. 1–2.

Ratsimamanga, S.U., *Eugenia Jambolana: Madagascar*, Malagasy Institute of Applied Research, Antananarivo. Available at: http://ssc.undp.org/uploads/media/Eugenia_Jambolana _Madagascar.pdf (Accessed on March 21, 2017).

Rinaldi, R., and Shetty, P., 2015. Traditional medicine for modern times: Facts and figures. Available at: http://www.scidev.net/global/medicine/feature/traditional-medicine-modern-times-facts-figures.html (Accessed on March 27, 2017).

Robinson, M.M. and Zhang, X., 2011. The world medicines situation 2011. Traditional medicines: Global situation, issues and challenges. Available at: http://digicollection.org/hss/documents/s18063en/s18063en.pdf (Accessed on November 9, 2017).

Rukangira, E. 1996. *Medicinal Plants and Traditional Medicine in Africa: Constraints and Challenges.* Conserve Africa International. Sustainable Development International, pp. 179–184.

Sackey, E.K.A., and Kasilo, O.M.J., 2010. Intellectual property approaches to the protection of traditional knowledge in the African Region. Special Issue on Decade of African Traditional Medicine (2001–2010). *African Health Monitor,* 14(1):89–102. Available at: http://apps.who.int/medicinedocs/documents/s21374en/s21374en.pdf (Accessed on April 15, 2017).

Sambo, L., 2003. Integration of traditional medicine into National Health Systems in the African Region—The journey so far. Special Issue on Traditional Medicine: Our culture, our future. *African Health Monitor,* 4(1):8–11. Available at: http://apps.who.int/medicinedocs/fr/m/abstract/Js21375en/ (Accessed on April 12, 2017).

Simpore, J., Nikiema, J.B., Sia, D., 2003. Country reports: Evaluation of Traditional Medicines for the management of HIV/AIDS: The experience of Burkina Faso. Special Issue on Traditional Medicine: Our culture, our future. *African Health Monitor,* 4(1):29–32. Available at: http://apps.who.int/medicinedocs/fr/m/abstract/Js21375en/ (Accessed on April 12, 2017).

The Government of Ghana, 2007. The Second Edition of the Ghanaian Herbal Pharmacopoeia. Published by Science and Technology Policy Research Institute, Council for Scientific and Industrial Research in Accra. Available at: https://openlibrary.org/books/OL16817515M/Ghana_herbal_pharmacopoeia (Accessed on March 25, 2017).

The Government of Nigeria, 2008. *Nigerian Herbal Pharmacopoeia. Federal Ministry of Health,* Printed in Abuja, Nigeria, in collaboration with WHO Regional Office for Africa, Brazzaville, Republic of the Congo.

The Government of South Africa, 2013. Draft national policy for intellectual property rights.

Traoré, M., Diallo, A., Nikièma, J.B., Tinto, H., Dakuyo, Z.P., Ouédraogo, J.B., Guissou, I.P., Guiguemdé, T.R., 2008. In vitro and in vivo antiplasmodial activity of 'Saye', an herbal remedy used in Burkina Faso traditional medicine. *Phytotherapy Research,* 22:550–551.

UNAIDS, 2000. Collaboration with traditional healers in HIV/AIDS prevention and care in sub-Saharan Africa: A literature review. UNAIDS best collection practice, pp. 1–58. Available at: http://data.unaids.org/publications/irc-pub01/jc299-tradheal_en.pdf (Accessed on November 9, 2017).

UNAIDS, 2006. Collaborating with Traditional Healers for HIV Prevention and Care in sub-Saharan Africa: Suggestions for Programme Managers and Field Workers. UNAIDS best collection practice, pp. 1–54. Available at: http://data.unaids.org/publications/irc-pub07/jc967-tradhealers_en.pdf (Accessed on November 9, 2017).

United Nations General Assembly Special Session on HIV/AIDS (UNGASS) on AIDS, New York, 2006. Available at: http://www.aidsfocus.ch/en/platform-aidsfocus.ch/basics/political-declarations-to-hiv-aids/united-nations-general-assembly-special-session-on-hiv-aids-ungass (Accessed on November 9, 2017).

Wachtel-Galor, S., and Benzie, I.F.F., 2011. Herbal medicine. An introduction to its history, usage, regulation, current trends and research needs. In: I.F.F. Benzie and S. Wachtel-Galor (Eds.), *Herbal Medicine: Biomolecular and Clinical Aspects,* 2nd ed. CRC Press, Boca Raton, FL. Chapter 1. Available at: www.ncbi.nlm.nih.gov/books/NBK92773 (Accessed on March 22, 2017).

Wambebe, C., Khamofu, H., Momoh, J.A.F., Ekpeyong, A.B.S., Njoku, O.S., et al. 2001. Double-blind, placebo controlled, randomized cross-over clinical trial of NIPRISAN in patients with sickle-cell disorder. *Phytomedicine*, 8(4):252–261.

Wambebe, C., 2003. Accelerating local production of traditional medicines in Africa. Special Issue on Traditional Medicine: Our culture, our future. *African Health Monitor*, 4(1):19–21. Available at: http://apps.who.int/medicinedocs/fr/m/abstract/Js21375en/ (Accessed on April 12, 2017).

West African Health Organization, 2013. *WAHO Herbal Pharmacopoeia for Economic Community of the West African States (ECOWAS)*, KS Printkraft Ghana, Ltd, Bobo Dioulasso.

World Bank, 2003. Traditional medicine practice in contemporary Uganda. Indigenous Knowledge Notes. No. 54. Available at: http://www.academia.edu/205701/ Traditional_Medicine_Practicein_Contemporary_Uganda (Accessed on March 27, 2017).

World Health Organization, 1978. The promotion of and development of traditional medicine. *Report of a WHO Meeting*. WHO, Geneva, Switzerland.

World Health Organization, 2001. Promoting the role of traditional medicine in health systems: A strategy for the African Region (document AFR/RC50/9). WHO Regional Office for Africa, Temporary location, Harare, Zimbabwe, pp. 1–25.

World Health Organization, 2002. *WHO Traditional Medicine Strategy 2002–2005*. WHO, Geneva, Switzerland. Document reference, WHO/EDM/TRM/2002.1. Available at: http://apps.who.int/medicinedocs/en/d/Js2297e/4.2.html (Accessed on April 27, 2017).

World Health Organization, 2002. WHO regional expert committee on traditional medicine. *Final Report of the First Meeting*. Harare, Zimbabwe, Temporary Location, 16–19 November 2001. WHO Regional Office for Africa (Document reference, AFR/TRM.01.02).

World Health Organization, 2003a. Regional meeting on integration of traditional medicine in health systems: Strengthening collaboration between traditional and conventional health practitioners, Harare, Zimbabwe, November 26–29, 2001. *Final Report*. WHO Regional Office for Africa, Brazzaville, Republic of the Congo (Document reference AFR/TRM/03.2).

World Health Organization, 2003b. Special issue, on traditional medicine: Our culture, our future. *African Health Monitor*, 4(1). Available at: http://apps.who.int/medicinedocs/fr/m/abstract/Js21375en/ (Accessed on April 12, 2017).

World Health Organization, 2003c. WHO guidelines on good agricultural and collection practices (GACP) for medicinal plants, WHO, Geneva, Switzerland. Available at: http://apps.who.int/iris/bitstream/10665/42783/1/9241546271.pdf (Accessed on April 22, 2017).

World Health Organization, 2004a. *Guidelines for Clinical Study of Traditional Medicines in WHO African Region*. WHO Regional Office for Africa, Brazzaville, Republic of the Congo (Document AFR/TRM/04.4). Available at: http://apps.who.int/medicinedocs/fr/m/abstract/Js21350en/ (Accessed on April 22, 2017).

World Health Organization, 2004b. *Guidelines for Registration of Traditional Medicines*. WHO Regional Office for Africa. Brazzaville, Republic of the Congo (Document, AFRO/EDM/TRM.2004.01). Available at: http://apps.who.int/medicinedocs/en/d/Js20127en/ (Accessed on May 4, 2017).

World Health Organization, 2004c. Final Report of Regional workshop on Research and Development of Traditional Medicine and Intellectual Property Rights held in Johannesburg, South Africa, November 25–27. WHO Regional Office for Africa, Brazzaville, Republic of the Congo (Document, AFR/TRM/04.2).

World Health Organization, 2004d. Regional Meeting on Institutionalization of Traditional Medicine in Health Systems. *Final Report*, Ouida, Benin, September 13–15. WHO Regional Office for Africa, Brazzaville, Republic of the Congo (Document AFR/TRM/04.6).

World Health Organization, 2004e. *Guidelines on Developing Consumer Information on Proper Use of Traditional, Complementary and Alternative Medicine*. World Health Organization, Geneva, Switzerland. Available at: http://apps.who.int/medicinedocs/pdf/s5525e/s5525e.pdf (Accessed on March 24, 2017).

World Health Organization, 2005a. National policy on traditional medicine and regulation of herbal medicines. *Report of a WHO Global Survey*. Available at: http://apps.who.int/medicinedocs/en/d/Js7916e/9.1.html#Js7916e.9.1 (Accessed on April 28, 2017).

World Health Organization, 2005b, Local production of essential medicines, including anti-retrovirals: Issues, challenges and perspectives in the African Region (Document, AFR/RC55/10), *Regional Committee for Africa, 55th Session*, Maputo, Mozambique, August 22–26 (AFR/RC55/10). Available at: http://apps.who.int/medicinedocs/en/d/Js20136en/ (Accessed on April 28, 2017).

World Health Organization, 2005c. *WHO Eastern Mediterranean Region. Countries that responded to the survey: Eastern Mediterranean Region*. In: *National Policy on Traditional Medicine and Regulation of Herbal Medicines*. Report of a WHO global survey. WHO, Geneva, Switzerland, pp. 92–93.

World Health Organization, 2007. Declaration on Traditional Medicine, *Fifty-Seventh Session of the WHO Regional Committee for Africa*, Brazzaville, Republic of the Congo, August 27–31, pp. 1–4.

World Health Organization, 2011a. Progress report on decade of traditional medicine in the African Region (Document AFR/RC61/PR/2), *Sixty-first Session of the WHO Regional Committee for Africa*, Yamoussoukro, Côte d'Ivoire, August 28–September 2, pp. 1–5.

World Health Organization, 2011b. Message of the WHO Regional Director at the occasion of the ninth African Traditional medicine day, August 31. Available at: www.afro.who.int/../3280-message.en/rdo/speeches/3280-message-on-the-occasion of-af (Accessed on March 27, 2017).

World Health Organization, 2012. Final Report of Regional workshop on Research and Development of Traditional Medicine and Intellectual Property Rights, Harare, Zimbabwe, May 21–23. WHO Regional Office for Africa, Brazzaville, Republic of the Congo.

World Health Organization, 2013. Enhancing the role of traditional medicine in health systems: A strategy for the African Region (Document AFR/RC63/6), *Sixty-Third Session of WHO Regional Committee for Africa, September 2–6*, Brazzaville, Republic of the Congo. Available at: http://www.afro.who.int/en/sixty-third-session.html.

World Health Organization, 2014a. Traditional medicine. *Report by the Secretariat to the 134th session of the Executive Board, Provisional Agenda Item 9.1 (EB134/24 A67/26)*, WHO, Geneva, Switzerland.

World Health Organization, 2014b. *Final Report of the WHO/CIDA Regional Stakeholders Workshop on Traditional Medicine and Malaria, February 25–29*. WHO Regional Office for Africa, Brazzaville, Republic of the Congo.

World Health Organization, 2016a. *WHO Regional Regulatory Framework for Regulation of Traditional Medicine: Practitioners, Practices, and Products*. WHO Regional Office for Africa, Brazzaville, Republic of the Congo (Document AFRO/EDM/TRM/2015.5) (NLM Classification: WB 55).

World Health Organization, 2016b. *Regional Framework for Collaboration between Practitioners of Traditional Medicine and Conventional Medicine.* WHO Regional Office for Africa, Brazzaville, Republic of the Congo. (Document AFRO/EDM/ TRM/2016.6) (NLM Classification: WB 55).

World Health Organization. Traditional medicine: For definitions. Available at: http://www.who. int/medicines/areas/traditional/definitions/en/index.html (Accessed on April 21, 2017).

World Health Organization Guidelines, 2016c. *Module on Traditional Medicine for Training of Health Sciences Students and Conventional Medicine Practitioners.* WHO Regional Office for Africa, Brazzaville, Republic of the Congo (Document AFRO/EDM/ TRM/2016.1).

World Health Organization, 2016d. *Module for Training of Traditional Medicine Practitioners in Primary Health Care.* WHO Regional Office for Africa, Brazzaville, Republic of the Congo (Document AFRO/EDM/TRM/2016.2) (NLM Classification: WB 55).

World Health Organization, 2016e. *WHO Regional Policy Guidance on National Policy for the Protection of Indigenous Knowledge in African Traditional Medicine.* WHO Regional Office for Africa, Brazzaville, Republic of the Congo (Document AFRO/ EDM/TRM/2016.3) (NLM Classification: WB 55.A3).

World Health Organization, 2016f. *Sui Generis Legislative Framework for Protection of Indigenous Knowledge in African Traditional Medicine.* WHO Regional Office for Africa, Brazzaville, Republic of the Congo (Document AFRO/EDM/TRM/2016.4) (NLM Classification: WB 55.A3).

World Health Organization, 2015. *Final Report of the Regional Workshop on Development of Work Plans for Implementation of the Regional Strategy on Traditional Medicine.* Harare, Zimbabwe, November 11–14, 2014. WHO Regional Office for Africa, Brazzaville, Republic of the Congo.

Zhang, X., 2004. Traditional medicine: Its importance and protection. In: S. Twarog and P. Kapoor (Eds.), *Protecting and Promoting Traditional Knowledge: Systems, National Experiences and International Dimensions.* United Nations Conference on Trade and Development, United Nations, New York and Geneva, UNCTDA/DIT/TED/10, pp. 3–6.

Zion Market Research, 2017. Dietary Supplements Market by Ingredients (Botanicals, Vitamins, Minerals, Amino Acids, Enzymes) for Additional Supplements, Medicinal Supplements, and Sports Nutrition Applications—Global Industry Perspective, Comprehensive Analysis and Forecast, 2016–2022. Available at: https://globenewswire. com/news-release/2017/01/11/905073/0/en/Global-Dietary-Supplements-Market-will- reach-USD-220-3-Billion-in-2022-Zion-Market-Research.html (Accessed on December 24, 2017).

# CHAPTER 2

# Intellectual Property Rights and Traditional Medical Knowledge in Africa
## *Issues and Development*

Wend Wendland and Fei Jiao

## CONTENTS

## 2.1 INTRODUCTION

Communities in Lesotho and South Africa have, for generations, produced tinctures from the roots of two naturally grown species of the *Pelargonium* plant to treat respiratory infections and diseases, such as tuberculosis. In 1897, an English boy suffering from tuberculosis was sent to South Africa. He was cured through the use of a traditional treatment using the *Pelargonium* plant, and subsequently the remedy was commercialized in Great Britain (African Centre for Biosafety, 2008:3–4). In 2007, a patent was granted by the European Patent Office on a method for producing extracts of the two plant species and on the use of these extracts for the treatment of acute and chronic inflammatory diseases and infections (African Centre for Biosafety, 2008:8). The patent application mentioned that the plant is still being used traditionally for medicinal purposes in South Africa, for gastrointestinal disorders and respiratory diseases. Two nongovernmental organizations and three commercial companies opposed the patent in 2008, claiming that the invention lacked novelty and an inventive step (African Centre for Biosafety, 2008:9). In 2010, the European Patent Office revoked the patent because the techniques referred to in the patent application to extract ingredients from the roots of the plant native to South Africa were well known in South Africa (African Centre for Biosafety, 2010).

The *Pelargonium* case is emblematic of what are colloquially referred to as cases of "biopiracy," or, less colorfully, cases in which traditional medical knowledge and associated genetic resources are claimed to have been "misappropriated."

Using the *Pelargonium* case as a springboard, discussed in this chapter is the relationship between intellectual property law and traditional medical knowledge, in particular, the role that intellectual property rules and principles can play in protecting traditional medical knowledge against misappropriation.

First, we clarify the meanings of "protection" of traditional medical knowledge and of "traditional" in this context. Then, since the conventional intellectual property system cannot fully protect traditional medical knowledge, described are *sui generis* initiatives at national and regional levels in Africa, and at the international level, with an emphasis on the ongoing text-based negotiations of the World Intellectual Property Organization (WIPO) Intergovernmental Committee on Intellectual Property and Genetic Resources, Traditional Knowledge and Folklore (IGC). Defensive measures, such as traditional knowledge databases, may also be useful to protect traditional medical knowledge, and the pros and cons of traditional knowledge documentation are identified.

## 2.2 TRADITIONAL MEDICAL KNOWLEDGE

Traditional medicine describes a group of health-care practices and products with a long history of use, and frequently refers to knowledge developed by indigenous and local cultures that incorporate plant, animal, and mineral-based medicines, spiritual therapies, and manual techniques (WIPO, 2014:3). Traditional medicine tends to be practiced outside of allopathic medicine (also known as biomedicine, conventional, or Western medicine), which is the dominant system of medicine in the developed world (WIPO, 2014:3). In many cultures, traditional medicine functions as a comprehensive system of health care refined over hundreds or even thousands of years (WIPO, 2014:3). As well as being accessible and affordable, traditional medicine is often part of a wider belief system, and considered an integral part of everyday life and well-being. Populations throughout Africa, Asia, and Latin America widely use traditional medicine to help meet their primary health-care needs, and there is an increase in the use of these medicines in many developed countries as well.

Malaria, as a case in point, is one of the most common infectious diseases and a major public health problem in many developing countries. Half of the world's population is at risk of malaria, and an estimated 207 million cases led to nearly 0.6 million deaths in 2012. Around 80% of malaria cases occur within the African region (WHO, 2013:xiii). Traditional medicines and associated genetic resources are the sources of the two main groups of modern antimalarial drugs (artemisinin and quinine derivatives). Artemisinin was isolated in 1971 as the active ingredient of the plant *Artemisia annua*, relying upon the Chinese traditional medical text, *Handbook of Prescriptions for Emergencies*, written in the third century A.D. *Artemisia annua* had been used to treat malaria in China for thousands of years (WHO, 2010:ix).

As this one example shows, traditional medical knowledge is useful, both in day-to-day health care and also in modern medical research and development. It is particularly in the latter context—modern research and development (R&D)—that intellectual property questions and options arise. For example, one-third to one-half of pharmaceutical drugs are originally derived from plants, such as aspirin which was isolated from willow bark (WIPO, 2014:10). This intellectual property dimension is the focus of this chapter.

Traditional medicine is also an important source of income for many indigenous peoples and local communities (WIPO, 2014:5). Some economic activities, such as "the wild collection, domestication, cultivation and management of medicinal plant resources," support many indigenous peoples and local communities (WIPO, 2014:5).

Traditional medical knowledge sometimes forms an integral part of the identity of indigenous peoples and local communities. For instance, traditional African medicine "embraces people, animals, plants and inanimate objects in an inseparable whole from which all beings derive their life force," and may also involve spiritual healing, which means to mediate through spiritual or divine powers (WIPO, 2014:6). In Zimbabwe, therapeutic herbs, which are considered as having supernatural and magical properties, only become effective when "a healer incorporates a system of rituals, divinations and symbols into treatment" and "the entire local society plays a role in the effectiveness of the healing magic" (WIPO, 2014:6).

## 2.3 SOME KEY CONCEPTS: THE "PROTECTION" OF "TRADITIONAL" MEDICAL KNOWLEDGE

Various reasons lie behind calls for the "protection" of traditional medical knowledge. For instance, some traditional healers in Africa believe that traditional medical knowledge ought to be protected to preserve and promote traditional medicine as complementary to modern health practices because traditional medical knowledge can play a role in curing or treating various illnesses, including HIV/AIDS (WIPO 2001:87).

In some cases, the very survival and integrity of traditional medical knowledge is under threat, as external social and environmental pressures, migration, the encroachment of modern lifestyles and the disruption of traditional ways of life weaken the traditional means of maintaining or passing traditional medical knowledge on to the future generations. There might even be a risk of losing the very language that sustains and transmits the knowledge. Either through acculturation or diffusion, some traditional medical knowledge has been irretrievably lost. Thus, a primary need is to preserve such knowledge (WIPO 2005:7–9). Preservation has two broad elements—first, the preservation of the living cultural and social context of traditional medical knowledge, so that the customary framework for developing, passing on and governing access to traditional medical knowledge is maintained; and second, the preservation of traditional medical knowledge in a fixed form, such as when it is documented. Preservation may have the goal of assisting the survival of traditional medical knowledge for future generations of the original community and ensuring their continuity within an essentially traditional or customary framework, or the goal of making it available to a wider public (including scholars and researchers), in recognition of its importance as part of the collective cultural heritage of humanity.

Intellectual property protection of traditional medical knowledge is different from its "preservation" or "safeguarding." Intellectual property protection aims to protect traditional medical knowledge from unauthorized use by third parties. However, "protection" and "preservation" are not mutually exclusive. Having different objectives, they may be implemented in conjunction with one another and be mutually-supportive. They may, however, also conflict. For example, when traditional medical knowledge is documented for preservation, it has to be ensured that such documentation does not inadvertently facilitate the misappropriation or illegitimate use of the knowledge. Whether documentation helps or harms, from an intellectual property standpoint, depends on who undertakes the documentation and why and how it is undertaken.

What does "traditional" mean in this context? There is perhaps a misconception that "traditional" means "old." However, what makes medical knowledge "traditional" is that it has been, and is, created in a manner that reflects and embodies the traditions of a people or community. This means the knowledge is often inter-generational and created, maintained and developed collectively. "Traditional," therefore, is less about *when* the knowledge was developed and more about *how* it was and is developed, preserved and transmitted.

The collective, communal character of traditional knowledge is essential to its being "traditional." This does not mean that individuals, such as *sangomas* in South Africa, do not play a part—indeed, individuals are often the custodians, preservers and practitioners of the knowledge. They may also innovate, building and improving upon the collective heritage of their ancestors. What makes their innovations "traditional," however, is that they are regarded as community held and not "owned," in the Western property sense, by an individual (WIPO 2013[2]:1).

A last word on "protection." Protection, in the intellectual property context, can mean two different things:

- Positive protection—Two aspects of positive protection by intellectual property rights can be explored, one concerned with preventing unauthorized use and the other concerned with active exploitation of traditional medical knowledge by its holder. For instance, positive rights in traditional medical knowledge may prevent others from gaining illegitimate access to traditional medical knowledge or using it for commercial gain without prior and informed consent and/or equitably sharing the benefits, but it may also be used by its holders to build up their own enterprises based on their knowledge (WIPO 2013[2]:2).

• Defensive protection—Defensive protection refers to a set of strategies to ensure that third parties do not gain illegitimate or unfounded intellectual property rights over traditional medical knowledge. Defensive protection of traditional medical knowledge includes measures to preempt or to invalidate patents that illegitimately claim pre-existing traditional medical knowledge as inventions (WIPO 2013[2]:2). A preeminent example of the defensive approach is the Traditional Knowledge Digital Library (TKDL) of India (see further below).

## 2.4 CONVENTIONAL INTELLECTUAL PROPERTY PROTECTION

Generally, and although other forms of intellectual property are relevant, the most important type of intellectual property rights for medicines is patent protection. A patent grants an inventor a set of exclusive rights for a limited time. Patents allow their right holders to prevent others from making, using, selling, offering for sale or importing a patented invention without permission. To obtain a patent, inventions must generally fulfill three requirements: novelty, inventive step and industrial applicability.

On the one hand, pharmaceutical companies can successfully patent traditional medical knowledge-based drugs as long as the three patentability requirements are fulfilled. For example, isolated and purified compounds can be patented in some countries. Examples of patents based on traditional medical knowledge include patents granted in the United States of America based on *maca*, a traditional Peruvian food and medicine first cultivated by the Incas, and a European patent based on Kava, a medical plant first domesticated in the Republic of Vanuatu (WIPO 2013[2]:2). In China, patent law protects new traditional medicine-based products and processes and new uses of traditional medicine, including herbal preparations, extracts from herbal medicines, foods containing herbal medicines, methods for preparing herbal formulas and new medical indications for traditional formulas (WIPO 2013[2]:2).

However, on the other hand, traditional medical knowledge holders are presented with significant obstacles when obtaining patents in respect of the knowledge as such. The most significant challenge may be the requirement for novelty. For example, in Article 33 of the Patent Cooperation Treaty (PCT), novelty is defined as follows: "[f]or the purposes of the international preliminary examination, a claimed invention shall be considered novel if it is not anticipated by the prior art as defined in the Regulations." Rule 64.1(a) of the Regulations under the PCT defines "prior art" as "everything made available to the public anywhere in the world by means of written disclosure (including drawings and other illustrations) shall be considered prior art provided that such making available occurred prior to the relevant date." The European Patent Convention (EPC) gives an even broader definition of what constitutes prior art/state of the art. According to Article 54 (2), the state of the art comprises "everything made available to the public by means of a written or oral description, by use, or in any other way, before the date of filing of the European patent application." Eventhough "traditional" does not necessarily mean the knowledge is "old," in some jurisdictions, if an invention becomes publicly available in any way before a patent application is filed, the application will be rejected. Making the invention publicly available may include selling the invention, disseminating information about the invention, or documenting the invention so that it can be accessed by a third party. Because many traditional medicines have been used for generations, disseminated in local communities and/or documented in publicly available sources, these medicines may fail to qualify for patent protection for lack of novelty (WIPO 2014:25).

The requirement for inventive step is also a significant barrier to patenting traditional medicines as such. Inventive step, also referred to as "non-obviousness," relates to whether the invention would have been obvious to a person skilled in the art (WIPO 2008:20). Because herbal medicines typically comprise natural products in their raw form, it may be difficult to claim that these remedies are novel and involve an inventive step. It can also be problematic with traditional medicine to differentiate between prior art and a claimed invention, yet ascertaining that difference is a prerequisite for assessing inventive step (WIPO 2014:25).

In addition, patent protection is limited in duration, but the holders of traditional medical knowledge may believe that their knowledge should be protected retroactively and/or indefinitely (WIPO 2014:25). The identification of inventors is needed for patent applications, but it may be difficult to identify the inventor(s) of traditional medical knowledge (Von Lewinski 2008:97–100). Furthermore, applying for a patent is a financial and human resource consuming process, and the high costs may impair the ability of traditional medical knowledge holders to obtain patent protection (WIPO 2014:26).

Moreover, collective ownership of traditional medical knowledge may be difficult to accommodate within the patent system (WIPO 2014:29–30). However, indigenous peoples and local communities can start a business entity and control intellectual property rights through such entity. In addition, indigenous peoples and local communities may collectively control intellectual property rights through licensing (WIPO 2014:30).

## 2.5 *SUI GENERIS* INITIATIVES

The limitations inherent in conventional patent systems have led to the exploration and development of *sui generis* systems for the protection of traditional knowledge at the national, regional, and international levels. This chapter focuses mainly on the international level, especially the work being done at WIPO.

First, however, what do we mean by *sui generis*? We use this term here to refer to laws and other mechanisms that provide for intellectual property-like protection that is specially adapted and designed to accommodate the particular features of traditional knowledge and the interests of its bearers and practitioners. As we see it, a *sui generis* approach to the legal protection of traditional knowledge draws upon the values, principles, and rules of the conventional intellectual property system to establish a system that provides bespoke protection to traditional knowledge. This means that the *sui generis* system that the WIPO IGC (see further discussion later in this chapter) is trying to design would provide for the same kind of protection as conventional intellectual property systems (so, not for "preservation" and "safeguarding," but for protection against the misappropriation of the intellectual content of the knowledge). It also means that it would be founded upon the same kinds of exceptions and limitations that conventional intellectual property systems use to strike balances between the competing interests of the patent holder, other innovators, and consumers. For example, the fact that most protected intellectual properties fall into the public domain after their term of protection has expired is a key feature of that balance.

## 2.5.1 The National Level

African countries have been active at the national level, with some countries having adopted *sui generis* systems to protect traditional knowledge. WIPO has prepared a useful database of *sui generis* laws from all regions, including Africa (available at: http://www.wipo.int/tk/en/databases/tklaws/).

Some countries have adopted special *sui generis* laws and measures, specifically to protect traditional medical knowledge. For example, the United Republic of Tanzania adopted the Traditional and Alternative Medicine Act No. 23 of 2002 to make provision for the promotion, control, and regulation of traditional and alternative medicines practice, to establish the Traditional and Alternative Health Practice Council, and to provide for related matters. Ghana adopted the Traditional Medicine Practice Act in 2000 to regulate the practice of traditional medicine and to provide for the registration of traditional practitioners and license practices.

## 2.5.2 The Regional Level

The African region as a whole has also been active. We recall, as examples, the groundbreaking African Model Legislation for the Protection of the Rights of Local Communities, Farmers and Breeders, and for the Regulation of Access to Biological Resources (African Model Law), adopted in 1998. Recently, the Swakopmund Protocol on the Protection of Traditional Knowledge and Expressions of Folklore (Swakopmund Protocol) was adopted by the African Regional Intellectual Property Organization (ARIPO) in 2010. The latter, which came into force on May 11, 2015, is aimed at protecting the rights of the holders of traditional knowledge and expressions of folklore against misappropriation, misuse, and illegal use outside the traditional context (Section 1 of the Swakopmund Protocol). The holders of traditional knowledge are granted the exclusive right to authorize their use (Section 7 of the Swakopmund Protocol). The fair and equitable sharing of benefits arising from commercial or industrial use, by mutual agreement of the parties, is captured in Section 9 of the Swakopmund Protocol. Both the African Model Law and the Swakopmund Protocol recognize the role of customary laws and practices in protecting traditional knowledge: indeed, customary laws and practices play an important role in the protection of traditional medical knowledge. For example, in Zimbabwe, only a select group of indigenous peoples know exactly how to identify, prepare, and use traditional herbs, know the system for diagnosing and treating illness, and can give lessons in cultural and social practices. Elders select their successors and grant access to traditional medical knowledge "through ceremonies where knowledge is revealed as a gift" (WIPO, 2014:6).

### 2.5.3 The International Level

In 1992, the Convention on Biological Diversity (CBD) was adopted to promote "the conservation of biological diversity, the sustainable use of its components and the fair and equitable sharing of the benefits arising out of the utilization of genetic resources" (Article 1 of the CBD). The provision on the respect and recognition of traditional knowledge—Article 8(j)—is a key element of the CBD. It refers to the respect, preservation, and maintenance of "knowledge, innovations and practices of indigenous and local communities embodying traditional lifestyles relevant for the conservation and sustainable use of biological diversity"; the promotion of "their wider application with the approval and involvement of the holders of such knowledge, innovations and practices"; and "equitable sharing of benefits arising from the utilization of such knowledge, innovations and practices" (Article 8[j] of the CBD).

The Nagoya Protocol on Access to Genetic Resources and the Fair and Equitable Sharing of Benefits Arising from Their Utilization was adopted in 2010 and came into force on October 12, 2014, to ensure "the fair and equitable sharing of the benefits arising from the utilization of genetic resources, including by appropriate access to genetic resources and by appropriate transfer of relevant technologies, taking into account all rights over those resources and to technologies, and by appropriate funding, thereby contributing to the conservation of biological diversity and the sustainable use of its components" (Article 1 of the Nagoya Protocol on Access to Genetic Resources and the Fair and Equitable Sharing of Benefits Arising from Their Utilization).

With specific reference to intellectual property, in 2000, WIPO member states decided that a distinct body should be established within WIPO to facilitate discussions among the member states on the relationship between intellectual property and traditional knowledge, traditional cultural expressions, and genetic resources. To this end, the IGC was established. The IGC was conceived as part of a larger and structured endeavor by WIPO to move toward a modern, responsive intellectual property system that could embrace "traditional" forms of creativity and innovations, be comprehensive in terms of beneficiaries, and be fully consistent with developmental, cultural, and environmental goals.

Participants of the IGC comprise WIPO member states and a wide array of observers:

- Although representatives from the intellectual property offices of WIPO member states constitute a substantial part of the government delegations, the cross-cutting nature of the issues under discussion encourages and calls for a very diverse spectrum of participation. Intellectual property office representatives frequently need to coordinate their views with government experts who are specialized in environment, agriculture, trade, foreign affairs, food, education, science and technology, health, and culture issues, to mention only some (WIPO, 2012:2).

- The observers include relevant intergovernmental organizations, such as the secretariats of the CBD, the World Trade Organization, United Nations Educational, Scientific and Cultural Organization (UNESCO), and the United Nations Food and Agriculture Organization, and numerous accredited nongovernmental organizations (NGOs) (WIPO, 2012:2). Indigenous peoples and local communities in particular need to be able to participate, express their views, and have their voices heard in the IGC decision-making process, in accordance with the 2007 UN Declaration on the Rights of Indigenous Peoples, as the outcome will affect their rights (WIPO, 2012:2). In April 2001, a fast-track accreditation procedure was put in operation, with almost 300 *ad hoc* observers presently registered, many of whom represent indigenous peoples and local communities. In 2004, the IGC decided that its sessions should be preceded by panel presentations chaired by and composed of representatives of indigenous and local communities, whose participation is funded by WIPO. Another significant step was the creation of the WIPO Voluntary Fund for Accredited Indigenous and Local Communities in 2005, which is designed to finance their participation. Since then, almost 70 representatives of various indigenous people and local communities have been funded through this mechanism, funded by voluntary contributions made by states and foundations (WIPO PR/2017/803, 2017).

The IGC is currently undertaking text-based negotiations with the objective of reaching agreement on a text (or texts) of an international legal instrument (or instruments) relating to intellectual property, which will ensure the effective protection of traditional knowledge and traditional cultural expressions, and address the interface between intellectual property and access to and benefit-sharing in genetic resources.

The significance of the IGC cannot be overstated: the negotiations in the IGC are perhaps the first comprehensive international intellectual property norm-setting process initiated and led mainly by developing countries. A substantive agreement in the IGC would represent a momentous and profound shift in intellectual property policy, law, and practice.

Regarding specifically traditional knowledge, what the IGC seeks to do is, at the international level, clarify which new intellectual property-like rights, measures, and mechanisms for the intellectual property-like protection of traditional knowledge might be necessary and appropriate. While the current IGC negotiating text makes no specific reference to traditional medical knowledge, the scope of the negotiations on "traditional knowledge" applies equally to traditional medical knowledge.

The IGC has, as at the time of writing, met 34 times, and expectations are high for concrete outcomes. Yet, the challenge is significant. The issues are legally, politically, culturally, and operationally complex, and there are a number of foundational questions on which there is not yet clarity and agreement. A seminal question is as follows: What are the precise objectives of the IGC's negotiations that all member states might agree upon? Then, there are a number of outstanding technical and policy issues that still require further discussion and convergence. Examples of such issues include the definition of "traditional" knowledge, the identification of beneficiaries, and the crafting of the scope of protection, including appropriate exceptions and limitations. Cross-cutting outstanding issues (issues that cut across all three themes of the negotiations, namely, traditional knowledge, genetic resources, and traditional cultural expressions) include the meaning and role of the "public domain," the meaning of "misappropriation," and how to deal with traditional knowledge and cultural expressions that are already "publicly available." For example, the IGC's discussions address concepts such as the following:

- "Public domain": This fundamental concept is usually seen as integral to the balance inherent in the intellectual property system. Exclusive rights are balanced against the interests of users, other innovators and creators, and the general public, with the intent to foster, stimulate, and reward innovation and creativity. Within the IGC, some argue that the public domain is essential to give rise to further creativity and that without a rich and robust public domain, creativity would be stifled. Hence, the scope of protection of traditional knowledge should be limited in order not to encroach too far on or imperil the public domain. In contrast, some contend that the protection of traditional knowledge overrides concerns about the public domain, and that robust protection against misappropriation and misuse is essential.
- "Publicly available": When defining the scope of protection, it has been proposed by some member states in the IGC that different kinds or levels of rights or measures would be available to right holders depending on the nature and characteristics of traditional knowledge and based on how, by whom, why, and where it is used. This leads to a suggestion to differentiate publicly available traditional knowledge from other kinds of traditional knowledge, such as secret traditional knowledge and traditional knowledge with restricted access and use, and to accord tiered layers of rights to different kinds of traditional knowledge.

## 2.6 PRACTICAL OPTIONS FOR PROTECTING TRADITIONAL MEDICAL KNOWLEDGE

While the negotiations of the WIPO IGC are aimed at the development of international legal instruments, which could eventually be implemented through the national legislation of ratifying and acceding countries, there are also practical (non-legislative) options that we mention briefly.

### 2.6.1 Documentation

Documenting traditional knowledge includes recording it, writing it down, taking pictures of it, or filming it—anything that involves recording traditional knowledge in a way that preserves it and could make it available for others to learn about it. This is different from the traditional ways of preserving and passing on knowledge within the community. Documentation is especially important, because it is often the way people beyond the traditional circle get access to traditional knowledge.

Today, the cultural survival of many indigenous peoples and local communities is threatened, and some traditional systems of disseminating knowledge may already be lost. Documenting traditional medical knowledge may help preserve knowledge. Documenting traditional medicinal knowledge may also improve the use of the knowledge. Documentation can also be a vital step in facilitating research on traditional medical knowledge safety and efficacy. Given the important role traditional medicine plays in providing health care, documenting traditional medical knowledge may help improve public health. Documentation may also promote commercialization of traditional medical knowledge (WIPO, 2014:32).

Depending on how documentation is carried out, it can promote a community's interests or damage those interests. This is because important intellectual property rights may be lost or strengthened when traditional medical knowledge is documented. Documentation is necessary to obtain certain types of intellectual property protection, which may help knowledge holders to market traditional medical-based products and services. The WIPO Traditional Knowledge Documentation Toolkit helps the holders of traditional knowledge and the custodians of genetic resources to become aware of the issues and options and manage their interests, if they decide to document their traditional knowledge (WIPO, 2017).

Documentation may also facilitate investment and innovations related to traditional medicine. Traditional medical knowledge can "be useful for bioprospecting, and may facilitate basic research on the healing properties of medicinal plants" (WIPO, 2014:32).

Documenting traditional medical knowledge may also be useful for defensive protection of traditional medicine, which, as explained earlier, means to prevent third parties from improperly obtaining intellectual property rights over traditional medical knowledge (WIPO, 2014:32). For example, the Indian government presented documentation of the traditional use of *Neem* to the European Patent Office to invalidate a patent granted on the antifungal properties of *Neem*, and the patent was revoked in 2008 (WIPO, 2014:32). India's Traditional Knowledge Digital Library (TKDL) is a pioneering digital knowledge repository for traditional knowledge, designed to prevent misappropriation of India's traditional medicinal knowledge and reduce biopiracy. The TKDL project involves digital documentation of the ancient texts on Indian systems of medicines—that is, Ayurveda, Siddha, Unani, and Yoga—that are currently available in the public domain, in five international languages, namely, English, German, French, Japanese, and Spanish, and in a format that is understandable and searchable to patent examiners at international patent offices (IPOs). The TKDL is a collaborative project between the Council of Scientific and Industrial Research (CSIR), Ministry of Science and Technology, and the Department of AYUSH, Ministry of Health and Family Welfare, of India, and is being implemented at the CSIR. An interdisciplinary team of traditional medicine (Ayurveda, Unani, Siddha, and Yoga) experts, patent examiners, information technology experts, scientists, and technical officers were involved in the creation of TKDL.

In addition, there are some documentation initiatives in African countries. For example, the Department of Botany of Makerere University, Kampala, Uganda, has done broad ethnobotanical research among the *Batwa, Bakonjo,* and *Bamba* communities in the southwest of Uganda. The department's research activities have included documentation of the communities' knowledge concerning the nutritional, medicinal, and other properties of the plant genetic resources. The documented knowledge has been made publicly available by the university for academic research (WIPO, 2001:89).

However, the act of documentation does not necessarily protect the knowledge itself or prevent third parties from using the knowledge. Documenting traditional medical knowledge "may expose knowledge to third parties," and if traditional medical knowledge "is freely available it may become part of the public domain." At this point, knowledge holders "generally cannot obtain trade secret or patent protection" for traditional medical knowledge (WIPO, 2014:33). In addition, public disclosure may facilitate the unauthorized use of traditional medical knowledge that knowledge holders wish to protect (WIPO, 2014:33). Knowledge holders have limited control over traditional medical knowledge that is publically available. While this information may have initially been released for altruistic purposes, third parties are able to commercialize traditional medical knowledge in ways knowledge holders may find objectionable (WIPO, 2014:33). For instance, a foreign manufacturer might wish to put on the market "a traditional herbal medicine for traditionally contraindicated symptoms." Notwithstanding safety issues, "such marketing efforts may negatively affect the reputation of the traditional medicines or groups involved" (WIPO, 2014:33).

So as to avoid loss of intellectual property protection, misappropriation of resources, and legal challenges to ownership, the following considerations would need to be taken into account:

- Ownership of many forms of traditional medical knowledge
- The goal and likely effects of documentation
- The most appropriate form of documentation
- How and under what conditions to permit access to documentation (WIPO, 2014:33)

### 2.6.2 Other Options

Contracts are another tool that can be used to protect traditional medical knowledge. Suitable contractual agreements can address intellectual property issues and regulate access to traditional medical knowledge and benefit sharing. For example, recently an agreement has been signed between indigenous *San* and *Khoi* peoples and the pharmaceutical company Cape Kingdom Nutraceuticals. The agreement acknowledged the *San* and the *Khoi*'s medical knowledge and recognized that the *San* and the *Khoi* peoples are entitled to a fair and equitable share of the benefits that result from the commercial development of their knowledge (Lee, 2013). Contracts, such as confidentiality agreements, licensing agreements, and material transfer agreements, can also be used in some cases where the holders of traditional medical knowledge collaborate with outside individuals or organizations for the purposes of protecting their intellectual property rights or commercialization of their knowledge (WIPO, 2014:36–37). For example, in 1995, the University of Zimbabwe signed an agreement with the University of Lausanne to collaborate on traditional medicine research, which made provision for joint patent applications. The University of Lausanne, however, filed a patent on its own for the antifungal properties of the plant, *Swartzia madagascariensis*. When details of the patent application and these agreements were made public, the University of Lausanne was criticized. In 2003, the University of Lausanne agreed to renegotiate the controversial agreement (WIPO, 2014:38).

Other practical tools, such as guidelines and protocols, may also be valuable for the protection of traditional medical knowledge. For example, the WIPO Guide on Intellectual Property Issues in Access and Benefit-Sharing Agreements (forthcoming 2018) provides guidance on the intellectual property aspects of mutually agreed terms for fair and equitable benefit-sharing related to genetic resources and associated traditional knowledge (WIPO, 2013a).

## 2.7 CONCLUDING REMARKS

Returning to the *Pelargonium* case, views are divided on how important traditional knowledge really is to the pharmaceutical industry and to drug discovery. For some, traditional knowledge subsidizes the pharmaceutical industry. For others, it has no relevance for present and future drug discovery, and cases such as *Pelargonium* are not that common and their significance is overstated. Dutfield asserts that the truth lies somewhere in between—while there is enough evidence to demonstrate that loss of traditional knowledge means cutting off access to a potentially huge and priceless stock of substances that scientists are unlikely to find on their own, one should not overestimate the value of traditional knowledge (Dutfield, 2011:237–243). As Dutfield points out, "the debate on the role of traditional knowledge in drug discovery and the extent to which this is exploitative is one characterized more by heat than light" (Dutfield, 2011:243).

This is part of the context in which the WIPO negotiators continue to try to reach agreement on new intellectual property standards relating to access to and use of traditional knowledge, including medical knowledge. These might include "positive" and/or "defensive" measures. It is critical that, somehow, this process overcomes its many challenges, including for the legitimacy and perhaps even sustainability of the conventional intellectual property system as a whole. To achieve this, key concerns as to unintended consequences that new international norms could create, such as uncertainty in the intellectual property system and impeding innovation and the achievement of economic benefits, would need to be addressed. How to address "publicly available" traditional knowledge lies at the center of these concerns. Ultimately, an international outcome should be one that provides clarity, equity, legal predictability, and an appropriate degree of flexibility for all stakeholders.

## REFERENCES

About TKDL, Available at: http://www.tkdl.res.in/tkdl/langdefault/common/Abouttkdl. asp?GL=Eng (Accessed on March 11, 2017).

African Centre for Biosafety, 2008. Knowledge not for sale: Umckaloabo and the *Pelargonium* patent challenges. Available at: https://www.publiceye.ch/fileadmin/files/documents/ Biodiversitaet/Paper_knowledge_not_for_sale.pdf (Accessed on December 21, 2016).

African Centre for Biosafety, 2010. Joy as *Pelargonium* patent revoked. Available at: http:// acbio.org.za/joy-as-pelargonium-patent-revoked/ (Accessed on December 21, 2016).

Dutfield, G., 2011. A critical analysis of the debate on traditional knowledge, drug discovery and patent-based biopiracy. *European Intellectual Property Review*, 33(4), 237–243.

Lee, R., 2013. Recognizing indigenous rights. Available at: http://www.osisa.org/indigenous-peoples/south-africa/recognising-indigenous-rights (Accessed on December 21, 2016).

Von Lewinski, S., 2008. *Indigenous Heritage and Intellectual Property: Genetic Resources, Traditional Knowledge and Folklore*. 2nd ed. Kluwer Law International, The Hague.

WHO, 2010. *WHO Guidelines for the Treatment of Malaria*. 2nd ed. World Health Organization, Geneva, Switzerland.

WHO, 2013. *World Malaria Report 2013*. World Health Organization, Geneva, Switzerland.

WIPO, 2001. *Intellectual Property Needs and Expectations of Traditional Knowledge Holders: WIPO Report on Fact-finding Missions on Intellectual Property and Traditional Knowledge (1998–1999)*. World Intellectual Property Organization, Geneva, Switzerland.

WIPO, 2005. *Intellectual Property and Traditional Knowledge*. World Intellectual Property Organization, Geneva, Switzerland.

WIPO, 2008. *WIPO Intellectual Property Handbook*. World Intellectual Property Organization, Geneva, Switzerland.

WIPO, 2012. Background Brief No. 2: The WIPO Intergovernmental Committee on Intellectual Property and Genetic Resources, Traditional Knowledge and Folklore. Available at: http://www.wipo.int/publications/en/details.jsp?id=3861&plang=EN (Accessed on December 21, 2016).

WIPO, 2013a. Draft Intellectual Property Guidelines for Access to Genetic Resources and Equitable Sharing of the Benefits Arising from Their Utilization. Available at: http://www.wipo.int/export/sites/www/tk/en/resources/pdf/redrafted_guidelines.pdf (Accessed on December 21, 2016).

WIPO, 2013b. Background Brief No. 6: Intellectual Property and Traditional Medical Knowledge. Available at: http://www.wipo.int/publications/en/details. jsp?id=3871&plang=EN (Accessed on December 21, 2016).

WIPO, 2014. Documenting traditional medical knowledge (prepared by ABBOTT R.). Available at: http://www.wipo.int/export/sites/www/tk/en/resources/pdf/medical_ tk.pdf (Accessed on December 21, 2016).

WIPO PR/2017/803, 2017. Australian Donation Means New Life for Fund That Involves Indigenous Peoples in International Negotiations, Geneva/Canberra, March 1, Jointly released by WIPO and Australia's Ministry for Industry, Innovation and Science. Available at: http://www.wipo.int/pressroom/en/articles/2017/article_0001.html (Accessed March 10, 2017).

WIPO, 2017. Documenting Traditional Knowledge—A Toolkit. Available at http://www.wipo. int/publications/en/details.jsp?id=4235 (Accessed on December 12, 2017).

WIPO, and ABS Capacity Development Initiative, 2018. A Guide to Intellectual Property Issues in Access and Benefit-Sharing Agreements.

# CHAPTER 3

# African Medicinal Plants and Traditional Medical Knowledge

## Access and Benefit Sharing in the Context of Research and Development

Gerard Bodeker, Emma Weisbord, Drissa Diallo, Robert Byamukama, Yahaya Sekagya, and Charlotte I.E.A. van't Klooster

## CONTENTS

## 3.1 INTRODUCTION

Drawing on a series of country studies in Africa, the World Health Organization Global Atlas on Traditional Complementary and Alternative Medicine reports that 80% or more of the population of most African countries rely on traditional medicinal practices for primary health care (Bodeker et al., 2005). This has been reinforced by more recent reports (WHO-AFRO, 2010), where the use of traditional medicine in Africa is reported as being as high as 85% in sub-Saharan African populations (Stanley, 2011). Often this is the only health-care system that is within people's means, especially in rural areas. In many African countries, the number of traditional health practitioners (THPs) outnumbers doctors. Ghana and Swaziland have reported 25,000 and 10,000 patients, respectively, for every medical doctor, while for every THP there are approximately 200 and 100 patients, respectively (WHO-AFRO, 2010). These figures underscore the need to maintain and support the well-established reliance on traditional medicine (TM), traditional healers, and producers throughout the continent. There has been increasing recognition for these traditions through international, regional, and national policies; research promotion; capacity building; and local development. Some of the achievements in modernizing African traditional medicine have led to the development of pharmacology based on documented traditional knowledge (TK).

There have also been continued calls for incentives for the sustainable cultivation and development of medicinal plants in an effort to produce traditional African products for African consumers (Bodeker et al., 1997; Bodeker et al., 2003; Stanley, 2011).

Aside from the intrinsic importance of these health traditions, the global economic value of TM is projected to reach US$114 billion by 2015 (PRWeb, 2012). Some countries have begun to take advantage of the potential in this developing market. In Ghana in 2010, for example, it is estimated that 950 tonnes of raw medicinal plants were sold nationally, valued at GH$7.8 million, not including the value of exported medicinals, reported to be over GH$15 million in 2008, all supplied by 30,000 wild collectors (GhanaWeb, 2013). The consumer market is estimated at over 500 million customers who make use of traditional medicinal plants (Stanley, 2011). While important economic development possibilities exist within this field, traditional producers lack organizational capacity and are generally not included in industry development or decision making at government levels.

These developments are not without their challenges and risks for individuals, communities, and governments. Intellectual property rights (IPRs) relating to traditional medical knowledge is a relatively new topic, and some countries are starting to integrate legislation to protect stakeholders as well as sign on to international agreements that protect the rights of knowledge holders.

The knowledge that is used as the basis for development of drugs, nutraceuticals, pharmacological products, and general medical products is often based on historical and purposeful use of a plant by a community or region. Under international legal covenants such as the Convention on Biological Diversity (CBD) and regional frameworks such as the African Union Model Law on Traditional Knowledge, this knowledge is legally owned by its TK holders. Ownership can exist at various levels—be it in the public domain, across a continent, region, community, family, or at the individual scale. Examples of these levels of ownership are found across Africa.

Along with well-founded fears of overexploitation of plant resources by outside users for commercial markets, THPs and TK holders worry that their knowledge and resources will be used without their consent.

As has been evidenced in several accounts of modernization efforts using African medicinal plants, there are underlying inequalities and injustices that arise when using TK without the free prior informed consent (FPIC) of THPs or knowledge holders and accompanying equitable benefit-sharing agreements in place.

Any commercial development of TM needs to raise questions of who owns the knowledge and who will benefit from the product and its proceeds. It is necessary that access and benefit sharing (ABS) questions be posed at the outset of planning for research and development (R&D).

During the second half of the twentieth century, the commercial interest for African plants rose, initially with no concept of ownership of the traditional knowledge of their use, which was assumed to be in the common domain. The cases of commercial exploitation of *Prunus africana* (Hook.f.) Kalkman (Rosaceae), *Hoodia gordonii* (Masson) Sweet ex Decne. (Apocynaceae), and *Agasthoma betulina* (P.J. Bergius) Pillans (Rutaceae) epitomize how the modernization and commercialization of TK can create conflicts between THPs, TK holders, and industrial interests when ABS and ownership rights are not accounted for. Much of the modernization of TM in Africa has happened in the absence of international frameworks that aim to protect TK holders.

Discussions of ABS, IPRs, and ethics have been mainly handled in academic forums where the perspective relied mainly on the context of the CBD. While these discussions are important, they often lack the perspective of community action and lessons learned from real case studies. This chapter aims to fill this gap in the literature, using case studies from the African continent and providing practical examples of how communities have managed to work within these frameworks to claim their TK and set forth legal arguments for the use of their resources, whether genetic or cultural. These examples from across Africa illustrate how communities, THPs, local governments, and commercial interests can work together to create win-win scenarios of knowledge and benefit sharing.

But first, it is important to understand the legal context within which discussions on IPR protection for TK and consideration of FPIC and ABS agreements can take place.

## 3.2 REGULATION OF ACCESS TO GENETIC RESOURCES AND BENEFIT SHARING IN AFRICA

Access and benefit sharing of genetic resources have been part of many debates in the last decades of the previous century leading to new regulations on access to genetic resources and the development of benefit-sharing principles, which are presented in this section.

In 1992, the UN Conference on Environment and Development led to the establishment of the CBD, which entered into force in 1993 to promote the conservation of biological diversity, the sustainable use of its components, and the fair and equitable sharing of benefits arising out of the utilization of genetic resources (Secretariat of the CBD, 2011a). The CBD was the first instrument addressing biological diversity in a comprehensive way, shifting away from the concept of common heritage of mankind to the concept of ownership of biodiversity by indigenous communities and individuals, thereby giving them the right to protect their genetic resources and the knowledge associated with these genetic resources (Bodeker, 2003). Articles related to access to genetic resources and benefit sharing of the CBD are Article 8(j), 10(c), 15, 16, and 19. Although the CBD entered into force in 1993, it was not until 1999 that the provisions were operationalized, which resulted first in providing information on basic issues, legal instruments, and policy proposals regarding ABS (Seiler and Dutfield, 2001) and led to the development of the Bonn Guidelines on Access to Genetic Resources and the Fair and Equitable Sharing of Benefits Arising Out of Their Utilization. The Bonn Guidelines were adopted in 2002 by the Conference of the Parties (COP) of the CBD in order to provide guidance in respect of implementation of relevant provisions under the above mentioned Articles of the Convention related to access to genetic resources and benefit sharing. The voluntary guidelines were developed to assist parties, governments, and other stakeholders in developing overall ABS strategies and in identifying the steps involved in the process of obtaining access to genetic resources and benefit sharing (Secretariat of the CBD, 2002).

Following the CBD, the UN Food and Agriculture Organization (FAO) abandoned the 1983 International Undertaking, which was based on the universally accepted principle that plant genetic resources (PGRs) are a common heritage of mankind and consequently should be available without restriction, to shift to the new global thinking of fair and equitable benefit sharing (McManis, 2003). This development resulted in the FAO's new International Treaty on Plant Genetic Resources for Food and Agriculture (ITPGRFA), which was adopted in 2001 and came into force in 2004. The objectives of the treaty are the conservation and sustainable use of PGRs for food and agriculture and the fair and equitable sharing of the benefits arising out of their use, in harmony with the CBD for sustainable agriculture and food security (FAO, 2009). The ABS goals are dealt with in Part IV of the treaty and are to be achieved through a multilateral system of exchange of genetic resources.

By ratifying the treaty, member countries agree to make their genetic diversity and related information about the crops stored in their gene banks available to all through this multilateral system, in order to facilitate access to PGRs for food and agriculture, and to share the benefits in a fair and equitable way (FAO, 2013). Users who have access to genetic materials through this multilateral system agree that they will share new developments with others for further research. In case they want to keep the developments to themselves, they will agree to pay a percentage of any commercial benefit they derive from their research into a common fund to support conservation and further development of agriculture in the developing world (FAO, 2013). The governing body of the treaty will set the conditions for ABS in a Material Transfer Agreement.

In 2010, the Nagoya Protocol on Access to Genetic Resources and the Fair and Equitable Sharing of Benefits Arising from Their Utilization to the Convention on Biological Diversity was adopted by the COP to the CBD at its 10th meeting in Nagoya, Japan, in order to effectively implement Article 15 (Access to Genetic Resources) and 8(j) (Traditional Knowledge) of the Convention and its three objectives (Secretariat of the CBD, 2011b). The overall objective of the Nagoya Protocol is the fair and equitable sharing of benefits arising from the utilization of genetic resources, which includes appropriate access to genetic resources and appropriate transfer of relevant technologies, taking into account all rights over those resources and to technologies, and appropriate funding, thereby contributing to the conservation of biological diversity and the sustainable use of its components. However, the protocol should not only apply to genetic resources within the scope of Article 15 of the CBD and the benefits arising from the utilization of such resources but also to the TK associated with genetic resources within the scope of the convention and to the benefits arising from the utilization of such knowledge (Article 3).

To date, 92 parties have signed the protocol, and 26 have ratified it (Secretariat of the CBD, 2013a). Only 90 days after 50 parties ratify the protocol will it enter into force. When ratified, the protocol will provide greater legal certainty and transparency for both providers and users of genetic resources. By strengthening the opportunities for fair and equitable sharing of benefits, the Nagoya Protocol will create new incentives to conserve and sustainably use genetic resources, and therefore will further enhance the contribution of biodiversity to sustainable development and human well-being (Secretariat of the CBD, 2013b). The Nagoya Protocol forms the latest approach to developing an international instrument complementing other previously developed ABS instruments.

At the regional level, the African Model Legislation for the Protection of the Rights of Local Communities, Farmers and Breeders, and for the Regulation of Access to Biological Resources (2000) was developed by the Organization of African Unity (OAU, now African Union [AU]). The African Model Legislation forms an important regional instrument with the overall aim to ensure the conservation, evaluation, and sustainable use of biological resources, including agricultural genetic resources, and knowledge and technologies in order to maintain and improve their diversity as a means of sustaining all life support systems (OAU, 2000). Two specific objectives (c and d) are formulated on ABS, which are providing an appropriate system of access to biological resources, community knowledge, and technologies subject to the prior informed consent (PIC) of the state and the concerned local communities, and promoting appropriate mechanisms for a fair and equitable sharing of benefits arising from the use of biological resources, knowledge, and technologies. Part III deals particularly with access to biological resources, which include genetic resources, organisms or parts thereof, populations, or any other component of ecosystems, including ecosystems themselves, with actual or potential use or value for humanity (OAU, 2000).

With the Nagoya Protocol coming into force, new challenges will arise for African countries on ABS regulation and implementation. First, existing national and regional regulations will have to be re-examined in view of their conformity with the provisions of the protocol. Second, new ABS regulations need to be drafted in accordance with new international legal requirements. National ABS focus points, competent national authorities, and stakeholders in this field need to better understand the concerns of IPR negotiators and national IPR authorities and *vice versa* for the effective implementation of national and subregional ABS provisions that are ultimately linked to IPR (ABS Capacity Building Initiative, 2011).

In the context of this legal background, it will be instructive to consider a few prominent examples of IPR, FPIC, and ABS pertaining to the exploitation and development of African traditional medicinal knowledge.

## 3.3 CASE 1: *HOODIA* AND THE SAN PEOPLE

One of the most well-known cases of bioprospecting is that of *Hoodia gordonii*, a cactus-like plant that grows primarily in the semi-deserts of South Africa, Botswana, Namibia, and Angola. The San People have lived in the Kalahari Desert for approximately 120,000 years (Chennells, 2007) and have used the bitter flesh of *Hoodia* as sustenance during long trips across the hot, arid, and vast Kalahari (Martin and Vermeylen, 2005). It is this traditional use as a food and water substitute that led the South African Council for Scientific and Industrial Research (CSIR) to include *Hoodia* in investigations of edible wild plants in the region (Wynberg et al., 2009).

After nearly a decade of undisclosed research, in 1995 CSIR filed an application to patent the active components of *Hoodia* for their appetite suppressant properties (Wynberg et al., 2009). Three years later, CSIR licensed the *Hoodia* patent to Phytopharm, a UK-based herbal company, along with exclusive global manufacturing and marketing rights to any intellectual property relating to this cactus species (Wynberg et al., 2009). Phytopharm further tested, developed, and commercialized the patented product through a program called P57, named for *Hoodia*'s specific appetite-suppressing glycoside compounds (van Heerden, 2008).

Subsequently, Phytopharm partnered with Pfizer, who purchased the worldwide marketing rights from Phytopharm for a reported $32 million to develop and market diet pills based on the traditionally known hunger-suppression properties of *Hoodia* (Alikhan and Mashelkar, 2009). Phytopharm had earned over $10 million while the San were still waiting for benefits (Alikhan and Mashelkar, 2009). Pfizer finally decided not to pursue this development and sold the license back to Phytopharm for a nominal amount.

Still optimistic about the compound's marketability, Phytopharm partnered with Unilever to develop a *Hoodia*-based weight management product, licensed in the European Union as a functional food—the SlimFast shake (Wynberg and Chennells, 2009). However, this partnership collapsed 4 years later, reportedly due to safety and efficacy concerns on the part of Unilever, which media speculated to be from worries over digestive problems due to active compounds being metabolized too quickly (Starling, 2008). Subsequently, Phytopharm decided to exit the functional food business and then returned the patent on P57 to CSIR, completing a full circle in which the company had earned substantial revenues through R&D funding and the sale of licensing rights, while the San were still waiting for products to appear on which they could claim their long-anticipated royalties (Makoni, 2010; American Botanical Council, 2011).

A legal challenge was launched on behalf of the San People, as customary owners. An out-of-court settlement resulted in a benefit-sharing agreement, which provided for the San to obtain 8% of payments received from the licensee by CSIR and 6% of royalties from sales of the final product (Martin and Vermeylen, 2005). The San population founded the "San Hoodia Benefit Sharing Trust," which was created to ensure that the monies received were used for "the general develop-ment and training of the San community." The San's immediate plans included buying land, building clinics, and investing in education and development projects (Secretariat of the CBD, 2008). It was reported by the lawyer representing the San, Roger Chennels, that the San had received about 500,000 Rand (US$73,000) over a 7-year period from the agreement with CSIR "and are happy with the arrangement" (SciDevNet, 2010).

What this case highlights is that it is possible for a company to keep making money from a product through the R&D process while the customary owners await benefits from product development. A system of up-front benefits paid by CSIR and the various corporate partners for the right to conduct R&D would have better served the San's needs than the many years of hope, waiting, and disappointment that was ultimately their experience. And an additional clause could have ensured that the San benefited not just from the potential sale of products, but also from all commercial earnings related to their knowledge, such as the sale of the development rights to Pfizer. Had this latter point been included, the San would have earned 6% of the $10 million ($600,000) from the Pfizer sale, plus additional revenues from Phytopharm's Unilever licensing agreement—that is, at least 10 times more than the rather modest $75,000 that they actually received.

## 3.4 CASE 2: *PRUNUS AFRICANA*

Without adequate ABS agreements, threats such as local extinction, forest clear-ing, desertification, and loss of quality in wild populations of medicinal plants risk affecting their sustainable and continued use. These risks are evidenced in another well-documented case of bioprospecting: that of the *Prunus africana* tree, from Equatorial Africa. While the conservation and cultivation dimension of the trade in *P. africana* has been much discussed in literature, no research appears to have focused on the traditional resource rights and related ethical dimensions of this trade in African TM. The bark of *P. africana* was exploited from the 1960s for use in pros-tate medication by French and Spanish companies. This resulted in a vast depletion of wild stocks of the species across Central Africa. Had consideration been given to (1) the traditional ownership of forest resources and (2) the traditional and cus-tomary ownership of the medical knowledge associated with the use of the species, harvest rates would have been monitored, local communities could have benefited from royalties rather than as from being mere bark collectors, and monitoring of the harvest would have been a feature of sustainable production. However, none of this was the case, and *P. africana* stands today as a textbook case for the consequences of ABS agreements not being applied—species loss, exploitation of traditional medical knowledge, and exploitation of local labor, rather than creation of local microenter-prises (Bodeker et al., 2014).

## 3.5 CASE 3: BUCHU

A case that is considered to be a landmark decision between two parties is that of *Agathosma betulina*, colloquially called buchu in the Western Cape mountains. On August 19, 2013, a momentous agreement was struck between Cape Kingdom Nutraceuticals and the San and Khoi people, recognizing their indigenous knowledge and their legal entitlement to a share of the benefits from the commercial use of the buchu plant (OSISA, 2013). Traditionally the Khoi and San people use buchu for renal and digestive conditions (Moolla and Viljoen, 2008).

Cape Kingdom Nutraceuticals has commissioned clinical trials and laboratory research focused on developing buchu extracts that address lifestyle diseases such as obesity, diabetes, and hypertension.

The agreement stipulates that 3% of payments for the plant products, as well as knowledge of the plant's commercial use will be shared with the San and Khoi people (OSISA, 2013). While this amount is significantly less than the Hoodia/P57 agreement with CSIR for the San to obtain 8% of payments received from the licensee by CSIR and 6% of royalties from sales of the final product, perhaps there is more chance that a product will be developed.

While these three cases are quite well known and documented, it is instructive to consider other more successful cases in order to draw wider lessons for the equitable and sustainable use and development of medicinal plants.

## 3.6 COUNTRY EXAMPLES

### 3.6.1 Ghana's Sacred Groves

Between 2000 and 2007, an Australian mining company was granted legal exploration rights for gold in Northern Ghana, unknown to the local communities who had not been consulted on the decision. The prospect of gold mining led to an onslaught of legal and illegal mining activities in the area, causing a degradation of natural resources and threatening the sacred groves of the Tanchara community.

These sacred groves are home to varied species, including the shea tree (*Vitellaria paradoxa* C.F. Gaertn, Sapotaceae), a species that is indigenous to Africa and is a traditional African food plant. The shea fruit contains nutritious pulp and an oil-rich seed from which shea butter is extracted. Some of the constituents of shea butter are reported to have anti-inflammatory, emollient, and humectant properties (Pobeda and Sousselier, 1999). In Ghana, shea butter is used as lotion to protect the skin during the dry season (Goreja, 2004), while in Nigeria shea butter is used for the management of sinusitis and relief of nasal congestion (Tella, 1979).

Local communities revere these sacred groves as the belief is that the spirits of their ancestors reside among the indigenous trees, shrubs, and medicinal plants. Ten of the community's spiritual leaders who traditionally own and protect the groves united with the purpose of protesting the mining. Assisted by Ghana's Centre for

Indigenous Knowledge and Organizational Development (CIKOD), the community took action to protect their resources, both natural and cultural.

The process implemented by CIKOD and the Tanchara community through the leadership of the spiritual leaders, the Tingandem, can be studied as an example of how to incorporate IPR of TK holders into an ethical development process that is community driven and based on local values, visions, and resources. As well, the process used in this case allowed local community members to communicate their values and vision to external actors, ensuring that open, transparent communication is carried out with government agencies and development organizations. CIKOD has also carried out follow-up studies and monitored the evolution of endogenous development capacity. What was discovered after several years were the great gains in community mobilization thanks to the recognition achieved through community organizational development processes, components of which were the empowerment of women through economic participation and the increased respect and appreciation for biological diversity, the sacred groves. and their traditional protectors—the Tingandem.

The community's increasing capacity to mobilize, communicate, and negotiate with external actors allowed Tanchara to take on the threat from the gold mining activities. The process championed by CIKOD with Tanchara community members can be divided into several key steps (IIED, 2012):

- Train the trainers. The CIKOD staff underwent sensitization training to discuss how to work within the community's worldviews and addressed the expected challenges.
- PIC and awareness raising. CIKOD staff met with the local chief and elders first and then with the wider community to explain the process and gain PIC.
- Team training. The community selected male and female representatives to identify traditional knowledge and institutions used by the community, and questions were translated into the local language.
- Training the community team. Tools for Participatory Rural Appraisal were introduced to the team members, and community consultation allowed the development of a timetable for collection.
- Community institutions and resource mapping (CIRM). The natural, spiritual, and cultural resources of the community were assessed, with information reviewed by a third party to identify gaps in data.
- Community reporting. The collected information was verified at a community meeting, with the report being adopted as a community document.
- Community vision. The community developed a resource map as the basis for a discussion on how development should progress, with responses recorded by CIKOD and presented to Tanchara as a vision statement.
- Action plan. Activities relating to development were itemized and prioritized, and a community contract was developed.

Community also developed a biocultural community protocol (BCP) to be used as a negotiation tool for Tanchara to assert its property rights. BCPs are used by indigenous communities to increase their capacity to locally implement international or national environmental legislation and are developed through community consultation to "outline their core ecological, cultural and spiritual values and customary laws relating to their TK and resources, based on which they provide clear terms and conditions to regulate access to their knowledge and resources" (Natural Justice, 2009).

The challenges in creating the BCP were as follows (IIED, 2012):

- There is a lack of legally binding support for customary laws and the BCP.
- The younger generations are impacted by Western influences and do not necessarily follow customary laws.
- There is a lack of legal knowledge by the local community relating to their regional, national, and international community rights.
- There is uncertainty relating to understanding the importance of having a BCP in order to negotiate with external actors.

By the end of 2011, the BCP had yet to be recognized as legally binding, and the legality was vaguely understood (IIED, 2012). CIKOD involved experts to identify community rights under customary, national, and international laws (IIED, 2012). The CBD's Nagoya Protocol recognizes customary laws in Ghana and will be an important legal support for Tanchara (IIED, 2012). Once finalized, the BCP will be signed by the local Chief, his female counterpart the Pognaa, the Tingandem, and ideally by the District Chief Executive and Paramount Chief (IIED, 2012).

The main lesson to be taken from this case study is the importance of strengthening and supporting development that is community driven and that builds on local culture, knowledge, resources, and institutions. This practice, also known as *endogenous development*, aims to incorporate members from the community, without targeting specific subsections such as youth or women (Natural Justice, 2009). This important aspect of the case study highlights the necessity of accounting for the traditional leadership that constitutes a key component of African governance.

The act of recording Tanchara's resources is a key factor in developing a communal value and an awareness of their importance to local culture, as well as ensuring community members' roles as stewards. This case study also demonstrates the importance of national and international recognition of the BCP. Tanchara effectively engaged local stakeholders and government agencies in asserting their rights against the mining company and resulted in pushing prospecting back to 2013 (IIED, 2012).

This case demonstrates how a community is able to take hold of their development future and dictate the terms of progress based on their values. With the help of CIKOD, Tanchara has envisioned an endogenous development plan that conserves the sacred groves and supports sustainable use of communal resources through alternative socioeconomic activities like shea nut harvesting and ecotourism.

### 3.6.2 South Africa's K2C

In South Africa lies one of the world's largest biospheres, the Kruger to Canyons (K2C) Biosphere Reserve. Its four million hectares contain much more than important biodiversity hot spots. K2C is also home to some of the most culturally and linguistically diverse groups in the region (IIED, 2012). The southern region of this biosphere reserve is densely populated by the Bushbuckbridge communities that suffer from high levels of unemployment and depend on a cash economy and state grants (IIED, 2012).

Within these groups, THPs are responsible for people's physical, cultural, and spiritual health. These practitioners are the communities' TK holders for medicine, cultural ceremonies, and indigenous medicinal plants (Traditional Health Practitioners Bushbuckbridge, 2010). Healers use traditional harvesting practices for sustainable use of these culturally important plants; however, many species are now threatened by larger-scale commercial harvesting (IIED, 2012). In response to this overexploitation, the government has restricted access to certain protected zones, and traditional healers struggle to obtain the plants that are key to their communities' cultural identities (IIED, 2012). In addition to concerns stemming from restricted access to important areas due to cases of bioprospecting, community healers also fear the use of their knowledge without their FPIC.

The managing committee of K2C invited the nongovernmental organization Natural Justice to come and discuss ABS mechanisms that are community based, such as BCPs. Following this introduction to community engagement and empowerment, a group of healers met to examine the possibility of developing a BCP among THPs.

The process originated with a small assembly of practitioners, K2C managing directors, and members of Natural Justice to discuss the healer's worries of biopiracy and illegal medicinal plant harvesting. This initial gathering was followed by regular meetings between traditional healers where they were able to openly discuss concerns, learn about conservation law for medicinal plants, discuss TK protection, and develop a newfound sense of identity and community where distance and culture had once prevented this.

Through learning about ABS laws under the CBD and the South African Biodiversity Act, the traditional healers were able to develop a BCP and unite as the Kukula Traditional Health Practitioners Association, now 300 members strong (Natural Justice, 2012).

A facilitated workshop in mid-2009, comprising Kukula's elected executive team, the K2C management team, and Natural Justice, determined six priorities for developing the BCP (IIED, 2012):

- Build credibility, trust, and mutual respect among traditional healers.
- Identify the healers' concerns and values and ensure that they are fully understood by asking probing questions and reflections.
- Facilitate consensus among the healers by ensuring that all opinions are heard and considered.
- Make sure that all participants are part of the process and ensure they feel part of a shared vision for the BCP.
- Capture and reflect to the group decisions that are owned by the healers.
- Ensure participatory and fair practices throughout the process. Encourage all members of the association to express their views and be involved.

Throughout this facilitation process, several key factors were ensured (IIED, 2012):

- The legal frameworks within which the healers work were clearly explained.
- There were summaries at the end of each facilitated meeting of decisions and processes to date.
- Tasks for in between meetings were clearly stated, and each follow-up meeting began with opportunity for feedback about these tasks.

The BCP was drawn up and presented for comment to a wider audience within the association. It sets out the following (IIED, 2012):

- Biocultural values
- The connection of communities through culture to biodiversity
- Details of traditional knowledge
- Threats to livelihoods from biodiversity loss and the impact of no ABS agreements
- Community plans for improving conservation and sustainability of medicinal plants
- Information for people wanting to access TK and medicinal plants
- Links between values, concerns, and rights of healers under national and international law

The process of creating the BCP empowered the traditional healers and gave them a sense of community identity. The Kukula Traditional Health Practitioners Association has since developed its own constitution and has been registered under South African law as a not-for-profit since 2011 (IIED, 2012). After many open discussions, the Kukula members agreed to combine some traditional knowledge and shared this with a local, small cosmetic company, with the understanding that any resulting benefits from the use of their knowledge flows back to the association (IIED, 2012). A nondisclosure agreement signed in 2011 permits the research of the utility of some of their genetic resources and TK, and the group aims to negotiate an ABS agreement should the research result in developing cosmetic products (IIED, 2012). Education, openness, and awareness on the part of the government regarding the realities of commercial overharvesting versus traditional harvesting have allowed Kukula members to negotiate limited access to once restricted areas. Local groups agree that access to medicinal plants on communal land has increased while overharvesting has decreased, a change attributed to increased education on traditional practices for harvesting (IIED, 2012). As well, there is now a coordinated effort with local farmers to access their fields to harvest medicinals before ploughing commences (IIED, 2012).

The continuation of the BCP has been the development of a code of ethics for members to improve service to patients and help members through the process of registering as traditional health practitioners (Natural Justice, 2012).

In summary, the BCP has been a crucial technique for the Kukula Traditional Healers of Bushbuckbridge to help in identifying themselves as a community with shared concerns and values. The protocol defines their conservation vision for the sustainability of medicinal plants based on the community's traditional knowledge.

The association of traditional healers has grown and now works toward asserting their resource and knowledge rights.

The Bushbuckbridge BCP serves to illustrate how the benefits from the traditional knowledge commons can be used by an entire group. This example is recognized as being a success due to the integrity of the process and the continued community engagement and representation that occurred throughout the development. It is understood that the BCP is not an end product but an important step on the path to developing and maintaining a sustainable and healthy society.

## 3.7 EXPERIENCES OF THE DEPARTMENT OF TRADITIONAL MEDICINE, BAMAKO, MALI

Mali is unusual in enjoying a high level of government support for research and development of TM. The Department for Traditional Medicine (DMT), within the National Institute for Research on Public Health (part of the Ministry of Health), was founded in 1968, originally as the National Institute of Phytotherapy and Traditional Medicine. Since 1979, one of its aims has been the development of standardized "Médicaments Traditionnels Améliorés" (MTAs, or improved traditional medicines) (Willcox et al., 2012).

Economic benefits that have accrued to the DMT from the production of improved traditional medicines include the following:

- Average revenue of 25 million francs CFA7/year
- Job creation (recruitment of five youth with diplomas)
- Creation of a network for production and sales of medicinal plants

A national workshop on intellectual property, scientific research, and innovation for technological development was conducted which showed that

- There was insufficient protection for traditional knowledge by conventional protection methods.
- There is evidence of illicit appropriation of TK.
- Mistrust exists between researchers and traditional health practitioners.
- There is a trend toward economic exploitation of TK.

Benefit sharing between the DMT and the Malian Federation of Associations of Traditional Therapists and Herbalists (FEMATH) has included:

- Organization of THPs and of the TM sector
- Distribution of dictionaries for medicinal plants in collaboration with the association, Tradition and Medicine, Geneva, distribution of prizes for THPs with value around 100,000 FCFA (Dictionary and multilingual monographs of the medicinal potential of African plants of West Africa)
- Development of TM through local production of standardized medicines
- Establishing of texts relating to benefit sharing in the future

Benefits shared with the various Associations of Traditional Health Practitioners participating in the DMT's projects included:

- Building infrastructure to enable the production of raw material for production of phytomedicines
- Assistance in the production of phytomedicines (improved traditional medicines)
- Construction of over 20 centers for associations of THPs
- Construction of a drying and storage hall for the association of THPs
- Identification of a medicinal plant field and fencing off of this field for production
- Construction of an herbalist's shop in one region (Kolokani) with 21 rooms, and a center for the sale of medicinal plants by women
- Construction of orthopedic beds for THPs working in trauma
- Distribution of model skeletons for THPs working in trauma

Individual THPs who were involved in projects of the DMT received ongoing benefits, including:

- Training of their children on production of improved phytomedicines.
- Creation of a medicinal plant garden: "green pharmacy." The DMT also provided to communities a set of medicinal plants useful for managing common illnesses.
- Development of a sales point for their products.
- Cash benefits.

We now give a case study of the development of one particular improved traditional medicine for malaria. In the context of a search for candidates for new antimalarials, a population survey was conducted in Mali regarding the use of plant-based antimalarials. From the 66 plants identified as being used for the treatment of malaria in the two districts studied in Mali, alone or in various combinations, the one associated with the best outcomes was a decoction of *Argemone mexicana* L. (Papaveraceae) (Diallo et al., 2006; Willcox et al., 2011a). The survey showed that all patients who used this decoction of *Argemone mexicana* for uncomplicated malaria reported a complete cure with very few side effects.

Comparing this species with *Artemisia annua* L. (Compositae), the source of artemisinin and the associated class of antimalarials (artesunate, artether, etc.), it was noted that *A. annua*, while currently being grown on both experimental and commercial bases in Africa, does not grow well in dry areas where *A. mexicana* grows well.

Widespread use, reported clinical benefits, and ease of cultivation and availability led to a research and development program being established by the DMT to explore the potential to develop *A. mexicana* as an improved traditional antimalarial medicine (Willcox et al., 2007, 2011b; Graz et al., 2010).

The research team developed a consultative process to ensure that there was an ethical approach to IPR protection at the local level before the R&D phase began (Willcox et al., 2015). The research into *A. mexicana* began with a commitment to equitable benefit sharing and the involvement of THPs. One in particular, who had been using *A. mexicana* in the management of malaria, assisted in conducting an ethnobotanical study into the use of the plant for malaria and subsequently in scientific articles about *A. mexicana*. He was also involved in the standardization of phytomedicines.

The procedure began with ensuring that a benefit-sharing agreement was in place. This entailed obtaining informed oral consent from the village council for the research into *A. mexicana* and agreement for sharing of benefits during and after the research. In addition, there was a verbal agreement with the THP in response to his request that "Each time that you talk about this medicine, my name needs to appear." During the research, the THP was paid 60,000 FCFA/month. The THP also received a 25% share of a prize of 500,000 FCFA at the National Forum of Invention and Technological Innovation. Other benefits included that his son was sent for training as a health-care assistant; a consultation room, powered by solar panels, was built for the village; and a medicinal plant garden was created. These actions were done in order to follow international best practice guidelines, although they were not required by law. In the future it would be good to enshrine in the law the need to share benefits.

## 3.8 UGANDA'S MAKERERE UNIVERSITY AND PROMETRA UGANDA: MEMORANDUM OF UNDERSTANDING (MOU) FOR PARTNERSHIP ON THE MUTHI PROJECT

Uganda has a long history of research into TM. As far back as the 1960s a government team, led by Mr. Nasani Mubiru, began documenting the traditional medicine knowledge of many of Uganda's 111 districts. A monumental task, this national ethnomedical survey continued for almost 30 years and has resulted in a comprehensive written record of the national TM heritage. It is currently stored as a set of typed volumes at both Makerere University and at the National Chemotherapeutics Research Institute, both of which are in the capital, Kampala.

During the 1990s, Uganda was one of the first countries in Africa to engage THPs in combating HIV transmission and also in evaluating traditional herbal remedies used to manage AIDS-related conditions. Other research has focused on malaria and also on a range of common illnesses. In this report, as part of the EU-funded Multi-University Initiative on Traditional Healthcare (MUTHI) Makerere University collaborated with Mbarara University in Southwest Uganda and an association of THPs, PROMETRA Uganda, to create a legal framework to partner in investigating important traditional medicines for scientific evaluation.

MUTHI, which ran from 2010 to 2014, was a Coordination and Support Action project under the EC's Seventh Framework Programme (Health). Its overall objective was to create sustainable research capacity and research networks between the participants in Africa (Mali, South Africa, and Uganda), collaborating neighboring institutions, and the European project participants, to obtain improved health in Africa (UiO, 2011).

The process started with the launch of the MUTHI project in Cape Town, South Africa, in January 2011 (UiO, 2011). Ethnobotanical research was to be carried out by Makerere University partners to establish plants being used in the management of malaria and/or HIV/AIDS. From the outset, it was recognized that if the research team were to wait for the ethnobotanical results to select for plants for further laboratory analysis, the project would be delayed. It was therefore agreed that each of the partner organizations would work with herbalists, traditional healers, or any other group working with herbal medicines on malaria to select the plants to work on.

Several people involved in herbal medicine were met individually; some were individuals while others were groups of general traditional healers by calling them in a meeting at Makerere University. For example, PROMETRA Uganda deals with all aspects—herbals, physical therapies, and spiritual healing. Most THPs were ready to work with the Makerere team. However, they did harbor fears as is the often-realistic concern of traditional knowledge holders in general, that the researchers could steal their medicinal formulae and profit from this.

Most THPs informed the Makerere research group that they had previously worked with people, even some from national laboratories, who they claimed had stolen their medicinal knowledge and profited from this.

The Makerere team expressed interest in partnership and assured the THPs that the main objective of the project was to contribute to improving TM, particularly herbal medicine. It was explained how this would benefit them by putting safe and standardized herbal medicines on the open market and by being able to register these with National Drug Authority (an organization responsible for regulating drugs/medicines in Uganda).

The Makerere research team explained to the THPs that the research would generate information needed to register the herbal medicine with national regulatory bodies.

What the MUTHI project would contribute was explained, including:

* Determination of the efficacy
* Isolation and structural characterization of the compounds
* Safety
* Taxonomic identification of the plants to confirm the exact species being used

This interested the THPs, and most of them were then willing to work with the MUTHI project. The researchers also mentioned other countries they were working with through MUTHI and how far ahead they are, especially Mali. The THPs were also informed that the researchers would keep visiting them with their MUTHI collaborators when they were in Uganda. Training workshops would involve the THPs, and all these formed nonmonetary benefits and the THPs were interested in these.

A further explanation was given to the THPs individually about the complexity of structure elucidation and the lack of equipment in the country and the need to rely on collaborators, all of which could take a long time and can cause delays. This was done to ensure that the groups did not think that the project objectives would be achieved in a short period. The THPs were also assured that the research team would do a literature search on the plants and share with them the findings. For example, one group was using *Aristolochia elegans* Mast. (Aristolochiaceae), yet this has been reported by the World Health Organization (WHO) as a poisonous plant. The MUTHI researchers from Makerere shared these reports with the THPs. Also, care was taken to hold several separate meetings with individuals or groups so that there would be no concerns about stealing information from one another.

The major selection criterion for identifying the THP group to work with was the criterion of using a single plant for malaria, HIV/AIDS, and tuberculosis diseases. This was for simplicity of analysis under the research framework of the MUTHI project.

While most THPs reported using a mixture of medicinal plants, one of the groups, PROMETRA Uganda, mentioned that they were using single plants, so it was decided to work with this group. In addition, it was also a big group of traditional herbalists, spiritual healers, bone setters, etc. PROMETRA Uganda is the local chapter of an international organization of traditional medicine associations (PROMETRA, 2017).

The next step was to ask PROMETRA Uganda whether the healers were ready to supply the plant material for research. PROMETRA Uganda had a series of discussions within the practitioners themselves and finally agreed to supply the plant materials for research. At this point, the research team agreed to write Materials Transfer Agreements (MTAs). By this time, planning was underway for an ethnobotanical training workshop of MUTHI. When the consortium asked Uganda to host the workshop in Kampala, the Makerere MUTHI team involved PROMETRA Uganda as participants. One of the days of the workshop was to visit the group in Mpigi at their field headquarters.

A diverse delegation from various countries allowed for a very good interaction during the visit. The group of THPs directly raised all their concerns to the delegates, and these concerns were thoroughly discussed. After this workshop, the THPs developed trust in the researchers and agreed to supply the plant material as the process began of writing the MoU. The Makerere team, PROMETRA Uganda, and the MUTHI Project were very much concerned about the IPR issues. It was explained that the MUTHI project had it that one of the project milestones for each African partner was writing a MoU.

An IPR workshop was also planned and participants from PROMETRA Uganda were selected for training. After the training, the MoU was drafted by the Makerere side and sent to PROMETRA for their input. PROMETRA agreed with most of the suggestions and also had questions on patenting. On the PROMETRA side, the problem of patenting was brought into question relating to what would happen if the MoUs were not renewed. The team resolved this quandary by agreeing to hold the patents jointly if they were obtained during the time that the MoU is valid.

Another problem from the perspective of PROMETRA is the continuing monitoring of royalties. This was solved by agreeing that both parties can participate in monitoring activities. However, as the public university is often faced with funding shortages, PROMETRA Uganda would be in a more appropriate position to engage the PROMETRA International Network to supervise these financial flows.

The MoU was presented at an IPR workshop in Kampala in February 2013 where PROMETRA participants were part of this workshop and the team received advice from international IPR experts who were facilitating the workshop. The MoU was then modified to incorporate the feedback from the workshop. This was then submitted to the legal department of Makerere University through the vice chancellor. The legal department incorporated correct legal terminology into the MoU and advised the research team to discuss it further with PROMETRA Uganda. PROMETRA Uganda held an internal workshop with its THPs to review the draft MoU, and once they agreed to the proposed changes, to then go ahead with signing the MoU. This was sent to PROMETRA Uganda, and they informed Makerere that they needed to consult PROMETRA International for advice. PROMETRA International was consulted and agreed with the proposed changes, and a final MoU was signed by both parties. From the Makerere side, the legal department insisted that PROMETRA needed someone to witness the MoU. The key terms of the MoU have been articulated in the preamble of the document and describe the importance of using a multidisciplinary approach through collaborative research to improve traditional medicines.

The process involved in generating this MoU was lengthy and slow but convincing to both parties. However, time and attention to detail, respectful consideration of the views of the THPs, and the needs of the research team were necessary components of the process. They were the key requirements for eventually arriving at a mutually satisfactory MoU to commence the herbal research program.

## 3.9 CONCLUSION

In order to increase the capacity of all to gain access to the beneficial resources in these African plants and to ensure the equitable and fair use of TK, WHO's regional office in Africa has proposed five courses of action (WHO-AFRO, 2010).

First, legislation to protect knowledge must account for the communal and locally innovative aspect of TK. A complete framework will actively strive to document TK, develop applications for it, encourage innovation within communities, and protect biodiversity and TK from privatization trends. Second, institutional capacity building must be ensured to protect TK. This should include regional administration and enforcement for cross-boundary and multiethnic TK and support structures at the country level for developing databases. Third, cooperation between stakeholders will create a united front and foster mutually beneficial partnerships. Fourth, educate THPs and communities about their rights, responsibilities, and options as TK holders. Last, African regional governments should prioritize the integration of traditional medicine into the formal health system.

What is clear from the examples presented in this chapter is that the way forward in combining research, development, and ethics in the development of African medicinal plants and herbal medicines is to develop an inclusive R&D framework, with full engagement at all stages by THPs. This needs to be guided by a values system that seeks not to offer the bare minimum in benefits to customary owners and maximum profits to the developers. Rather, as stated by the International Society for

Ethnobiology (ISE) in their Ethical Guidelines (Box 3.1): "It involves an approach of working collaboratively, in ways that support community driven development of indigenous people's cultures and acknowledge indigenous cultural and intellectual property rights. Central to this is an approach characterized by what ISE terms 'mindfulness'—that is, a continual willingness to evaluate one's own understandings, actions, and responsibilities" (ISE, 2006).

## BOX 3.1 TWELVE GUIDELINES IN ISE CODE OF ETHICS

1. Understanding local community institutions, authority, and protocols
2. Establishing educated prior informed consent
3. Full disclosure and mechanisms to ensure mutual understanding
4. Communication, consultation, approval, and permission
5. Good faith commitment and respect for cultural norms and dignity
6. Standards for mutually agreed upon terms and conditions
7. Clarity and agreement of objectives, conditions, and mutually agreed upon terms
8. Compliance with moratoriums
9. Educational uses of research materials
10. Treatment of existing project materials
11. Ecosystem harms
12. Considerations in collaborative, interdisciplinary, cross-cultural research

## ACKNOWLEDGMENTS

Work on this chapter was funded by the European Union Research Directorate through the MUTHI project, FP7 Grant Agreement No: 266005. Helpful editorial input from Dr. Merlin Willcox, Department of Primary Care Health Sciences, University of Oxford, is acknowledged with appreciation.

## REFERENCES

ABS Capacity Building Initiative, 2011. Expert Meeting on "ABS and Intellectual Property Rights" hosted by the Ethiopian Institute of Biodiversity Conservation, September 5–9, Addis Ababa.

Alikhan, S., and Mashelkar, R.A., 2009. *Intellectual Property and Competitive Strategies in 21st Century.* Kluwer Law International.

American Botanical Council, 2011. Phytopharm returns *Hoodia gordonii* right to South African R&D Company. *HerbalEGram*, 8(3). Available at: http://cms.herbalgram.org/heg/volume8/03March/PhytopharmHoodiaTransfer.html?ts=1391609963&signature=f78a4b81b7cfc90b9a2bafac5eb496b6&ts=1391610062&signature=f411359c6a873914c04ea1456074b7cf (Accessed on February 27, 2017).

Bodcker, G., 2003. Traditional medical knowledge, intellectual property rights and benefit sharing. *Cardozo Journal International and Comparative Law*, 11(2):785–814.

Bodeker, G. et al., 1997. Medicinal Plants for Forest Conservation and Health Care. UN Food and Agriculture Organization, Rome.

Bodeker, G., Burley, J., Bhat, K.K.S., Vantomme, P., 2003. *Medicinal Plants for Forest Conservation and Healthcare.* UN Food and Agriculture Organization, Rome, Italy.

Bodeker, G., Ong, C.-K., Grundy, C., Burford, G., and Shein, K., 2005. *World Health Organization Global Atlas of Traditional, Complementary and Alternative Medicine.* WHO, Geneva, Switzerland.

Bodeker, G., van't Klooster, C., Weisbord, E., 2014. *Prunus africana* (Hook.f.) Kalkman: The overexploitation of a medicinal plant species and its legal context. *Journal of Alternative and Complementary Medicine*, 20(11):810–822.

Chennells, R., 2007. San Hoodia Case. A Report for GenBenefit. Available at: https://www.uclan.ac.uk/research/explore/projects/assets/cpe_genbenefit_san_case.pdf (Accessed on February 27, 2017).

Diallo, D., Graz, B., Falquet, J., Traore, A.K., Giani, S., Mounkoro, P.P., Berthe, A., Sacko, M., Diakite, C., 2006. Malaria treatment in remote areas of Mali: Use of modern and traditional medicines, patient outcome. *Transactions of the Royal Society of Tropical Medicine and Hygiene*, 100:515–520.

FAO, 2009. *International Treaty on Plant Genetic Resources for Food and Agriculture.* UN Food and Agriculture Organization, Rome, Italy.

FAO, 2013. International treaty of plant genetic resources on food and agriculture. Available at: http://www.fao.org/plant-treaty/en/ (Accessed on February 27, 2017).

GhanaWeb, 2013. Health News: Let's promote traditional medicine industry. Available at: http://www.ghanaweb.com/GhanaHomePage/health/artikel.php?ID=291506 (Accessed on February 27, 2017).

Goreja, W.G., 2004. *Shea Butter: The Nourishing Properties of Africa's Best-Kept Natural Beauty Secret.* TNC International Inc., Stone Mountain, Georgia, USA, p. 5.

Graz, B., Willcox, M.L., Diakite, C., Falquet, J., Dackuo, F., Sidibe, O., Giani, S., Diallo, D., 2010. *Argemone mexicana* decoction versus artesunate-amodiaquine for the management of malaria in Mali: Policy and public-health implications. *Transactions of the Royal Society of Tropical Medicine and Hygiene*, 104:33–41.

International Institute for Environment and Development (IIED), 2012. *Participatory Learning and Action: Biodiversity and Culture: Exploring Community Protocols, Rights and Consent.* Issue 65, IIED, London, UK.

International Society of Ethnobiology (ISE), 2006. International Society of Ethnobiology Code of Ethics (with 2008 additions). Available at: http://www.ethnobiology.net/what-we-do/core-programs/ise-ethics-program/code-of-ethics/ (Accessed on February 27, 2017).

Makoni, M., 2010. *San People's Cactus Drug Dropped by Phytopharm.* SciDevNet. Available at: http://www.scidev.net/global/indigenous/news/san-people-s-cactus-drug-dropped-by-phytopharm-1.html (Accessed on February 27, 2017).

Martin, G., and Vermeylen, S., 2005. Intellectual property, indigenous knowledge, and biodiversity. *Capitalism Nature Socialism*, 16(3):27–48.

Mcmanis, C.R., 2003. Intellectual property, genetic resources and traditional knowledge protection: Thinking globally, acting locally. *Cardozo Journal International and Comparative Law*, 11:547–583.

Moolla, A., and Viljoen, A.M., 2008. "Buchu"—*Agathosma betulina* and *Agathosma crenulata* (Rutaceae): A review. *Journal of Ethnopharmacology*, 119(3):413–419.

Natural Justice, 2009. Bio-cultural community protocols: A community approach to ensuring the integrity of environmental law and policy. Available at: http://www.unep.org/communityprotocols/PDF/communityprotocols.pdf (Accessed on February 27, 2017).

Natural Justice, 2012. Kukula healers review 2012 and plan for 2013. Available at: http://natural-justice.blogspot.co.uk/2012/12/kukula-healers-review-2012-plan-for-2013.html (Accessed on February 27, 2017).

OAU, 2000. *African Model Legislation for the Protection of the Rights of Local Communities, Farmers and Breeders, and for the Regulation of Access to Biological Resources.* Organization of African Unity, Algeria.

Open Society Initiative for Southern Africa (OSISA), 2013. Recognising indigenous rights. Available at: http://www.osisa.org/indigenous-peoples/south-africa/recognising-indigenous-rights (Accessed on February 27, 2017).

Pobeda, M., and Sousselier, L., 1999. Shea butter: The revival of an African wonder. Available at: http://www.ceci.ca/assets/uploads/PDF-FR/Karite/SheaButterRevivalAfricanWonder.pdf (Accessed on February 27, 2017).

PROMETRA, 2017. PROMETRA—Uganda. Available at: http://prometra.org/chapters/uganda (Accessed on February 27, 2017).

PRWeb, 2012. Global traditional medicine market to reach US$114 billion by 2015, according to a new report published by Global Industry Analysts, Inc. Available at: http://www.prweb.com/releases/alternative_medicine/homeopathy_chinese/prweb9087888.htm (Accessed on February 27, 2017).

San people's cactus drug dropped by Phytopharm. SciDevNet, December 20, 2010. http://www.scidev.net/global/indigenous/news/san-people-s-cactus-drug-dropped-by-phytopharm-1.html. Accessed November 07, 2017.

Secretariat of the Convention on Biological Diversity, 2002. *Bonn Guidelines on Access to Genetic Resources and Fair and Equitable Sharing of the Benefits Arising Out of Their Utilization.* Secretariat of the CBD, Montreal, Canada.

Secretariat of the Convention on Biological Diversity, 2008. Access and benefit-sharing in practice: Trends in partnerships across sectors. Montreal, Canada. Technical Series, No. 38.

Secretariat of the CBD, 2011a. *Convention on Biological Diversity.* Text and annexes. United Nations Environment Programme. Secretariat of the CBD, Montreal, Canada.

Secretariat of the CBD, 2011b. *Nagoya Protocol on Access to Genetic Resources and the Fair and Equitable Sharing of Benefits Arising from Their Utilization to the Convention on Biological Diversity.* United Nations Environment Programme. Secretariat of the CBD, Montreal, Canada.

Secretariat of the CBD, 2013a. Nagoya Protocol signatories. Available at: https://www.cbd.int/abs/nagoya-protocol/signatories/ (Accessed on February 27, 2017).

Secretariat of the CBD, 2013b. *Press Release (1 Oct. 2013). Landmark treaty on Genetic Resources Reaches Halfway Mark to Entry into Force.* United Nations Environment Programme. Secretariat of the CBD, Montreal, Canada.

Seiler, A., and Dutfield, G., 2001. Regulating access and benefit sharing. Basic issues, legal instruments, policy proposals. Study commissioned by the Federal Republic of Germany in preparation for the first meeting of the Ad Hoc Working Group on access and benefit sharing in Bonn, October 2001. UNEP/CBD/WG-ABS/1/INF/4. Convention on Biological Diversity.

Stanley, B., 2011. *Recognition and Respect for African Traditional Medicine.* International Development Research Council. Available at: http://www.idrc.ca/EN/Resources/Publications/Pages/ArticleDetails.aspx?PublicationID=713 (Accessed on December 2013).

Starling, S., 2008. Unilever drops *Hoodia*—Nutraingredients. Available at: http://www. nutraingredients.com/Industry/Unilever-drops-hoodia (Accessed on February 27, 2017).

Tella, A., 1979. Preliminary studies on nasal decongestant activity from the seed of the shea butter tree, *Butyrospermum parkii*. *Journal of Clinical Pharmacology*, 7(5):495–497.

Traditional Health Practitioners Bushbuckbridge, 2010. Biocultural protocol of the traditional health practitioners of Bushbuckbridge. Available at: http://community-protocols.org/ wp-content/uploads/documents/South_Africa-Bushbuckridge_Biocultural_Protocol. pdf (Accessed on February 27, 2017).

University of Oslo (UiO), 2011. Multi-disciplinary University Traditional Health Initiative (MUTHI). Available at: http://www.mn.uio.no/farmasi/english/research/projects/ muthi/ (Accessed on February 27, 2017).

van Heerden, F.R., 2008. *Hoodia gordonii*: A natural appetite suppressant. *Journal of Ethnopharmacology*, 119(3):434–437.

Willcox, M., Diallo, D., Sanogo, R., Giani, S., Graz, B., Falquet, J., Bodeker, G., 2015. Intellectual property rights, benefit-sharing and development of "improved traditional medicines": A new approach. *Journal of Ethnopharmacology*, 176:281–285.

Willcox, M., Sanogo, R., Diakite, C., Giani, S., Paulsen, B.S., Diallo, D., 2012. Improved traditional medicines in Mali. *Journal of Alternative and Complementary Medicine*, 18:212–220.

Willcox, M.L., Graz, B., Diakite, C., Falquet, J., Dackouo, F., Sidibe, O., Giani, S., Diallo, D., 2011b. Is parasite clearance clinically important after malaria treatment in a high trans-mission area? A 3-month follow-up of home-based management with herbal medi-cine or ACT. *Transactions of the Royal Society of Tropical Medicine and Hygiene*, 105:23–31.

Willcox, M.L., Graz, B., Falquet, J., Diakite, C., Giani, S., Diallo, D., 2011a. A "reverse phar-macology" approach for developing an anti-malarial phytomedicine. *Malaria Journal*, 10:S8.

Willcox, M.L., Graz, B., Falquet, J., Sidibe, O., Forster, M., Diallo, D., 2007. *Argemone mexi-cana* decoction for the treatment of uncomplicated falciparum malaria. *Transactions of the Royal Society of Tropical Medicine and Hygiene*, 101:1190–1198.

World Health Organization African Regional Office (WHO-AFRO), 2010. The African Health Monitor Special Issue: African Traditional Medicine Day. Special Issue 14, August 31. Available at: http://ahm.afro.who.int/special-issue14/ahm-special-issue-14. pdf (Accessed on February 27, 2017).

Wynberg, R., and Chennells, R., 2009. Green diamonds of the South: An overview of the San-Hoodia case. In: R. Wynberg, D. Schroeder, and R. Chennells (Eds.), *Indigenous Peoples, Consent and Benefit Sharing: Lessons from the San Hoodia Case*. Springer, Berlin, pp. 89–124.

# CHAPTER 4

# Using Appropriate Methodology and Technology for Research and Development of African Traditional Medicines

Philippe Rasoanaivo, Merlin Wilcox, and Bertrand Graz

## CONTENTS

## 4.1 INTRODUCTION

There is no longer any doubt regarding the value of African traditional remedies. What is difficult is the conversion of these remedies into modern therapeutic agents in a sustainable and safe manner. Overall, despite the richness and the endemicity of the African plant biodiversity associated with a wealth of indigenous knowledge, the continent has only contributed 83 of the world's 1,100 leading commercial medicinal plants (Rasoanaivo, 2011). This chapter explores how African traditional medicine can contribute its legitimate share to the global therapeutic arsenal using appropriate science and technology tools.

One of the drawbacks of African traditional medicine is the linkage of its use with superstitions, religious practices, and magical rites. However, it has been established that about 80% of African traditional medicine relies wholly or essentially on the use of plant parts and rarely animal parts and minerals (Kasilo et al., 2010). The direct connection between phytoconstituents and therapeutics was attributed to a young German pharmacist. In 1804, the first isolation of a natural product was achieved by Friedrich Wilhelm Adam Sertürner, who purified morphine from opium (*Papaver somniferum*), and found that it largely reproduced the analgesic and sedative effects of opium. His success led others to seek "active principles" of medicinal plants. Since that breakthrough, pure bioactive natural compounds were found in many other plants by the application of modern scientific methods to the chemical and biological investigation of medicinal plants. In many cases, this has led to the identification, structural elucidation, and analysis of the mechanism of action of the bioactive constituents.

However, for other medicinal plants it has not been possible to isolate a single "active" compound (e.g., *Hypericum perforatum*, which is an effective antidepressant) (Williamson, 2001). Several plants contain multiple active ingredients that act synergistically (Rasoanaivo et al., 2011). There are also several examples of herbal medicines with excellent therapeutic effects, which subsequently produce disappointing results when evaluated in the laboratory with standard biological screenings, or when investigated for the identification of the active principles. Conversely, there are several bioactive compounds isolated from plants with excellent biological activity in the laboratory, which are ineffective or too toxic to use in human patients.

There are two opposite views in old Greek philosophy dealing with the two distinct approaches, namely, single-constituent drugs versus multicomponent phytomedicines. The underlying philosophy related to a single drug is that "every healing has its quintessence," and the second one related to multicomponent phytomedicines is that "nature does nothing without purpose or uselessly." The former approach forms the basis of today's dominating "single target–single compound" paradigm of drug discovery in pharmaceutical companies. In the latter approach, it is assumed that complex, multifactorial diseases may require multicomponent, multifunctional therapies, and complex molecular interactions produce effects that may not be achieved by a single component. There are thus two fundamental questions that should be considered before initiating research on medicinal plants: Is it relevant to put effort into isolating the active constituents in the hope of using them as a drug, or is it preferable to use traditional preparations and subsequently identify the bioactive ingredients?

African scientists should look for new possibilities, "thinking outside the box" on how to advance traditional medicines as sources of new drug leads and phytomedicines. Appropriate methodology and technology for research and development (R&D) should be creative enough to have the potential to tackle the problems from a different angle. This approach might subsequently make a substantial impact on a global health problem. A clearly defined process for traditional medicines and natural products research is urgently needed if this discipline is to advance and result in products of acceptable quality, efficacy, and safety profiles. In this chapter, we first examine the two research paradigms with implications to development and associated policies. Then we discuss some relevant innovative strategies for R&D of African traditional medicines.

## 4.2 THE PARADIGM OF SINGLE-CONSTITUENT DRUG PRODUCTS

Ethnomedical uses claimed for a traditional preparation generally correlate with the biological action of the isolated drugs. Farnsworth et al. (1985) made a correlation between the traditional uses of some plants with the pharmacological actions of the isolated drugs. They found that of the 119 plant-derived drugs, 88 (74%) were discovered as a result of scientific follow-up of their ethnomedical uses. At the present time, about 50% of the drugs approved for clinical use are natural products or inspired by natural products (Newman and Cragg, 2012). This is not surprising, because natural compounds offer structural diversity combined with surprising/unexpected biological properties, which cannot be rivaled by the creativity and synthetic ingenuity of medicinal chemists. In addition, they provide scaffold molecules for a much greater percentage of semi-synthetically and synthetically produced molecules.

The isolation of natural products is broadly classified into one of the following three categories: structure-directed isolation (searching new or novel structures); bioactivity-guided isolation (searching for bioactive constituents); or chemotaxonomy-oriented study (searching for the relationship between botanical classification and chemical constituents, or searching for known and abundant compounds as scaffolds for semi-synthesis). Each of these categories consists of different approaches and distinct isolation strategies. For example, the first and third approaches may use phytochemical screening, which is a simple, quick, and inexpensive procedure that gives the researcher a quick answer to the various types of constituents present in a mixture (Sasidharan et al., 2011).

## 4.3 BIOASSAY-GUIDED FRACTIONATION AND STRUCTURE ELUCIDATION

This type of research is carried out only when the plant is known as having strong ethnomedical data, or a biological activity under investigation is shown by the crude extract. The work is done to identify what ingredient(s) is(are) responsible for the relevant activity. The core objective is therefore the identification of the single "active principle" in medicinal plants, based on the assumption that they have one or a few ingredients that determine their therapeutic effects. Success of the single-constituent drug approach depends mainly on four factors:

- Appropriate extraction procedure
- Availability of bioassays
- Ability to elaborate appropriate strategy for fractionation
- Ability to elucidate diverse structures

The first three factors refer to bioassay-guided fractionation, which requires a strong collaboration between a biologist and a chemist, such that the desired active compounds are obtained efficiently. Extraction is the first step in the study of medicinal plants, because it is necessary to extract the desired chemical components from the plant materials for further investigation. The selection of a solvent system largely depends on the specific nature of the bioactive compound being targeted. If the plant is selected on the basis of traditional uses, then it is necessary to prepare the extract according to the traditional recipe. Different solvent systems are also available to extract the bioactive compound from natural sources. Other modern extraction techniques are also available, namely, solid-phase micro-extraction, supercritical-fluid extraction, pressurized-liquid extraction, microwave-assisted extraction, solid-phase extraction, and surfactant-mediated techniques, which possess certain advantages over traditional methods (Sticher, 2008). In bioassays, models have moved from a holistic approach using humans and later on animal models (also called multitarget functional bioassays) toward a reductionist approach (also called single-target specific bioassays) with enzymatic or receptor binding techniques that can be done at a nanoscale level (Figure 4.1).

The major demand of the pharmaceutical industry has become the discovery of a new drug entity that interacts with a single, well-defined molecular target, preferably without disturbing other cellular functions to avoid side effects.

Historically, Sertürner, who isolated morphine, tested it on himself and three 17-year-old children in order to establish that his crystals carried the pharmacological activity of raw opium. In view of its dream-inducing properties, he named his crystalline material "morphium," a word derived from "Morpheus," used for the god of dreams. Due to the tremendous progress of biology, a myriad of documents dealing with bioassays is routinely available through databases. And over the last two decades, a wealth of new technologies for bioactivity screening has emerged. Fractionation can be very simple, into a few fractions, or more advanced (Sticher, 2008), such as sophisticated hyphenated techniques (Wolfender et al., 2006).

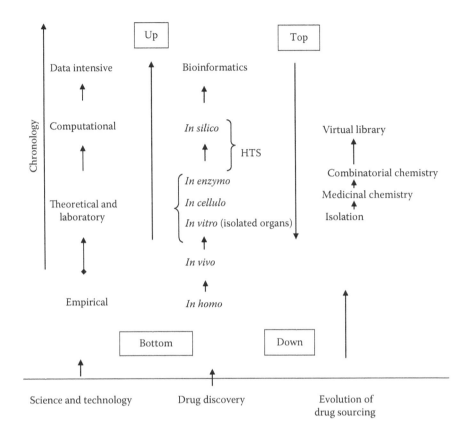

**Figure 4.1** Evolution of bioassays in drug discovery in parallel with the evolution of science and technology.

Structure elucidation is an area that has been revolutionized by advances in spectroscopic techniques, particularly mass spectrometry and nuclear magnetic resonance (Fukushi, 2006).

In summary, advances in analytical, preparative, and structural instrumentation for extraction, separation, and structure elucidation, coupled with the increasing availability of various bioassays, means that it is now possible to demonstrate biological activities from an extract, then isolate, identify, and determine the structure of the biologically active constituents.

## 4.4  ETHNOBOTANY-BASED VERSUS RANDOM COLLECTION SCREENING PROGRAMS IN AFRICA

We report here well-documented plant-based screening programs from African plants with the aim of discovering single active constituents, and in which bioactive constituents were isolated and chemical structures elucidated.

## 4.4.1 Screening of African Plants for Antimalarial Activities

Despite strong efforts to control it, malaria remains the most deadly parasitic disease in the world today. Malaria is a public health problem in tropical and subtropical areas, and particularly in sub-Saharan Africa, among the poorest and underprivileged communities, and the disease has severe social and economic impacts for these communities. For economic reasons and also attachment to cultural values, most affected populations in sub-Saharan Africa turn toward traditional medicine for their primary health care. Most research into African antimalarial plants has mainly followed the paradigm of single active constituents targeting mainly the erythrocytic stage of malaria parasites with the aim of finding an African equivalent to quinine or artemisinin.

At least three ethnobotanical screening programs have been conducted on South African plants, while there have been four studies adopting a more direct approach, where plants within a particular genus were screened for antiplasmodial activity. In addition, some plants were evaluated in individual studies. Overall, 222 species belonging to 61 families were tested for *in vitro* antiplasmodial activities (Pillay et al., 2008). Twenty-four antiplasmodial compounds belonging to various chemical types were isolated. They displayed good antiplasmodial activities in the *in vitro* model, but their development as potential antimalarial medicines was limited by inherent cytotoxicity and lack of selectivity. The authors reported that only six compounds, namely, three α, β-unsaturated sesquiterpene lactones and three phenolic diterpenes (Figure 4.2), were considered to be hits for a potential advanced investigation. They could also be used as scaffolds for structure–activity relationship studies.

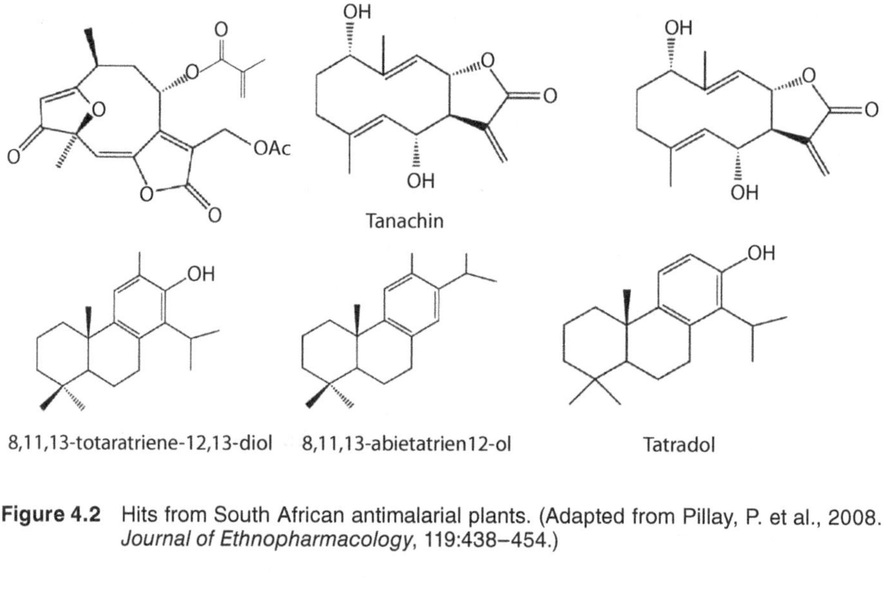

Tanachin

8,11,13-totaratriene-12,13-diol    8,11,13-abietatrien12-ol        Tatradol

**Figure 4.2**  Hits from South African antimalarial plants. (Adapted from Pillay, P. et al., 2008. *Journal of Ethnopharmacology*, 119:438–454.)

Similarly, 217 different species have been cited for their use as antimalarials in folk medicine in Cameroon. The authors reported that about a hundred compounds have been isolated from 26 species, some of which are potential leads for development as new antimalarials. Crude extracts and/or essential oils prepared from 54 other species were also found to show a wide range of activity on *Plasmodium* spp. (Titanji et al., 2008).

Other examples of antimalarial screening were those done in Madagascar (Rasoanaivo et al., 1999, 2004). In the first screening 50 plants were screened for antiplasmodial activity and chloroquine potentiating effects. The most important result was the identification of a dehydroaporphine, dehydrodicentrine, with strong antiplasmodial activity ($IC_{50} = 0.08$ μg/mL). In the second screening, 190 plants, of which 51 are used to treat malaria in traditional medicine, were submitted to a screening program for antiplasmodial activity. Thirty-nine plants, of which 12 are used as herbal antimalarials, were found to display *in vitro* antiplasmodial activity ($IC_{50} < 5$ μg/mL).

## 4.4.2 Screening of South African Plants for Anticancer Activities

A total of 7,500 plant extracts representing 700 plant species were screened for *in vitro* anticancer activity against breast MCF7, renal TK10, and melanoma UACC62 human cell lines between 1999 and 2006. This investigation indicated that 50 plant extracts (representing 41 plant species) had moderate anticancer activity, and these were screened by the NCI against a panel of 60 human cancer cell lines. A hit rate of 5.9% was thus obtained based on the number of species with moderate activity expressed as a percentage of the 700 plant species tested (Fouche et al., 2008). The majority of aqueous extracts did not show any activity in the screen. The extracts of plant species with limited published information for their anticancer properties were subjected to bioassay-guided fractionation, and the active constituents were isolated and identified. Structures of the bioactive constituents are given in Figure 4.3.

## 4.4.3 Screening of Indian Ocean Plants for Antiviral Drugs against Chikungunya

Chikungunya is a debilitating infectious tropical disease that is caused by an arbovirus that is transmitted by mosquitoes of the genus *Aedes*. Currently, there is neither selective antiviral drug nor vaccine for the treatment or prevention of this viral disease. The sudden emergence of chikungunya virus (CHIKV) infections in the Indian Ocean islands in the mid-2000s has created a serious public health problem in the region. In response to this, the French Institution CRVOI (*Centre de Recherche et de Veille sur les Maladies Emergentes dans l'Océan Indien*) was established in 2007 to organize, among other projects, multidisciplinary research programs dedicated to the fight against emerging infectious diseases in the Indian Ocean region. The recent outbreak of CHIKV has stimulated renewed interest in

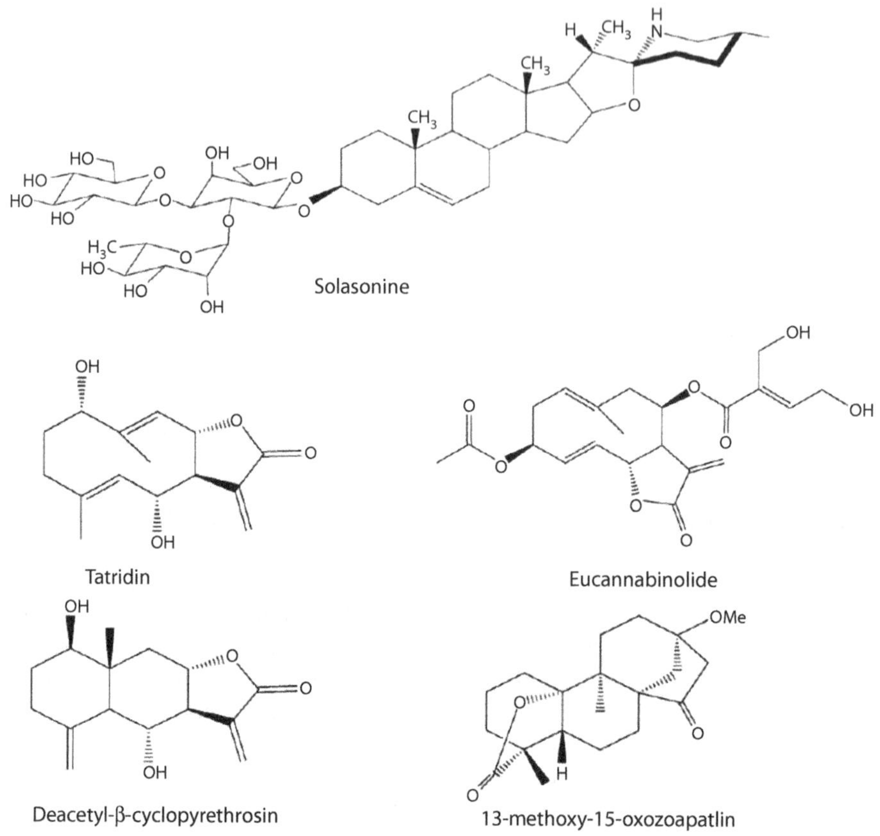

Solasonine

Tatridin

Eucannabinolide

Deacetyl-β-cyclopyrethrosin

13-methoxy-15-oxozoapatlin

**Figure 4.3** Bioactive constituents form the anticancer screening program. (Adapted from Fouche, G. et al., 2008. *Journal of Ethnopharmacology*, 119(3):455–461.)

developing selective antiviral agents as countermeasure to this pathogen. To this end, the CRVOI launched a call for proposals.

In 2008, in response to the CRVOI call for proposals, a North-South collaborative network of natural product chemists and biologists was created. The project called **PHYTOCHIK** had as its overall objective the discovery and characterization of selective antiviral compounds derived from the vast Indian Ocean plant biodiversity. Such bioactive compounds should be capable of fighting emerging viral diseases such as Chikungunya. In addition, plants from New Caledonia were included in the project. The results of this investigation have been published (Leyssen et al., 2014).

The outcome of the project indicated that 53 out of 972 plants collected from the three islands indicated good preliminary results. Furthermore, more than 50 pure compounds were isolated from the plants. However, it was frustrating to note in most cases the loss of the antiviral activities after test reconfirmation of the active extracts, or during bioassay-directed fractionation of the promising extracts. Furthermore, most of the studied extracts that possess potent anti-CHIKV activities did not lead

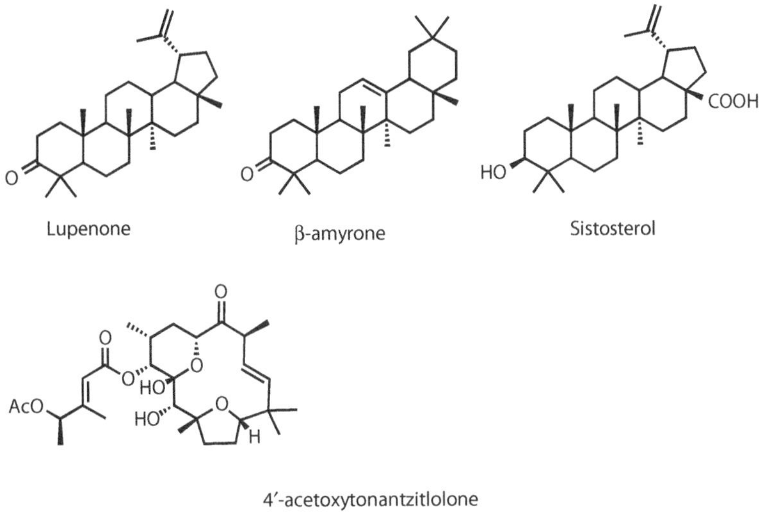

Lupenone                 β-amyrone                    Sistosterol

4′-acetoxytonantzitlolone

**Figure 4.4**  Four pure compounds with inhibitory activity in the CHIK virus-cell-based assay. (Adapted from Leyssen, P. et al. 2014. Biodiversity as a source of potent and selective inhibitors of chikungunya virus replication. In: A. Gurib-Fakim (Ed.), *Novel Plant Bioresources: Applications in Food, Medicine, and Cosmetics.* Hoboken, NJ: Wiley-Blackwell, pp. 151–161.)

to active products, and only a few of them gave known compounds with a moderate antiviral activity (Figure 4.4).

## 4.5  CRITICAL ANALYSIS OF THE ETHNOBOTANY-BASED DRUG DISCOVERY IN AFRICA

We collected published data on biological testing of African medicinal plants from regional journals as well as major natural product journals through HINARI, ARDI, and other databases. We came up with three main conclusions.

### 4.5.1  Use of *In Vitro* Models: Between Simplicity and Realism

Although *in vivo* models were very useful in the past to demonstrate biological activities in reputed medicinal plants, the advent of the *in vitro* techniques has facilitated the biological screening of extracts. They are widely applied in current ethnopharmacological studies mainly because they facilitate bioassay-guided isolation of active principles. *In vitro* models fulfill the requirements for bioassay-directed fractionation of natural products, namely, simplicity (small-scale sample of 1–2 mg for each assay); rapidity (result must be available within a week, preferably within 2 days); reproducibility (same or similar data have to be obtained by the assay at different times, by different persons, and in different locations); and comparability (data must be clear-cut and quantitatively expressed). In some cases, the *in vitro* models have led to good results. But *in vitro* methods raise one relevant question: Do they explain or relate to the use of the activity of the plant? Furthermore, although it is difficult to predict an *in vivo* situation from *in vitro* results, several published papers have a tendency to extrapolate results from *in vitro* tests to justify the traditional uses of medicinal plants without taking into account the bioavailability, the traditional recipes for preparing the remedies, and the effects of other constituents. Synergistic, antagonistic, or additive effects can occur, which are extremely difficult to predict. Our own recent example was the investigation of the antimalarial activities of *Bivinia jabertii* (Salicaceae), traditionally used to treat malaria in Madagascar (Manjovelo, 2012). The aqueous extract showed *in vivo* and *in vitro* antimalarial activity in the primary screening. Bioassay-guided fractionation using a radiolabeled antiplasmodial test led to the isolation of three active compounds that were identified as phenol glycosides. One of them, bivinin A (Figure 4.5), has strong *in vitro* activity but lacks *in vivo* effects. A relevant paper described the limitations of *in vitro* tests (Houghton et al., 2007).

## 4.5.2 Isolation of Active Principles Is the Bottleneck of the Single-Constituent Drug Approach

Isolation of natural products is still the rate-limiting step in natural product chemistry despite the recent progress in analytical and preparative chromatographic methods. This may be due to differences in isolation methods from previous ones *vis-à-vis* source of material, quantity available, and particularly the person who is performing this isolation. Although the scientist may simply be repeating the known procedure, not one of them is identical to the previous ones.

Furthermore, other difficulties include the following:

- The variability of the source material should be considered, since plants showing promising biological activity in assay systems fail to have the activity confirmed on subsequent re-collections.

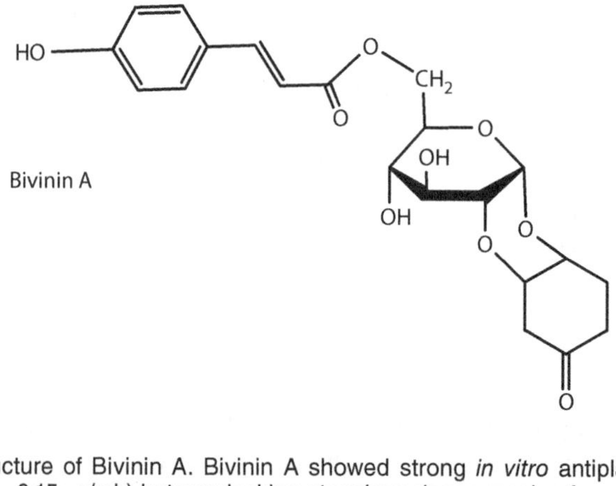

Bivinin A

**Figure 4.5** Structure of Bivinin A. Bivinin A showed strong *in vitro* antiplasmodial activity (IC = 0.15 µg/mL) but was lacking at various doses ranging from 20 to 150 mg/kg. (Adapted from Manjovelo, C.S., 2012. Nouvelles molécules isolées de plantes du Sud de Madagascar: *Bivinia jalbertii et Capuronianthus mahafalensis*. Thèse de Doctorat. Faculté des Sciences, Université de Toliara.)

- There is a possibility that the active compound is a known compound, thus leading to much wasted effort in the search for new bioactive compounds.
- Some compounds are labile under certain conditions, and progressive degradation occurs during the fractionation procedure.
- The fractionation procedure used to isolate the active ingredients is inappropriate, especially for hydrophilic compounds.
- If a combination of substances is needed for the effect, then the bioassay-guided fractionation, narrowing activity down first to a fraction and eventually a compound, is doomed to failure,
- Pharmacologists, rather than qualified phytochemists, work on isolation procedures. As a result, the active ingredients have not been correctly identified in some of the literature.

### 4.5.3 Follow-Up of the Results Is Not Straightforward

The investigation of many reputed African medicinal plants has led to the isolation of several new molecules, some of them showing good biological activities. Review articles were published on the subject (Abegaz et al., 1998; Hostettmann et al., 2000; Hou & Harinantenaina, 2010; Ntie-Kang et al., 2013). To the best of our knowledge, very few attempts have been made to bring bioactive compounds from African medicinal plants into advanced drug development. There are several reasons for this:

- Lack of contact with partners from the research-industry-investor communities to identify which research has potential commercial interest.
- Lack of knowledge in the process of patenting.
- Lack of knowledge on bringing research to market. What are the steps to take when commercialising research, and which are the best strategies to adopt?
- Lack of entrepreneurial skills.

To the best of our knowledge, none of the bioactive compounds isolated from the above-mentioned screening programs have been brought hitherto into advanced drug development. Moreover, most of them are known compounds or are derivatives of known compounds.

## 4.6 ETHNOBOTANY-BASED SINGLE DRUGS WITH SUCCESS STORIES IN AFRICA

We report here relevant bioactive constituents isolated from African medicinal plants, which have reached the stage of commercialization as single-drug ingredients, or at least the stage of patenting and preclinical development.

### 4.6.1 Libiguins, a New Class of Phragmalin Limonoids Causing Profound Enhancement of Sexual Activity

Erectile dysfunction (ED) is defined as the consistent or recurrent inability of a man to attain and/or maintain a penile erection sufficient for sexual activity. It is a common impairment among elderly men, and prevalence rates increase with age. It is also considered to be a significant public health problem, given its relationship to diabetes, vascular diseases, dyslipidemia, and hypertension. Erectile dysfunction has many different causes, often classified into four types: psychogenic, vasculogenic or organic, neurologic, and endocrinologic. In clinical situation, it is often difficult to delineate which factors are involved and in which order. Sexual dysfunction is not limited only to ED in males. A syndrome termed "Hypoactive Sexual Dysfunction Disorder" is common in females and is characterized by deficiency of sexual fantasies and receptivity of sexual activity. It is thus obvious that sexuality is a highly complex and multifaceted behavioral trait that needs further entry points for its study. The discovery of pharmacological agents that can influence sexual behavior may give new opportunities to understand the biological basis for sexual behavior, as well as new therapies for the treatment of sexual dysfunction.

A team at the *Institut Malgache de Recherches Appliquées* (Madagascar), in collaboration with scientists at Uppsala University (Sweden), investigated *Neobeguea mahafalensis*, a medicinal plant endemic to Madagascar, whose stem barks are used to treat ED in old men. It was found that the decoction of root barks displayed an unprecedented high potency and remarkably long duration in augmenting sexual activity in male rodents. The high-performance liquid chromatography (HPLC) profile of the crude extract was very complex. The isolation of the active constituents was therefore an extremely complicated procedure due to the presence of many compounds with closely similar chromatographic properties. However, unequivocal dedication to bioassay-guided fractionation led to the isolation of three pharmaco-active constituents, which turned out to be novel limonoids with unprecedented C-16/30 δ-lactone ring (Razafimahefa et al., 2014). This new class of substances was termed *libiguins*, and Figure 4.6 shows exemplary compounds of the series.

Libiguins were found to be highly lipophilic, which is presumably highly important for their pharmacological activities. *In vivo* pharmacological tests showed that

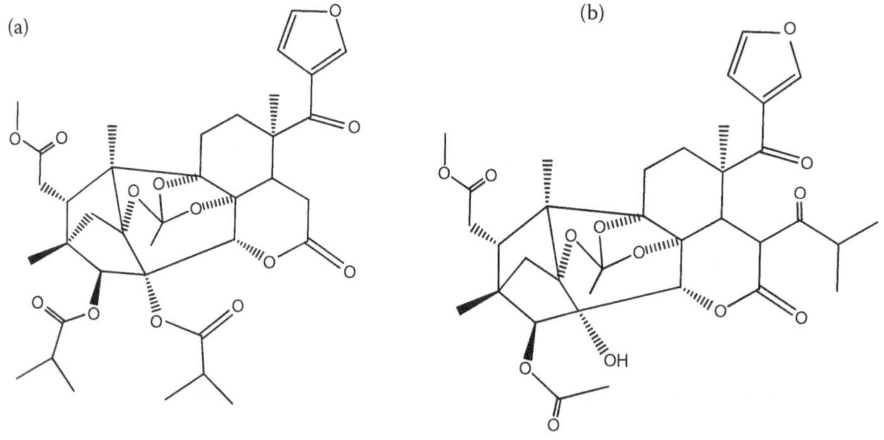

**Figure 4.6**  Structure of libiguins A and B.

libiguins dose-dependently (0.04–0.4 mg/kg by oral administration) delayed mating behavior in experimental animals for 3 days. The effects observed for the extract and pure limonoids suggest a mechanism at a central site, possibly the hypothalamus. The lipophilic nature of the active constituents is in support with a central site of action as the lipophilic compounds would then have the ability to pass the blood-brain barrier. These findings resulted in a new patent covering the potential use of the novel compounds for treatment of sexual dysfunction. A semi-synthetic derivative is now in the advanced stage of pharmacological evaluation. The studies open a new route for mapping the complex system involved in the regulation of mating behavior. This finding may also lead to new ways to treat sexual dysfunction.

## 4.7 PLANTS: THE PARADIGM OF MULTIPLE-COMPONENT PHYTOMEDICINE

Use complex mixtures of compounds of different structural classes to protect themselves against herbivores, bacteria, fungi, and viruses. These complex mixtures may contain constituents that are specific for a single target. A majority of metabolites, however, can interfere with several targets in a pleiotropic fashion. The composition of such extracts appears to be optimized, since the components are not only additive, but also apparently synergistic in their bioactivity. At this point, although each individual substance within these multicomponents has a low molar fraction, the therapeutic activity of these substances is established via a potentiation of their effects through combined and simultaneous attacks on multiple molecular targets.

In contrast to single-drug combinations, a botanical multicomponent therapeutic agent possesses a complex repertoire of chemicals that belong to a variety of substances. This may explain the frequently observed pleiotropic bioactivity spectra of these compounds, which may also suggest that they possess novel therapeutic potentials. Many diseases are not caused by the dysregulation of a single molecular target but have a multifactorial pathogenesis, and the observed effects often cannot be clearly assigned to specific chemical compounds (Jalencas and Mestres, 2013). Interestingly, considerable bioactive properties are exhibited not only by remedies that contain high doses of phytochemicals with prominent pharmaceutical efficacy, but also by preparations that lack a sole active principal component. This mechanistic view therefore explains why in many cases, the fractionation or isolation of principal constituents from extracts ends up with a loss of previously detected activities.

The launch of a new generation of botanical therapeutics, including plant-derived pharmaceuticals, multicomponent botanical drugs, and functional foods, results from a better understanding of the relationship between plants and human health. Many of these products have complemented conventional pharmaceuticals in the treatment, prevention, and diagnosis of diseases. A strong interest in multicomponent preparations is likely to arise from the observation that some of these multisubstance mixtures possess prominent pharmacological properties at low or nontoxic concentrations.

## 4.8 SYNERGY AND POSITIVE INTERACTIONS

Interactions between phytochemical components often modify the pharmaco-logical effects of phytomedicines. These interactions can either potentiate the effect of bioactive constituents or interfere with their activity. It is generally believed that there are two types of phytochemical interactions: endo-interactions that occur between components within a plant species and exo-interactions that occur between components from different plants or between plants and synthetic drugs. Interactions between complex mixtures may affect a wide range of biological processes such as synergistic action at different points of the same signaling cascade (multitarget effects), inhibition of binding to target proteins, metabolism, bioavailability, solubil-ity, activation of prodrugs, interference with cellular transport processes (uptake and efflux), and body clearance. Researchers should be prepared to demonstrate the poly-valence of traditional extracts, particularly when they can be backed up by *in vivo* or clinical studies, in an attempt to achieve a degree of paradigm shift in ways of think-ing about the basis for activity observed away from the "single active compound" model.

The general understanding of synergy is that it is an effect seen by a combination of substances being greater than would have been expected from a consideration of individual contributions. There are various ways to prove synergism:

Summation of effects: This is when the total effect of a combination is greater than expected from the sum of its effects.

Comparison of the effect of a combination with that of each of its components: This method is independent of any knowledge of the mechanism of action, and it seems logical.

Isobologram method (Berenbaum, 1989): This is the method of choice, and although more complicated, is independent of the mechanism of action and applies under most conditions. It also makes no assumptions as to the behavior of each agent and is therefore applicable to multiple-component mixtures.

## 4.9  GOING BEYOND THE STANDARD BIOLOGICAL
## TEST: EXAMPLE OF MALARIA

There are two well-recognized standard tests to prove the antimalarial efficacy of extracts or pure compounds: the *in vitro* radiolabeled microtest (Desjardins et al., 1979) and the *in vivo* 4-day suppressive test (Peters et al., 1975). They have been accepted scientifically for the testing of antimalarial activities of plants and isolated compounds, and as such they have been applied extensively to evaluate the antima-larial activities of medicinal plants as shown in the previously mentioned antimalarial screening programs. The emphasis has been on plants whose efficacy and mode of action are congruent with the conventions of standard pharmacology, and less atten-tion has been on those that do not lend themselves to simple tests to establish their effi-cacy. Researchers tend to impose invisible frameworks around problems or situations, whereas the solution may begin at some point outside that mental box or boundary.

South America and Asia have provided the two best antimalarials to date: quinine and artemisinin. In Africa, however, as most people living in malarial endemic areas use traditional medicine to fight this disease, why have new treatments not emerged recently from ethnobotany-oriented research? There are several examples of herbal medicines with reputedly excellent antimalarial activity, which subsequently produce disappointing results when evaluated in the laboratory. Conversely, there are several antiplasmodial compounds isolated from plants with excellent activity in the laboratory, which are ineffective or too toxic to use in human patients. The absence of an African antimalarial compound with nanomolar antiplasmodial activity should not be understood as a failure of the pharmacopoeia but rather a clue that the answer may be found in a different direction. We would like to exemplify it with a serendipitous discovery on malaria and the immune system.

In a continuing effort toward the discovery of new and potent antimalarial drugs from Madagascar biodiversity, a team at Institut Malgache de Recherches Appliquées (IMRA) found that an aqueous extract of a *Tabernaemontana* species endemic to Madagascar failed to demonstrate *in vivo* activities in the standard 4-day suppressive test, with 42% parasitemia at day 4. Surprisingly, at day 9 post-infection, the team observed a strong drop in parasitemia down to 0.8%, and the appearance of mononuclear cells assumed to be lymphocytes as well as platelets in treated mice while all control mice died. This serendipitous finding was the starting point for a new cross-disciplinary approach in malaria using a "cure + protection" approach. What curative antimalarial should be used in this approach? At this point, chloroquine has been the keystone of antimalarial drugs due to its efficacy, low cost, and suitability for both radical cure and prophylaxis. It was even thought to be a miracle drug. It remained effective for more than 40 years in Africa despite the chaotic clinical setting of underdosing, noncompliance, and indiscriminate use in treating all fevers. Despite the abandonment of chloroquine as antimalarial due to drug resistance, many efforts are still devoted to explore the therapeutic applications of this drug against other diseases because of its lysosomotropic and immunomodulatory effects. Interestingly, there is a renewed interest in the investigation of the effects of chloroquine in the immune system. Therefore, a subtherapeutic dose of chloroquine (curative) was combined with the aqueous plant extract of *Tabernaemonta* species (protective). Complete sterile immunity was observed with treated mice after adequate treatments. Treated mice survived during a normal lifespan despite monthly challenges with *Plasmodium yoellii* without treatment. A preliminary account of the studies was given in a patent (Rasoanaivo and Razafimahefa, 2012). The holistic approach of traditional medicine was evoked because complex, pleiotropic diseases such as malaria may require multicomponent, multifunctional therapies, and complex molecular interactions produce effects that may not be achieved by a single component. At present, it is difficult to answer the question of whether "old" chloroquine will be able to live a "second youth." However, since chloroquine is a slow-eliminating drug and a residual drug can last up to a month in humans after usage, it may have a considerable impact on host innate and adaptive immune responses. And *Tabernaemonta* refined extract is a "helping hand" in the process. This unexpected scientific discovery may pave the way for various new studies, and might open the door to a new avenue of investigation into immunity against malaria, and probably into other infectious diseases.

Because of strict regulations, *in vivo* tests are used less and less frequently in drug discovery. However, it can be concluded that in the case of many antimalarial plants and herbal combination therapies widely used in African pharmacopoeias, *in vivo* testing may represent the only relevant means of recognizing and measuring the efficacy of the traditional therapy.

## 4.10 PHYTOMEDICINES WITH SUCCESS STORIES IN AFRICA

We report here success stories that have reached the stage of commercialization at a large scale, with patenting.

### 4.10.1 Madeglucyl in the Treatment of Type II Diabetes

Diabetes mellitus is a metabolic disorder caused by inherited and/or acquired deficiency in the production of insulin by the pancreas, or by the ineffectiveness of the insulin produced. Such a deficiency results in increased concentrations of glucose in the blood, which in turn damage many of the body's systems, in particular the blood vessels and nerves. There are two types of diabetes: type 1 and type 2. Type 1, insulin-dependent diabetes mellitus, in which the body does not produce any insulin, most often occurs in children and young adults. People with type 1 diabetes must take daily insulin injections to stay alive. Type 1 diabetes accounts for 5%–10% of diabetes. Type 2, non-insulin-dependent diabetes mellitus, in which the body does not produce enough, or properly use, insulin, is the most common form of the disease, accounting for 90%–95% of diabetes. Type 2 diabetes is seriously approaching epidemic proportions, due to an increased number of elderly people. Diabetes is found in all parts of the world and is rapidly increasing in most parts of the world. It affects about 5% of the global population, and its treatment without any side effects is still a challenge to the medical system. Chronic hyperglycemia during diabetes causes glycation of body proteins that in turn leads to secondary complications affecting eyes, kidneys, nerves, and arteries. The therapeutic measurements include use of insulin and other agents like amylin analogues; alpha glycosidase inhibitors like acarbose, miglitol, and voglibose; sulfonylureas; and biguanides for the treatment of hyperglycemia. These drugs also have certain adverse effects like causing hypoglycemia at higher doses, liver problems, lactic acidosis, and diarrhea. Apart from currently available therapeutic options, many herbal medicines have been recommended for the treatment of diabetes. Traditional plant medicines are used throughout the world for a range of diabetic presentations. Herbal drugs are prescribed widely because of their effectiveness, less side effects, and relatively low cost. Therefore, investigation on such agents from traditional medicinal plants has become more important.

*Eugenia jambolana* (*Syzygium cumini*) is arguably one of the most highly studied plants. Historically, the tree was exclusive to the Indian subcontinent but is currently found growing throughout the Asian subcontinent, Eastern Africa, South Africa, and Madagascar. The fruits are the most important plant part. Relevant information on *Eugenia jambolana* was published in the Madagascar pharmacopoeia (*Syzygium cumini*, 2008). Mechanistic studies indicate that *Eugenia jambolana* possesses free radical scavenging and antioxidant effects, prevents lipid peroxidation, regenerates the beta-cells, prevents alterations in glycation status and formation of advanced glycation end products, improves glucose utilization and maintains glucose homeostasis, activates peroxisome proliferator-activated receptor (PPAR), inhibits α-glucosidases, and ameliorates dyslipidemia (Baliga et al., 2013). It is clear that attempts to identify the single active ingredients of *Eugenia jambolana* for such various activities have not been successful. The team at IMRA assumed that bioactive ingredients may be insoluble polysaccharides. To this end, the team devised an appropriate extraction protocol. A patented phytomedicine called Madeglucyl was produced by IMRA from the seeds of *Eugenia jambolana*. Madeglucyl had its efficacy proven by clinical data, obtained from studies in Madagascar, the United States, and Germany, where it demonstrated a good tolerability and a significant effect 15 days after starting the treatment. Toxicological and pharmacological data confirmed that Madeglucyl was devoid of any side effects and could contribute to maintaining normal sugar levels in several experimental conditions (Puri et al., 2010).

The overall figure of the effects of Madeglucyl can be summarized as follows:

- The South Reduction of glycemia in healthy volunteers (−20% at glucose peak time, 60 min after oral glucose load.
- Reduction of glycemia (−49%, after 90 days) in subjects diagnosed with type 2 diabetes.
- No hypoglycemic effect in healthy subjects without glucose load.
- Absence of hypoglycemia as a side effect in patients affected by type 2 diabetes.
- Good tolerability in all the treated subjects even at the highest dosages.

### 4.10.2 African Cactus *Hoodia gordonii* as Appetite Suppressant

There are several plants of commercial importance in South Africa (Street and Prinsloo, 2013). Among these, *Hoodia gordonii* (Asclepiadaceae) is a succulent plant, indigenous to South Africa, Namibia, and Botswana. It has been known as an appetite suppressant, and contains substances that suppress hunger, appetite, and thirst. *Hoodia* is well known to the San bushmen of South Africa who eat this plant to reduce hunger sensations.

It has been emphasized in the literature that the active components of *Hoodia gordonii* that suppress appetite are steroidal glycosides, of which the compound referred to as P57 or P57A53 (Figure 4.7) was reported to be the isolated appetite-suppressant principle (van Heerden, 2008). However, other unidentified constituents of *Hoodia* could contribute to its biological effects, and *Hoodia* may act on the body by mechanisms other than those already proposed in the scientific literature.

*Hoodia gordonii* is commercialized as a dietary supplement. Although the active ingredient is known, *Hoodia* phytomedicines contain whole aerial parts of the plant

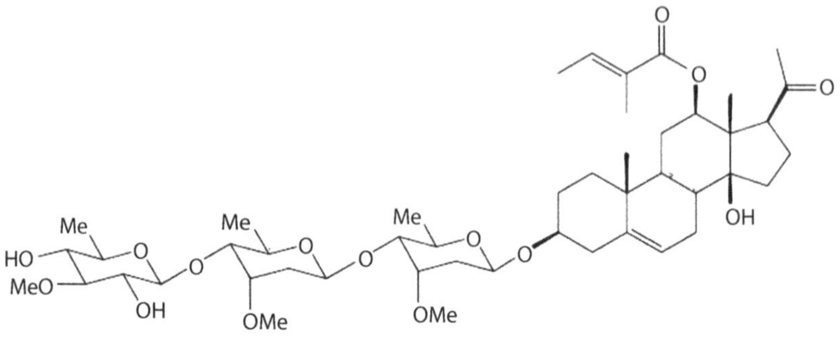

**Figure 4.7** The reported active principle of *Hoodia gordonii*.

in a powdered form, most often in capsules or tablets. Using *Hoodia* in this manner is close to the original folklore use by the San bushmen in South Africa.

## 4.11 REVERSE PHARMACOLOGY

### 4.11.1 Concept

The concept of "reverse pharmacology" was coined in India to develop pharmaceuticals from Ayurvedic medicines, and was also championed by the Chinese in the 1950s (Lei and Bodeker, 2004), but still involved a classical pathway of isolating compounds for further development (Patwardhan et al., 2009). The savings in time and cost come from the fact that the substantial experience of human use increases the chances that a remedy will be effective and safe, and that precautions will be known. However, as with classical drug discovery programs, there is no guarantee of successfully developing new treatments.

A "reverse pharmacology" approach was tested in order to develop a standardized phytomedicine against malaria in Mali (Willcox et al., 2011b). Clinical evaluation was prioritized from the start. Isolation of compounds was done only at the end of the pathway, mainly for the purposes of quality control, agronomic selection, and standardization (Figure 4.8).

### 4.11.2 Stage 1: Selecting the Most Promising Plant

The first step was to identify the most promising herbal remedy for further development. The classical way of identifying medicinal plants for further research is through ethnobotanical studies. Yet conventional ethnobotanical studies rarely involve clinicians. They could and should provide much more clinical information if the ultimate goal is to know which one, among numerous treatments for a given ailment, has the best effects (Graz et al., 2010a). Although identification of the plants is usually of a good standard, definition of the diseases that they treat is not. There is rarely sufficient questioning about the observed patient status and progress, perceived efficacy and limitations of the remedies, and whether these are indeed the "treatment of choice." Many plants are "supposed" to be good for one disease or another, but they are not actually the preferred treatment used in everyday life. In order to circumvent these problems, Graz et al. developed a new method called a retrospective treatment outcome (RTO) study (Graz et al., 2005). This simply adds two essential elements to the ethnobotanical method: clinical information and statistical analysis. Clinical information is collected retrospectively on the presentation and progress of a defined disease episode. Treatments and subsequent clinical outcomes are analyzed to elicit statistically significant correlations between them.

In the RTO, the first step was to understand local concepts and terms for diseases. For uncomplicated malaria, the definition was "fever with no other obvious cause during the rainy season," and for severe malaria, it was "fever with convulsions or loss of consciousness during the rainy season" (Diallo et al., 2006). The second step was to choose a representative random sample of households in the study area (by cluster sampling), and to ask in each sample unit whether anyone has had the disease of interest in the recent past. The timing was at the end of the malaria season. For uncomplicated malaria, a recall time of 2 weeks was used (as this is a common event, and there is a risk that information will be inaccurate if the recall period is too long) (Diallo et al., 2006). For severe malaria (which is rarer and more dramatic, so more likely to be remembered) a recall period of 6 months was used. The third step, if someone had the condition of interest, was to ask in detail what treatments the person had taken, in what order, at what stage the person had recovered from the illness, and if the cure was complete or with sequelae. In this way it was possible to understand what treatments patients were actually using in real life and with what results.

In Mali, use of this method resulted in a database of treatments taken for malaria cases in 952 households. The analysis was performed with the help of a statistician, starting with a test of correlation between reported clinical outcome and the plant preparations used. Since in some cases recipes contained more than one plant, a second step was to adjust for this in the analysis, in an attempt to determine whether individual components were associated with clinical outcomes. From the 66 plants used for the treatment of malaria in the two districts studied in Mali, alone or in various combinations, the one associated with the best outcomes was a decoction of *Argemone mexicana*. The clinical outcomes were not better when it was used in combination (Diallo et al., 2007). This remedy was selected for further study.

### 4.11.3 Stage 2: Observational Clinical Study

As patients were already using the remedy, and the literature search did not reveal any safety concerns about *Argemone mexicana* leaf decoction, an observational clinical study was organized with a small number of patients. It is a prerequisite to conduct such a study in an area where patients are already taking the remedy, so that one is not proposing a new treatment without some clinical evidence

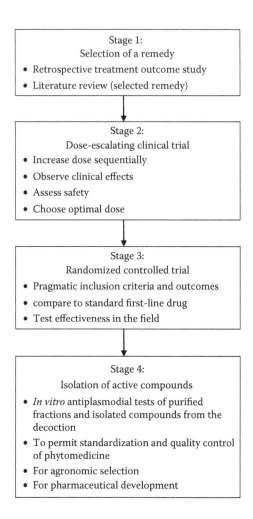

**Figure 4.8** Summary of the methodology used to develop an antimalarial phytomedicine by "reverse pharmacology." (Reproduced with permission from Willcox, M.L. et al., 2011b. *Malaria Journal*, 10:S8.)

of efficacy and safety. We observed patients being treated by a traditional healer with *Argemone mexicana* leaf decoction, and confirmed the diagnosis of uncomplicated malaria by clinical examination and blood film microscopy. Patients were followed up at regular intervals until day 28, with both clinical evaluation and blood tests. Because many patients in the first group did not seem to be improving, an increase in dose was agreed by the traditional healer and the study team, and this led to a marked improvement in treatment response (the rate of "adequate clinical response" increased from 35% to 73%) (Willcox et al., 2007). This dose was also safe, with no serious adverse effects observed clinically or on blood tests (hematology, biochemistry) or on electrocardiograms.

### 4.11.4 Stage 3: Randomized Controlled Trial (RCT)

As results from all previous stages were encouraging, the aim at this stage was to test the effectiveness of the phytomedicine in the field. In Mali, the objective was to develop a phytomedicine for home-based management of malaria (HMM), with the aims of symptomatic improvement and prevention of severe malaria. The vision was that, if effective, the plant could be recommended to communities to be cultivated and prepared locally as a first-line treatment for presumed malaria. Therefore, the inclusion criteria for the RCT reflected this: all patients with presumed malaria (history of fever during the last 24 hours, without another obvious cause, during the rainy season) were included. The comparison was Artesunate-amodiaquine (AsAQ), the first-line treatment for malaria recommended by the World Health Organization (WHO) and the Ministry of Health. The design was a "noninferiority" trial (Graz et al., 2010b).

The primary outcome measure was "clinical recovery" at day 28, without the need for a second-line treatment. An important secondary outcome measure was incidence of severe malaria, which is the most important outcome in public health terms. Large numbers of patients are needed in order to demonstrate noninferiority, because severe malaria is a relatively uncommon event. However, another approach is to see whether the incidence of severe malaria is kept below a prespecified level in both groups. In a previous study in a similar context, age-specific incidence (age <5 years) of severe malaria in untreated patients with presumed malaria was about 11%, and in patients treated at home with chloroquine (the standard treatment at that time) was about 5% per month (Sirima et al., 2003). The aim was, therefore, to keep the age-specific incidence of severe malaria (in patients aged <5 years) below 10%, and ideally ≤5%, in both groups.

Over 28 days, second-line treatment was not required for 89% (95% CI 84.1–93.2) of patients on *A. mexicana*, versus 95% (95% CI 88.8–98.3) on artesunate-amodiaquine. The observed age-specific incidence of severe malaria (in children aged 0–5 years) was 1.9% in both groups (*Argemone mexicana* and ACT) over the first 28 days of follow-up. The follow-up was extended to 3 months, and over this time the age-specific incidence of severe malaria was 2% per month in the herbal group and 1% per month in the ACT group. With 95% confidence, the age-specific incidence of severe malaria in both groups was <6% per month (Willcox et al., 2011a).

### 4.11.5 Stage 4: Isolation and Testing of Active Compounds

This is the last step of "reverse pharmacology." A phytomedicine can be developed without isolating an active ingredient, but it is useful to do this for two reasons: first, there needs to be a phytochemical marker for quality control and standardization of the herbal medicine, and also to permit agronomic selection of the best plants; and second, it is possible that a new modern drug could be developed in parallel by the pharmaceutical industry. However, it makes more sense to do this after the clinical safety and effectiveness have already been demonstrated, as chances may be higher that the isolated compound (or a derivative) will also be safe and effective. Much time and money are wasted in developing drugs that turn out to be unsafe or ineffective in humans (Verkman, 2004).

*Argemone mexicana* contains at least three protoberberine alkaloids in similar amounts (around 0.5% in the plants from Mali) with similar antimalarial activity: berberine, protopine, and allocryptopine ($IC_{50}$ *in vitro* = 0.32, 0.32, and 1.46 mcg/mL, respectively) (Simoes-Pires, 2009). Whereas all are active *in vitro*, the absorption of berberine is poor in some animal models, although it can be improved by P-glycoprotein inhibitors (Pan et al., 2002). It is not known whether *A. mexicana* contains any P-glycoprotein inhibitors, but if it does, their concentration would also be important. The pharmacokinetics of protopine and allocryptopine are now being studied in humans, so it is not yet known which of these is the best marker, or whether there is synergy between them (in which case maybe all should be used as markers). Unlike berberine, protopine and allocryptopine show a good selectivity for *Plasmodium,* and their cytotoxicities are low (Simoes-Pires, 2009). Since preliminary *in vivo* tests using freeze-dried AM decoction were unsuccessful both in mouse and in rat models (*Plasmodium berghei* and *Plasmodium chabaudi,* respectively, unpublished results), current research is focusing on the *in vitro* antiplasmodial activity of plasma samples from healthy volunteers to identify plant substances or metabolites involved in such activity.

While this research continues, the results of the first three stages of the project have already been widely disseminated to the community. People in the study area now know that, of the very many herbal remedies available, *Argemone mexicana* is one of the most effective against uncomplicated malaria. It is produced locally at no monetary cost. Families also know that any case that does not improve should seek modern health care rapidly, particularly if any signs of severe malaria develop. As a result of this work, we have documented a 3.5-fold increase in the use of *Argemone mexicana* for the treatment of uncomplicated malaria, and an 8-fold decrease in the consultation of traditional healers for severe malaria (Graz et al., 2010b). It is hoped that if this approach is scaled up, it could lead to substantial reductions in mortality from malaria and delay in the appearance of resistance to standard drugs such as artemisinin combination therapies.

## 4.12 INTEGRATED APPROACH FOR EVALUATING HERBAL REMEDIES

Based on outcomes described in this chapter, two fundamental questions must be taken into account before initiating research on plants used in traditional medicine. Is it desirable to invest substantial effort to discover pure compounds in the hope of using them as drugs per se, or is it preferable to use traditional preparations for therapeutic applications? African countries have an enormous wealth of information on medicinal plants, which are not only cheap and abundant but also culturally acceptable. However, most of them have neither a well-organized pharmaceutical industry nor the manufacturing capacity to isolate large quantities of active principles from plants. Thus, programs for drug discovery and development in these countries should not follow the Western approach. A flowchart for the investigation of medicinal plants is given in Figure 4.9. This flowchart focuses on the initial need to produce

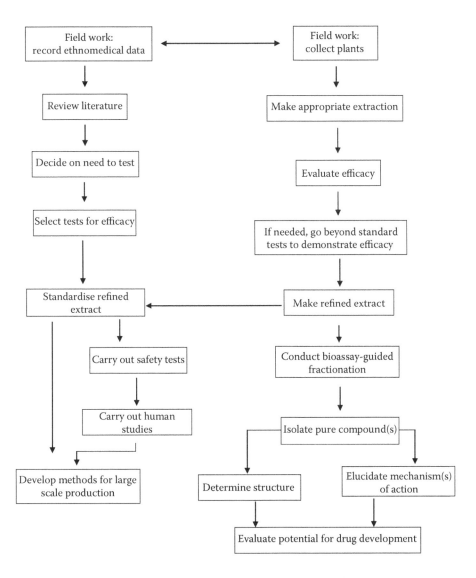

**Figure 4.9** A proposed flowchart for the investigation of medicinal plants.

safe and effective phytomedicine but includes the long-term objective of discovering the active principles, preferably in collaboration with a pharmaceutical industry.

## 4.13 CONCLUSION

Africa has abundant biodiversity that is still essentially untapped for its potential therapeutic uses as well as rich indigenous medical knowledge regarding therapeutic applications.

African scientists should focus on the diseases that affect their people and subsequently engage in the research and development of affordable products. At this point, we should not follow the Western approach of drug discovery in the initial stage of investigation of medicinal plants, but we should shift the paradigm in the evaluation of traditional medicines taking into account the message given by nature, and then translate the laboratory experiments into real clinical benefit. This approach cannot preclude any further long-term development if the possibility exists. In this regard, we should bear in mind that any drug cannot be developed without the active participation of a pharmaceutical industry.

## REFERENCES

Abegaz, B., Ngadjui, B., Bezabih, M., Mde, L.K., 1998. Novel natural products from marketed plants of Eastern and Southern Africa. *Lecture Presented at the Seventh International Chemistry Conference in Africa and 34th Convention of the South African Chemical Institute*, Durban, South Africa, July 6–10, pp. 919–1024.

Baliga, M.S., Fernandes, S., Thilakchand, K.R., D'souza, P., Rao, S., 2013. Scientific validation of the antidiabetic effects of *Syzygium jambolanum* DC (Black Plum), a traditional medicinal plant of India. *Journal of Alternative and Complementary Medicine*, 19(3):191–197.

Berenbaum, M.C. 1989. What is synergy? *Pharmacology Reviews*, 41:93–141.

Desjardins, R.E., Canfield, C.J., Haynes, J.D., Chulay, J.D., 1979. Quantitative assessment of antimalarial activity *in vitro* by a semiautomated microdilution technique. *Antimicrobial Agents and Chemotherapy*, 16(6):710–718.

Diallo, D., Diakite, C., Mounkoro, P.P., Sangare, D., Graz, B., Falquet, J., Giani, S., 2007. Knowledge of traditional healers on malaria in Kendi (Bandiagara) and Finkolo (Sikasso) in Mali. *LeMali Medical*, 22:1–8.

Diallo, D., Graz, B., Falquet, J., Traore, A.K., Giani, S., Mounkoro, P.P., Berthe, A., Sacko, M., Diakite, C., 2006. Malaria treatment in remote areas of Mali: Use of modern and traditional medicines, patient outcome. *Transactions of the Royal Society of Tropical Medicine and Hygiene*, 100(6):515–520.

Farnsworth, N.R., Akerele, O., Bingel, A.S., Soejarto, D.D., Guo, Z., 1985. Medicinal plants in therapy. *Bulletin of the World Health Organization*, 63(6):965–981.

Fouche, G., Cragg, G.M., Pillay, P., Kolesnikova, N., Maharaj, V.J., Senabe, J., 2008. In *vitro* anticancer screening of South African plants. *Journal of Ethnopharmacology*, 119(3):455–461.

Fukushi, E., 2006. Advanced NMR approaches for a detailed structure analysis of natural products. *Biosciences, Biotechnology and Biochemistry*, 70(8):1803–1812.

Graz, B., Diallo, D., Falquet, J., Willcox, M.L., Giani, S., 2005. Screening of traditional herbal medicine: First, do a retrospective study, with correlation between diverse treatments used and reported patient outcome. *Journal of Ethnopharmacology*, 101:338–339.

Graz, B., Falquet, J., Elisabetsky, E., 2010a. Ethnopharmacology, sustainable development and cooperation: The importance of gathering clinical data during field surveys. *Journal of Ethnopharmacology*, 130:635–638.

Graz, B., Willcox, M.L., Diakite, C., Falquet, J., Dackuo, F., Sidibe, O., Giani, S., Diallo, D., 2010b. *Argemone mexicana* decoction versus artesunate-amodiaquine for the management of malaria in Mali: Policy and public-health implications. *Transactions of the Royal Society of Tropical Medicine and Hygiene*, 104:33–41.

Hostettmann, K., Marston, K.A., Ndjoko, K., Wolfender, J.-L., 2000. The potential of African plants as a source of drugs. *Current Organic Chemistry*, 4:973–1010.

Hou, Y., and Harinantenaina, L., 2010. New and bioactive natural products isolated from Madagascar plants and marine organisms. *Current Medicinal Chemistry*, 17:1191–1219.

Houghton, P.J., Howesb, M.J., Lee, C.C., Steventon, G., 2007. Uses and abuses of *in vitro* tests in ethnopharmacology: Visualizing an elephant. *Journal of Ethnopharmacology*, 110:391–400.

Jalencas, X., and Mestres, J., 2013. On the origins of drug polypharmacology. *Medicinal Chemistry Communications*, 4:80–87.

Kasilo, O.M.J., Trapsida, J.-M., Mwikisa, C.N., Lusamba-Dikassa, P.S., 2010. An overview of the traditional medicine situation in the African region. *African Health Monitor*, 14(special issue):7–14.

Lei, S.H.-L., and Bodeker, G., 2004. Changshan (*Dichroa febrifuga*). Ancient febrifuge and modern antimalarial: Lessons for research from a forgotten tale. In: M. Willcox, G. Bodeker, and P. Rasoanaivo (Eds.), *Traditional Medicinal Plants and Malaria*. CRC Press, Boca Raton, FL, pp. 61–81.

Leyssen, P., Smadja, J., Rasoanaivo, P., Gurib-Fakim, A., Mahomoodally, F., Canard, B., Guillemot, J.-C., Litaudon, M., Guéritte, F., 2014. Biodiversity as a source of potent and selective inhibitors of chikungunya virus replication. In: A. Gurib-Fakim (Ed.), *Novel Plant Bioresources: Applications in Food, Medicine, and Cosmetics*. Wiley-Blackwell, Hoboken, NJ, pp. 151–161.

Manjovelo, C.S., 2012. Nouvelles molécules isolées de plantes du Sud de Madagascar: *Bivinia jalbertii et Capuronianthus mahafalensis*. Thèse de Doctorat. Faculté des Sciences, Université de Toliara.

Newman, D.J., and Cragg, G.M., 2012. Natural products as sources of new drugs over the 30 years from 1981 to 2010. *Journal of Natural Products*, 75:311–335.

Ntie-Kang, F., Lifongo, L.L., Meva'a Mbaze, L., Ekwelle, N., Owono, L.C., Megnassan, E., Judson, P.N., Sipp, W., Efange, S.M.N., 2013. Cameroonian medicinal plants: A bioactivity versus ethnobotanical survey and chemotaxonomic classification. *BMC Complementary and Alternative Medicine*, 13:147–171.

Pan, G.Y., Wang, G.J., Liu, X.D., Fawcett, J.P., Xie, Y.Y., 2002. The involvement of P-glycoprotein in berberine absorption. *Pharmacology and Toxicology*, 91:193–197.

Patwardhan, B., Mashelkar, R.A., Patwardhan, B., Mashelkar, R.A., 2009. Traditional medicine-inspired approaches to drug discovery: Can Ayurveda show the way forward? *Drug Discovery Today*, 14:804–811.

Peters, W., Portus, J.H., Robinson, B.L., 1975. The chemotherapy of rodent malaria, XXII. The value of drug resistant strains of *Plasmodium berghei* in screening for blood schizontocidal activity. *Annals of Tropical Medicine and Parasitology*, 69:155–171.

Pillay, P., Maharaj, V.J., Smith, P.J., 2008. Investigating South African plants as a source of new antimalarial drugs. *Journal of Ethnopharmacology*, 119:438–454.

Puri, M., Masum, H., Heys, J., Singer, P.A., 2010. Harnessing biodiversity: The Malagasy Institute of Applied Research (IMRA). *BMC International Health and Human Rights*, 10(Suppl 1):S9.

Rasoanaivo, P., 2011. Drugs and phytomedicines in Indian Ocean and Madagascar: Issues in research, policy and public health. *Asian Biotechnology and Development Review*, 13(3):7–25.

Rasoanaivo, P., Ramanitrahasimbola, D., Rafatro, H., Rakotondramanana, D., Robijaona, B. et al., 2004. Screening extracts of Madagascan plants in search of antiplasmodial compounds. *Phytotherapy Ressarch*, 18(9):742–747.

Rasoanaivo, P., Ratsimamanga-Urverg, S., Ramanitrahasimbola, D., Rafatro, H., Ratsimamanga, A.R., 1999. Criblage d'extraits de plantes de Madagascar pour recherche d'activité antipaludique et d'effet potentialisateur de la chloroquine. *Journal of Ethnopharmacology*, 64:117–126.

Rasoanaivo, P., and Razafimahefa, S., 2012. Compositions pharmaceutiques et leurs procedés de préparation pour le traitement des infections ou réinfections paludéennes. OMAPI Patent No. 2012/033.

Rasoanaivo, P., Wright, C., Willcox, M., Gilbert, B., 2011. Whole plant extracts versus single compounds for the treatment of malaria: Synergy and positive interactions. *Malaria Journal*, 10:S4.

Razafimahefa, S., Mutulis, F., Mutule, I., Liepinsh, E., Dambrova, M. et al., 2014. Libiguins A & B: Novel phragmalin limonoids isolated from *Neobeguea mahafalensis* causing profound enhancement of sexual activity. *Planta Medica*, 80:306–314.

Sasidharan, S., Chen, Y., Saravanan, D., Sundram, K.M., Latha, L.Y., 2011. Extraction, isolation and characterization of bioactive compounds from plants' extracts. *African Journal of Traditional, Complementary and Alternative Medicines*, 8(1):1–10.

Simoes-Pires, C.A., 2009. Investigation of antiplasmodial compounds from various plant extracts: *Argemone mexicana L.* (Papaveraceae), *Licania octandra* (Hoffmanns. ex. Roem & Schult) Kuntze (Chrysobalanaceae) *and Syzygium cumini* (L.) Skeels (Myrtaceae). PhD, Universite de Geneve.

Sirima, S.B., Konate, A., Tiono, A.B., Convelbo, N., Cousens, S., Pagnoni, F., 2003. Early treatment of childhood fevers with pre-packaged antimalarial drugs in the home reduces severe malaria morbidity in Burkina Faso. *Tropical Medicine and International Health*, 8:133–139.

Sticher, O., 2008. Natural product isolation. *Natural Product Reports*, 25:517–554.

Street, R.A., and Prinsloo, G., 2013. Commercially important medicinal plants of South Africa: A review. *Journal of Chemistry*, 2013:1–16.

*Syzygium cumini*, 2008. In: Vers une Pharmacopée Malagasy; monographies d'usage, 199–215, Ministry of Public Health of Madagascar.

Titanji, V.P.K., Zofou, D., Ngemenya, M.N., 2008. The antimalarial potential of medicinal plants used for the treatment of malaria in Cameroonian folk medicine. *African Journal of Traditional, Complementary and Alternative Medicines*, 5(3):302–321.

van Heerden, F.R., 2008. *Hoodia gordonii*: A natural appetite suppressant. *Journal of Ethnopharmacology*, 119:434–437.

Verkman, A.S., 2004. Drug discovery in academia. *American Journal of Physiology–Cell Physiology*, 286:C465–C474.

Willcox, M.L., Graz, B., Diakite, C., Falquet, J., Dackouo, F., Sidibe, O., Giani, S., Diallo, D., 2011a. Is parasite clearance clinically important after malaria treatment in a high transmission area? A 3-month follow-up of home-based management with herbal medicine or ACT. *Transactions of the Royal Society of Tropical Medicine and Hygiene*, 105:23–31.

Willcox, M.L., Graz, B., Falquet, J., Diakite, C., Giani, S., Diallo, D., 2011b. A "reverse pharmacology" approach for developing an anti-malarial phytomedicine. *Malaria Journal*, 10:S8.

Willcox, M.L., Graz, B., Falquet, J., Sidibe, O., Forster, M., Diallo, D., 2007. *Argemone mexicana* decoction for the treatment of uncomplicated falciparum malaria. *Transactions of the Royal Society of Tropical Medicine and Hygiene*, 101:1190–1198.

Williamson, E.M., 2001. Synergy and other interactions in phytomedicines. *Phytomedicine*, 8:401–409.

Wolfender, J.L., Queiroz, E.F., Hostettmann, K., 2006. The importance of hyphenated techniques in the discovery of new lead compounds from nature. *Expert Opinion in Drug Discovery*, 1(3):237–260.

# CHAPTER 5

# Development and Commercialization of Asiaticoside in Madagascar

Philippe Rasoanaivo, Alain Loiseau, Lucile Allorge-Boiteau, and Vinany Loharanombato

## CONTENTS

## 5.1 INTRODUCTION

*Centella asiatica* is found in subtropical regions (China, Malaysia, Australia, America, South Africa, and Indian Ocean islands). After the continental drift, *Centella asiatica* drifted to the middle of the Gondwanaland. It has been used as medicine in the Ayurvedic tradition of India for thousands of years for the treatment of leprosy, skin tuberculosis, wound healing, stomach aches, arthritis, varicose veins, high blood pressure, and as a memory enhancer. It is regarded as one of the most spiritual and rejuvenating herbs in Ayurveda and is used to improve meditation. It has gained worldwide reputation for its triterpene constituents used in the treatment of several illnesses. Several review papers were published on the chemistry, pharmacology, and clinical aspects of this species (Shukla and Kumar, 1997; Brinkhaus et al., 2000; Jamil et al., 2007; Singh et al., 2010; Chong and Aziz, 2011; Jahan et al., 2012; Shaival and Shaival, 2012).

Interestingly, it is the traditional use of *C. asiatica* to treat leprosy that attracted the attention of medical doctors in the nineteenth century. A summary of this story is given in the following paragraph. It turned out that the first scientific investigation of this plant and subsequent breakthroughs were undertaken in Madagascar during the period 1936–1947. Subsequently, outstanding work was done in France. Unfortunately, this pioneering work has received little emphasis and tends to be forgotten because of probably the difficult accessibility to, and availability of all old relevant documents. Furthermore, the first development of *C. asiatica* into the drug, Madecassol, was achieved by a renowned Malagasy scientist, Professor Albert Rakoto Ratsimamanga in collaboration with the pharmaceutical company, Laroche-Navarron Laboratories, in 1949. He also founded the *Institut Malgache de Recherches Appliquées* (IMRA) in 1958. IMRA is the first exporter of *C. asiatica* and remains the main supplier to the world market despite strong competition.

In this chapter, the pioneering work that was done by scientists in Madagascar first and then in France on this species will be highlighted. This review aims also to summarize the available information and contextualize the main aspects in order to establish the story of this exceptional plant. This is a relevant example of a success story on how to bring traditional knowledge into useful therapeutic applications with strong economic impact through commercialization and plant export.

## 5.2 *CENTELLA ASIATICA* AND LEPROSY IN THE NINETEENTH CENTURY

Boiteau et al. (1964:1215–1225) wrote an excellent and well-documented report on the story of *C. asiatica* and its use to treat lepromatous patients in the nineteenth century. It is worthwhile to make a summary of this report in order to contextualize the situation.

Apparently, Boileau, a medical doctor in Mauritius Island, was the pioneer of the use of *Centella asiatica* against leprosy. His life alone deserves a monograph. Boileau contracted leprosy while managing some leprosy patients. Subsequently, he voluntarily sequestered from society to a property called "La Paille" waiting for death to end his suffering. It was then that he learned about an American plant, referred to as "Cinchunchully," whose properties were praised particularly against leprosy. He wrote to all people he thought could collect the famous "Cinchunchully" and send it to him. Unfortunately, he apparently did not receive any response. However, while walking in his garden, his attention was attracted to a small plant whose leaf shape was significantly reminiscent of "Cinchunchully" as described in the published article. He prepared a tea of its plant and drank a few liters during 1 month. Surprisingly, Boileau found a significant reduction in pain and symptoms associated with leprosy. He then began to administer the treatment to 12 lepromatous patients. Based on favorable clinical outcomes, Boileau wrote an article in 1852 in a local newspaper, *Le Cernéen*, to announce his discovery. The article attracted the attention of a botanist in La Reunion Island who identified the plant as *Hydrocotyle asiatica*. He completed Boileau's article by adding comments on the botanical identity of the plant and its local uses.

J. Lepine, a pharmacist serving in Pondicherry (former French colony in India), was interested in the article. He started exchanging correspondence with Boileau. He made clinical trials of the plant on lepromatous patients in Pondicherry and Madras (now renamed Chennai, Capital of Tamil Nadu of the South India) and published his results in a local medical journal.

It was not surprising that other medical doctors were also interested in Boileau's discovery. A. Poupeau in 1853 applied the extract to patients in the central prison of Pondicherry. F. Houbert described in 1854 eight cases of leprosy and four cases of elephantiasis treated with *Hydrocotyle asiatica* in Pondicherry. In 1854, A. Hunter treated 79 cases of leprosy and 50 cases of various diseases with *Hydrocotyle asiatica* in Madras. Overall, all medical doctors came to the conclusion that leprosy was not cured by *Hydrocotyle asiatica*, but the plant could be usefully employed in many other diseases such as dermatosis and rheumatoid arthritis. Unfortunately, since then, no scientific follow-up was done on this plant.

## 5.3 DISCOVERY OF ASIATICOSIDE: PIONEERING WORK OF PIERRE BOITEAU

Physical searches for historical information used library resources at the Malagasy Academy and personal archive documentation provided by Lucile Allorge-Boiteau. In particular, the story of *C. asiatica* in Madagascar was published by Grimes and Boiteau (1945) in a document that is available only at the Malagasy Academy. Lack of appropriate indexing terms in early publications restricted the search for articles written before the availability of electronic databases.

After completing his engineering diploma in horticulture in 1931 at the *Ecole Nationale d'Horticulture de Versailles* (France), Pierre Boiteau did his military service in Madagascar from October 1932 to December 1933. He was first in charge of the "Green Space" in Antsirabe, and created there the *Parc de l'Est*. In 1935, he was appointed director of the *Parc Botanique et Zoologoqie de Tsimbazaza* in Antananarivo. Although he was a horticulturist by training, he manifested great interest in medicinal plants and traditional medicine. To facilitate contacts with the local populations, he learned the Malagasy language and obtained the *brevet supérieur de langue malgache* in 1937.

In 1936, Boiteau was kindly requested by Charles Grimes, Head of the Leprosy Hospital of Manankavaly located at 24 km from Antananarivo, to set up a vegetable garden around the hospital. On this occasion, his interest in medicinal plants led him to meet an old traditional healer who treated people with leprosy with six medicinal plants. His knowledge of the Malagasy language strongly helped him to establish a friendly relationship with the traditional healer, and to understand the use of the empirical recipe. Rapidly, he learned that five plants were just used as plaster to make the symptoms unrecognizable in order to escape the systematic control by the sanitary health personnel. The sixth plant named *Talapetraka* was administered differently. The plant was identified by Boiteau as *Centella asiatica* (synonymous *Hydrocotyle asiatica*) (Boiteau, 1945a,b). It was triturated with water for a long time and the water phase was successfully used as lotions for external lesions. This observation was the starting point of the chemical and clinical research on *C. asiatica* in Madagascar.

Grimes and Boiteau agreed to test clinically an alcoholic extract of *C. asiatica* on patients at the Leprosy Hospital of Manankavaly. The work was conducted in 1938. Remarkable results were obtained (Grimes, 1939). However, they observed that the therapeutic effect of the plant varied with the mode of preparation, the date of collection, and the dosage. Subsequently, Bontems (1941, 1942), pharmacist at the *Service de Prophylaxie de la Lèpre, Institut d'Hygyène Social de Tananarive*, undertook the phytochemical studies on *C. asiatica*, and isolated a crystalline compound he named *asiaticoside*. Grimes and Boiteau tested asiaticoside on lepromatous patients and found similar results with those obtained with alcoholic extract. They concluded that asiaticoside was the active constituent of *C. asiatica*. Boiteau mentioned (Boiteau et al., 1964) that he completely ignored previous works on *C. asiatica* reported in the previous paragraph when he initiated the work in Madagascar. In 1942, Devanne and Razafimahery pursued the phytochemical studies of *C. asiatica* and isolated a resinous compound they tentatively identified as the aglycone of asiaticoside. All the work in Madagascar was done under very difficult circumstances.

The work on *C. asiatica* was then discontinued for political reasons and World War II during the period 1941–1944. However, due to the tenacity of the pioneers of this work, it was resumed in 1944 with more clinical cases using asiaticoside. To this end, Boiteau was able to raise funds and to build an apparatus for the semi-industrial extraction of asiaticoside. Unfortunately, following the act of rebellion in 1947 and subsequent severe repressions by the French colonialist government, Boiteau, who defended the causes of the Malagasy People, was evicted from Madagascar and moved first to the Department of Agriculture in Limoges. He refused this proposal, and with the strong support of Professor Edgar Ledererat the *Muséun National d'Histoire Naturelle* in Paris, and Professor André Lwoff (Nobel Prize winner), he pursued his career at this institute. And the first part of the story of *C. asiatica* in Madagascar ended with this sad event.

## 5.4 DEVELOPMENT AND COMMERCIALIZATION OF ASIATICOSIDE

### 5.4.1 Pioneering Work of Albert Rakoto Ratsimamanga

Professor Albert Rakoto Ratsimamanga is a renowned Malagasy scientist. He was a medical doctor by training. He trained at the Faculty of Medicine of Antananarivo. He then pursued his doctoral duties in France, and defended his *doctorat d'état ès-sciences naturelles* (French system) in 1939 on the role of ascorbic acid on muscular labor (Ratsimamanga, 1939). He was thus the first Malagasy *docteur ès-sciences*. He published one book on ascorbic acid (Giroud and Ratsimamanga, 1942). He entered the *Centre National de Recherche Scientifique* (CNRS) in 1945 as *Maitre de Recherche* on a proposal from Frédéric Joliot, Research Director in CNRS and Nobel Prize in Chemistry, to whom Ratsimamanga came in contact during the Second War II because both belonged to a clandestine group of scientists who chose to remain resilient in France despite the German occupation. He was then promoted *Directeur de Recherches de classe excepptionnelle* from 1957 to 1972. He was the head of the *Laboratoire de Physiologie Nutritionnelle, des Hormones et des Vitamines* at the Faculty of Medicine in Paris, and appointed director of a laboratory at the *Ecole Pratique des Hautes Etudes*. One of his main areas of interest was the tissue (liver, spleen, adrenal-cortical gland) extracts. Particularly, he developed a drug named Surelen· which was based on adrenal-cortical gland extract. He was appointed Ambassador of Madagascar to France from 1960 to 1972. He knew Boiteau first by correspondences because they both were fervent defenders of the human rights and were close to Malagasy nationalists. Their relationship became closer following their political commitment and fight against Mussolini's aggression to Ethiopia in 1938.

The second part of the story of *C. asiatica* was at the *Muséum National d'Histoire Naturelle* in Paris. Boiteau pursued there the chemistry of *C. asiatica*. He made a preliminary structural analysis of asiaticoside, and made the acid hydrolysis of this compound leading to its aglycone which he named asiatic acid (Boiteau et al., 1949). Boiteau and Lederer then agreed that a young PhD doctorate, Judith Polonsky, should undertake the structural elucidation of asiatic acid for her thesis. Subsequently, she published several papers on the progress of the work (Polonsky, 1949a,b, 1950a,b, 1951, 1952a), and published a final paper on the complete structure (Polonsky, 1952b). Under the supervision of Polonsky, another PhD doctorate at *Muséum National d'Histoire Naturelle*, E. Sach, began the structural elucidation of asiaticoside which was subsequently solved (Polonsky et al., 1959).

Meanwhile, Boiteau was able to contact Professor Albert Rakoto Ratsimamanga. This first physical meeting opened a new and promising avenue to Ratsimamanga for the investigation of medicinal plants and traditional medicine of Madagascar, and it is in this area that he gained his reputation. He did a successful and fruitful work on the pharmacology of *C. asiatica*, and published several papers with Boiteau about the progress of the work. Two review papers summarized the overall pharmacological work (Boiteau and Ratsimamanga, 1956; Ratsimamanga and Boiteau, 1964). One paper gave an overview on the physiological role of triterpenoids (Ratsimamanga and Boiteau, 1964). Boiteau then left the *Muséum National d'Histoire Naturelle* to work fully in Ratsimamanga's laboratory. Boiteau et al. (1964) wrote an excellent book on triterpenoids and their role in animal and plant physiology.

One point that deserves attention was the involvement of an entrepreneur in the development of drugs. At this point, Ms Marguerite Navarron, pharmacist by training, and coming from a very rich family of the French extreme right-wing party, decided to marry a simple craftsman, Marcel Laroche. She was therefore rejected by her family. She conveyed her friends from India, Iran, Madagascar, and France for a meeting in which she asked them to describe what potential drugs they have to bring into commercialization. Ratsimamanga proposed Surelen. She then built a pharmaceutical company called Laroche Navarron Laboratories. The company started very small but grew rapidly. Later, Boiteau pushed Ratsimamanga to convince her to commercialize asiaticoside. She was first reluctant about "Ratsimamanga's herb," but finally accepted to launch asiaticoside in the market. A special drug patent under number 884 M was granted by the French Ministry of Industry. The drug was composed of pure asiaticoside in injectable form and began to enter the market in 1959 under the commercial name Madecassol, in honor of the country of origin of the medicine (i.e., Madagascar). Its first name was Madecasse, a word that originated from the Malayan language (Bavoux, 2002). With proceeds from the royalties from Surelen first, then from Madecassol, Ratsimamanga created the *Institut Malgache de Recherches Appliquées* in 1958. The philosophy behind this creation was the auto-centered development based on "African problems, African solutions."

As a very active and productive scientist, Boiteau coordinated the phytochemical investigation of *Centella asiatica* in Ratsimamanga's laboratory. At this point, a Malagasy PhD student, Thomas Rahandraha, chemical engineer by training, developed a chromatographic system for the analytical control of asiaticoside in view of the commercialization of Madecassol (Rahandraha et al., 1963a,b). This technique was also useful in the identification of another constituent of *C. asiatica,* which was named madecassic acid).

Simultaneously, the head of the Laroche Navarron Laboratories, Marguerite Laroche Navarron, recruited Henri Pinhas and Alain Loiseau (chemical engineers) for the industrial production of asiaticoside. She built a subsidiary company called SERDEX in charge of the industrial extraction as well as research for development. Pinhas, who was the head of the extraction unit at the Laroche Navarron Laboratories, elucidated the chemical structure of madecassic acid (Pinhas et al., 1967). Later, Pinhas et al. (1967) isolated another constituent named madecassoside and determined its structure (Pinhas and Bondiou, 1967). Like Madecassol, the names madecassic acid and madecassoside were derived from the word Madecasse. Many decades later, Loiseau et al. (2008) found that madecassoside was in fact a mixture of two isomers: cassoside and another novel glycoside named terminoloside. This molecule is a positional isomer of cassoside with an oleanan skeleton and has the same sugar series as asiaticoside and madecassoside—that is, a glucose-glucose-rhamnose series. Boiteau and Ratsimamanga devised the name *"cicatrisants majeurs"* (major wound healing drugs) for these triterpenoids, in occurrence asiaticoside, madecassoside, and terminoloside, and their respective aglycones, namely asiatic acid, medacassic acid, and terminolic acid. Their structures are shown in Figure 5.1.

As events progressed, it was shown that the mixture of triterpenoids was more active than asiaticoside alone. They act in synergy to promote wound healing. Madecassol ingredients became therefore a mixture of triterpenoids instead of asiaticoside alone. This drug is still used in modern medicine for the treatment of ulcers and venous insufficiency. Further investigations of the crude or purified

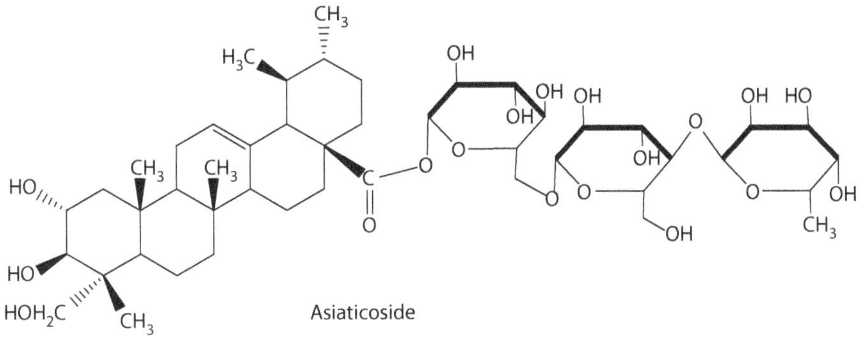

**Figure 5.1**   Structures of the three glycosides of *C. asiatica* originating from Madagascar.

**Table 5.1   Different Mixtures of the Triterpenoids of *C. asiatica* and their Areas of Applications**

| Active Principles | Chemical Compositions | Areas of Application |
|---|---|---|
| Asiatic acid | | Cosmetics |
| E.T.C.A.<br>Titrated extract of *C. asiatica* | Asiaticoside: 40%<br>Asiatic and madecassic acids: 60% | Wound healing<br>Venous insufficiency<br>Cosmetics |
| Glycosides of *C. asiatica* | Asiaticoside: ~20%<br>Madecassoside: ~55%<br>Others (not identified): ~25% | Cosmetics |
| Asiaticoside | | Cosmetics |
| EMACA | Asiaticoside: ≥55%<br>Asiatic acid: ≥5%<br>Madecassic acid: ≥10%<br>Others (not identified): ≤30% | Cosmetics |
| EPCA<br>Purified extract of *C. asiatica* | Asiaticoside: 14%–22%<br>Madecassoside: 14%–22%<br>Asiatic acid: 3%–6%<br>Madecassic acid: 3%–6%<br>NaCl: 20%<br>Others (not identified): ~40% | Cosmetics |
| ERCA<br>Refined extract of *C. asiatica* | Asiaticoside: ≥20%<br>Madecassoside: ≥20%<br>Asiatic acid: ≥4%<br>Others (not identified): ≤50% | Cosmetics |
| Aglycones | Asiatic acid: ~25%<br>Madecassic acid: ~55% | Cosmetics |

*Source:* Loiseau, A., 1998. Impieghi in cosmetologia di *Centella asiatica. Erboristeria Domani,*
6:64–69.

extracts of this species led to the discovery of their collagen regeneration properties. This has been exploited for cosmetic purposes, and it is in this area that
*C. asiatica* demonstrated its most profound applications. Different mixtures of the
triterpenoids of *C. asiatica* and their areas of applications are given in Table 5.1
(Loiseau, 1998).

## 5.5 EXPORT OF *CENTELLA ASIATICA* IN MADAGASCAR

*C. asiatica* is ranked as the second medicinal plant of economic value in Madagascar in terms of the annual quantity exported. Madagascar is one of the main suppliers to the world market. Bordeaux Tananarive was the first export company dealing with *C. asiatica*. Unfortunately, no data were available for the annual quantity exported by this company. As IMRA is a nongovernment, non-profit-making institution of applied research, it created a commercial branch called SOAMADINA. In 1972, IMRA, through its commercial branch, began the export of *C. asiatica*. Loiseau, chemical engineer at the Laroche Navarron Laboratories, moved to Ratsimamanga's laboratory in 1973, and then was transferred to IMRA in 1974 for full-time work. His main task was to supervise the quality control of *C. asiatica* for export. At this point, he analyzed the seasonal variations of the total triterpenoid extract according to time of harvesting. The quality index was ranked as Q1 for the top yield, Q2 for the medium yield, and Q3 for the low yield. The first results conserved in the IMRA archives are shown in Figure 5.2. The yield in active ingredients increases during the rainy season (December–April), attaining peak levels in February. It then falls during the drier, colder season (June–August), with a minimum yield in August–September. Similar results reported in Figure 5.3 were obtained by other authors (Rahajanirina et al., 2012).

In the last decade, it was observed that the exploitation of *C. asiatica* has started invariably in October to reach the maximal quantity collected in December, and then it has decreased slightly and progressively until May. Ecological requirements for good harvesting include therefore the hot and rainy seasons (October–April with peak in December–February) at around 900 m altitude. In such cases, they yield, and relative ratios of the relevant bioactive constituents reach the optimum values. Q1 quality is privileged for export; Q2 quality is acceptable for export; while Q3 quality is rejected. However, some companies do not take into consideration the yield in

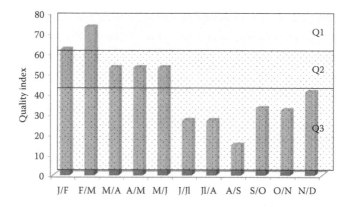

**Figure 5.2** Histogram showing 1 year seasonal variations of the total triterpenoids of *C. asiatica.*

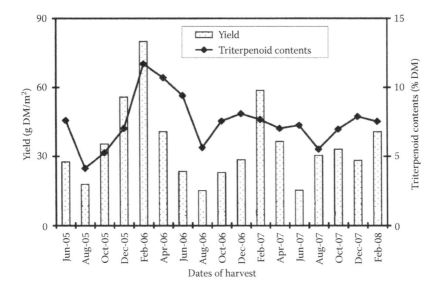

**Figure 5.3**  Every 2 months assessments of biomass yield and triterpenoid content.

total triterpenoids; instead they are interested in asiatic acid and madecassic acid for cosmetic purposes, and therefore they make indiscriminate collection.

The eastern regions of Madagascar fulfill the required ecological conditions for the best quality, and this is the main reason why *C. asiatica* originating from this part of Madagascar, if well harvested and processed, has all advantages for commercial purposes. Otherwise, under different ecosystems, such as in India, the yield of asiaticoside is much lower than that found in Madagascar (Rouillard-Guellec et al., 1997). Furthermore, the same authors demonstrated that extracts of *C.asiatica* from Madagascar were reported to have pronounced antiradical and antielastase activities compared to those from India, and these activities were not related to asiaticoside, thus justifying the use of total triterpenoids.

In 1973, IMRA initiated the cultivation of this species in the central highlands, at Andranovaky, 40 km west from Antananarivo (Ramiaramanana, 1984). However, the results were not successful because the cultivation was cost-prohibitive. Particularly, the water requirements are so high that this could not be done without sophisticated mechanical equipment. Furthermore, the yield decreased over the years, and this was also observed in Kenya (Loiseau, personal communication). Furthermore, it was observed that the plant was attacked by nematodes. Ecological requirements are therefore pivotal for the optimum yield of triterpenoids of *C. asiatica*.

Because of the specific contents in bioactive constituents that may act in synergy, importers seek for *C. asiatica* from Madagascar. IMRA-SOAMADINA was the first exporter of *C. asiatica* to the world market, but due to the increase in demand, other exporting companies entered the business. In 1995, a dozen companies were known to export this plant. Some abandoned the business while new ones appeared in the market. Annual quantities exported are shown in Figures 5.4 and 5.5.

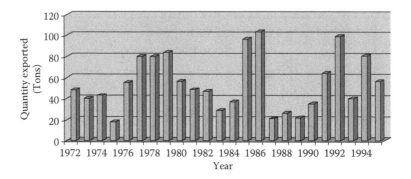

**Figure 5.4**  Histogram showing the annual quantities of *C. asiatica* exported for the period 1972–1995. (Adapted from the Ministry of Environment, Department of Forestry.)

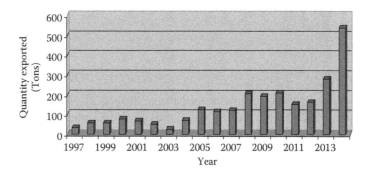

**Figure 5.5**  Histogram showing the annual quantities of *C. asiatica* exported for the period 1996–2014. (Adapted from the *Institut National de la Statistique*.)

## 5.6  CENTELLA-BASED PHYTOMEDICINES PRODUCED BY IMRA

*Centella asiatica* may be regarded as a remarkable plant by the users of its products. This species has many traditional uses. Consultations of electronic databases (Medline, HINARI, SciFinder) showed that this species displays several biological effects. Functional properties of this species were published (Seevaratnam et al., 2012).

As IMRA has grown, cutting-edge research and the commercial production of pharmaceutical products have remained tightly linked. To date, the institute has developed and formulated about 50 plant-based drugs for the treatment of a wide range of diseases in Madagascar, and the list is growing rapidly.

Innovation has long been based on the linear model. In its simplest form, this model postulates that innovation begins with new scientific research; proceeds sequentially through stages of product development, production, and marketing; and terminates with the successful sale of new products, processes, and services. As such, the linear model implies that the way to maintain leadership in markets for high-technology goods is to maintain leadership in basic scientific research.

Despite its pervasive use, the linear model suffers from several drawbacks that limit its applicability. Many innovations derive not from advances in science, but from exploiting existing scientific knowledge and from recognizing potential new markets for certain types of products, processes, or services.

Innovation capability is now seen less in terms of the ability to discover new technological principles, but more in terms of the ability to exploit the effects produced by new combinations that are well adapted to local realities and respond to local demands. This alternative model implies a more routine use of an existing technological base allowing for innovation without the need for particular breakthrough in science and technology, sometimes referred to as "innovation without research." Particularly, a natural model suggests it is usually a principle that nature has evolved to solve a particular problem or necessity in a given situation. That principle of analogy can be applied to solve scientific problems. It may help scientists to have confidence if they know that everything connects to everything else; then it is a matter of discerning, selecting, and combining.

Based on published ethnomedicinal uses of *C. asiatica* and their scientific validation (Jahan et al., 2012), IMRA has formulated various phytomedicines for therapeutic applications:

- ODY FERY: ointment comprising titrated extract of *C. asiatica* and essential oil of *Helichrysum faradifani* as wound healing phytomedicine.
- TOFA: powdered *C. asiatica* leaves combined with a medicinal plant for the treatment of gastric ulcers.
- FENOSOA: ointment including titrated extract of *C. asiatica* combined with essential oils of *Helichrysum bracteiferum* and *Cinnamosma madagascariensis* for the treatment of venous insufficiency and varicose veins.
- HUILE AMINCISSANTE: contains titrated *C. asiatica* extract for body care.
- TADIDY: titrated extract of *C. asiatica* combined with a titrated extract of a medicinal plant rich in resveratrol for the treatment of memory dysfunction.

It is also interesting to mention that the fresh *Centella* plant is commonly sold in the market in Madagascar for salads, vegetable, and tea drinks.

## 5.7 LESSONS LEARNED FROM THIS STORY

### 5.7.1 Leadership in Research and Development

The names of Boiteau and Ratsimamanga are unavoidably associated with *C. asiatica*. Boiteau had a strong belief in traditional medicine and medicinal plants, and this culminated in the publication of the 40-year work on the ethnobotany of Malagasy medicinal plants under the *Dictionnaire des Noms Malgaches dex Végétaux* with his wife and one daughter, also called the great Boiteau's achievement (Boiteau et al., 1999). It is because of his great motivation, enthusiasm, and tenacity that the first breakthrough discovery on *C. asiatica* was achieved in Madagascar. Leadership was then pivotal for the overall process. He was inspired by traditional medical knowledge that he acquired while in Madagascar to adopt a reverse pharmacology approach to investigate the plant. In fact, this approach refers to the traditional pathway of drug discovery, but was later termed *reverse pharmacology* with respect to the modern drug discovery paradigm. Boiteau made every effort to bring research initiative into useful applications. This is a good example on how to proceed in Africa to bring research into innovation, because some useful discoveries are just laboratory curiosities. At this point, the great Kenyan scientist T. Odhiambo said: "The knowledge acquired within four walls of our institutions does not bear any significant relevance with the practices of the larger society."

Because of his advantage of having an industrial partner, Laboratoires Laroche Navarron, Ratsimamanga was pivotal in coordinating the pharmacological work on asiaticoside, and bringing this compound into the market under the trade name Madecassol. This is a good example of how to translate research findings in academia into marketable products. In connection with this, H.A.M. Dzinotyiweyi, Minister of Science and Technology Development in Zimbabwe, said at a plenary lecture of the World Academy of Sciences (TWAS) for the advancement of sciences in developing countries in 2010: "It is now time to break the walls between science and commerce and to start building bridges instead."

Another point that deserves particular attention was the creation of the *Institut Malgache de Recherches Appliquées,* devoted to the useful applications of research. Ratsimamanga's goal was to create an institute that focused on understanding the mechanisms by which local medicinal plants and medical practices could serve as the basis for inexpensive, yet effective, treatments for the poor and less fortunate people of Madagascar. Such initiatives also generate income for the local communities and subsequently preserve Madagascar's unique natural flora. At its inception, IMRA was a nongovernmental organization, but since 1993 it has been granted status as a foundation termed *"FONDATION RAKOTO RATSIMAMANGA"* following a government decree. Since its creation, Ratsimamanga manifested his willingness to make IMRA as a foundation bearing his name. We would also like to mention the contribution of his wife, Suzanne Ratsimamanga, to the development of IMRA. It is by far the best-equipped center in Madagascar for natural products drug/phytopharmaceutical discovery and development as well as biodiversity conservation, and has a successful network of collaborations with institutes in the north and south, and strong south-north and north-south training exchange programs. IMRA is the oldest research institute in Madagascar but still is the leading institute in terms of research in medicinal and aromatic plants. This is a good example for African scientists in the Diasporas to build useful institutes for their countries of origin under the auto-centered development paradigm.

### 5.7.2 Single Drug versus Multicomponent Phytomedicine

Boiteau found that asiaticoside was the single biologically active constituent of *C. asiatica.* The first generation of Madecassol was therefore made with asiaticoside as a bioactive ingredient, keeping aside all other constituents. Later, it was found that in fact, the mixture of triterpenoids was more active than the single compound.

One lesson learned from *C. asiatica* and its triterpenoid contents was that in plant-based drugs, synergy with constituents may be taken into consideration. What are called medicinal plants are in fact complex chemical compositions, but traditional systems of medicines generally assume that a synergy of all ingredients of the plants will bring about the maximum therapeutic efficacy. Sometimes, the concentration of active ingredients in some herbal medicines is lower than therapeutic dosages, which has led to the suggestion that herbal therapeutic efficacy is due to placebo effects. In some cases, the total contents of a medicinal plant show a significantly better effect than an equivalent dose of a single isolated active ingredient. Furthermore, some diseases may be regulated by multiple factors. In these cases, separately targeting each individual factor is ineffective, and targeting multiple factors simultaneously may be effective for the treatment of such diseases.

### 5.7.3 Polypharmacology and Medicinal Plants

The advent of modern techniques, namely, combinatorial chemistry, high-through-put screening (HTS), bioinformatics, "omics" methods, and so on, with a "one drug, one target" philosophy has revolutionized drug discovery during the past 20 years. Unfortunately, biopharmaceutical companies attempting to increase productivity through these novel technologies have fallen short of achieving the desired results. The paradigm of drug discovery has shifted from "one drug, one target" to a more holistic approach based on "one drug, multiple targets," termed as polypharmacology (Medina-Franco et al., 2013). A direct application of polypharmacology is drug repurposing (also called drug repositioning), which is an increasingly growing approach to discover unknown off-target drugs by identifying a new clinical use for an existing approved drug (Ashburn and Thor, 2004). It is now generally admitted that polypharmacology is emerging as the next paradigm of drug discovery (Reddy and Zhang, 2013).

One relevant example of drug polypharmacology and drug repositioning is the plant-derived drug aspirin, often used as an analgesic to relieve minor pains or as an antipyretic to reduce fever, and also acts as an anti-inflammatory medication to treat rheumatoid arthritis, pericarditis, and Kawasaki diseases. Additionally, it has been used in the prevention of transient ischemic attacks, strokes, and heart attacks. Triterpenoids of *C. asiatica* are also a good example of drug polypharmacology and drug repositioning. First used as a wound healing drug, they became key compounds in the cosmetic industry (Loiseau and Mercier, 2000). It was speculated that "the origins of polypharmacology lie precisely at the heart of protein evolution" (Jalencas and Mestres, 2013), meaning that natural products preferentially target proteins, which are essential to an organism, because these are effective defense substances (Dancik et al., 2010). Polypharmacology thus reflects the mechanisms of adaptation of biological systems to increase the chances of survival in an adverse environment. As exemplified by *C. asiatica*, many medicinal plants have multipurpose applications. It is therefore worthwhile to investigate medicinal plants within the paradigm of polypharmacology. Serendipitous observations using reverse pharmacology may help in this approach. At the African Network for Drug and Diagnostic Innovation (ANDI) meeting in Nairobi in 2010, Bernard Munos said: "Innovation thrives from the interaction between innovators and users; the majority (59%) of drug innovation come not from drug companies, but from doctors trying to help patients for whom standard therapy had failed."

## ACKNOWLEDGMENTS

We are grateful to the Department of Forestry, Ministry of Environment, Ecology and Forests, as well as the National Institute of Statistics, for providing the data on *C. asiatica* export. We thank the World Health Organization for access to HINARI and the American Chemical Society for access to SciFinder.

## REFERENCES

Ashburn, T.T., and Thor, K.B., 2004. Drug repositioning: Identifying and developing new uses for existing drugs. *Nature Reviews Drug Discovery*, 3:673–683.

Bavoux, C., 2002. Des mots français pour nommer Madagascar et ses habitants: Problèmes et enjeux. *Langues et Linguistiques*, 28:1–26.

Boiteau, P., 1945a. *Travaux sur l'asiaticoside: Étude botanique*. Société des Amis du Parc Botanique et Zoologique de Tsimbazaza, 8th and 9th Annual Reports, pp. 71–75.

Boiteau, P., 1945b. *Travaux sur l'asiaticoside*. Rapport Annuel du Laboratoire de Botanique et de Technologie Végétale, pp. 26–40.

Boiteau, P., Boiteau, M., Allorge-Boiteau, L., 1999. *Dictionnaire des Noms Malgaches des Végétaux*. Editions Alzieu, La Maison du Livre, Fontanil Cornillon, France, Vols. 1–4.

Boiteau, P., Buzas, A., Lederer, E., Polonsky, J., 1949. Derivatives of *Centella asiatica* used to treat leprosy. *Nature*, 163:258.

Boiteau, P., and Chanez, M., 1967. Isolement d'un nouvel acide triterpénique de *Centella asiatica* L. (Urb) de Madagascar: l'acide madecassique. *Comptes-rendus de l'Académie des Sciences Paris, Sér D*, 264(2):407–410.

Boiteau, P., Pasich, B., Ratsimamanga, A.R., 1964. *Les triterpénoïdes en physiologie végétale et animale*. Gauthier-Villars, Paris.

Boiteau, P., and Ratsimamanga, A.R., 1956. L'asiaticoside extrait de *Centella asiatica* et ses emplois thérapeutiques dans la cicatrisation des plaies expérimentales et rebelles (lèpre, tuberculose cutanée et lupus). *Thérapie*, 2(1):125–151.

Bontems, J.E., 1941. Sur un hétérosde nouveau, asiaticoside, isolé à partir del'*Hydrocotyle asiatica* L (Umbelliferae). *Bulletin des Sciences Pharmacologiques*, 49:186–191.

Bontems, J.E., 1942. Sur un hétéroside nouveau: L'asiaticoside isolé à partir de *Hydrocotyle asiatica* (ombellifères). *Gazette Médicale de Madagascar*, 15:29–33.

Brinkhaus, B., Lindner, M., Schuppan, D., Hahn, E.G., 2000. Chemical, pharmacological and clinical profile of the East Asian medical plant *Centella asiatica*. *Phytomedicine*, 7(5):427–448.

Chong, N.J., and Aziz, Z., 2011. A systematic review on the chemical constituents of *Centella asiatica*. *Research Journal of Pharmaceutical, Biological and Chemical Sciences*, 2(3):445–459.

Dancik, V., Seiler, K.P., Young, D.W., Schreiber, S.L., Clemons, P.A., 2010. Distinct biological network properties between the targets of natural products and disease genes. *Journal of the American Chemical Society*, 132:9259–9261.

Giroud, A., and Ratsimamanga, A.R., 1942. *Acide Ascorbique. Vitamine C.* Editeur Hermann et Cie, Paris.

Grimes, C., 1939. Le traitement de la lèpre par l'*Hydrocotyle asiatica. Bulletin de la Société de Pathologie Exotique*, 32(6):692–700.

Grimes, C., and Boiteau, P., 1945. *Rapport sur la thérapeutique de la lèpre.* Société des Amis du Parc Botanique et Zoologique de Tsimbazaza, 8th and 9th Annual Reports, pp. 51–55.

Jahan, R., Hossain, S., Seraj, S., Nasrin, D., Khatun, Z., Das, R.P., Islam, M.T., Ahmed, I., Rahmatullah, M., 2012. *Centella asiatica* (L.) Urb.: Ethnomedicinal uses and their scientific validations. *American-Eurasian Journal of Sustainable Agriculture*, 6(4):261–270.

Jalencas, X., and Mestres, J., 2013. On the origins of drug polypharmacology. *Medicinal Chemistry Communications*, 4:80–87.

James, J.T., and Dubery, I.A., 2009. Pentacyclic triterpenoids from the medicinal herb, *Centellaasiatica* (L.) Urban. *Molecules*, 14:3922–3941.

Jamil, S.S., Nizami, Q., Salam, M., 2007. *Centella asiatica* (Linn.) Urban: A review. *Natural Product Radiance*, 6(2):158–170.

Loiseau, A., 1998. Impieghi in cosmetologia di *Centella asiatica. Erboristeria Domani*, 6:64–69.

Loiseau, A., and Mercier, M., 2000. *Centella asiatica* and skin care. *Cosmetics and Toiletries Magazine*, 15:63–67.

Loiseau, A., Sene, G., and Theron, E., 2008. Method for preparing a *Centella asiatica* extract rich in madecassoside and in terminoloside, United States of America Patent number US2008011581 A1.

Medina-Franco, J.L., Giulianotti, M.A., Welmaker, G.S., Houghten, R.A., 2013. Shifting from the single to the multitarget paradigm in drug discovery. *Drug Discovery Today*, 18:495–501.

Pinhas, H., Billet, D., Heitz, S., Chagneau, M., 1967. Structure de l'acide madécassique, nouveau triterpène de *Centella asiatica* de Madagascar. *Bulletin de la Société Chimique de France*, 6:1890–1895.

Pinhas, H., and Bondiou, J.C., 1967. Sur la constitution chimique de la partie glucidique du madecassoside. *Bulletin de la Société Chimique de France*, 6:1888–1890.

Polonsky, J., 1949a. Sur la constitution chimique de l'asiaticoside. *Bulletin de la Société de Chimie Biologique*, 31:46.

Polonsky, J., 1949b. Sur la constitution chimique de l'asiaticoside. *Comptes-rendus de l'Académie des Sciences Paris*, 228:1450–1451.

Polonsky, J., 1950a. Sur la constitution chimique de l'asiaticoside. *Comptes-rendus de l'Académie des Sciences Paris*, 230:485.

Polonsky, J., 1950b. Sur la constitution chimique de l'asiaticoside. *Comptes-rendus de l'Académie des Sciences Paris*, 230:1784.

Polonsky, J., 1951. Sur la constitution chimique de l'asiaticoside. *Comptes-rendus de l'Académie des Sciences Paris*, 232:1873.

Polonsky, J., 1952a. Sur la constitution chimique de l'acide asiatique. *Bulletin de la Société Chimique de France*, 19:649–654.

Polonsky, J., 1952b. Sur la constitution chimique de l'acide asiatique. *Bulletin de la Société Chimique de France*, 19:1015–1021.

Polonsky, J., Sach, E., Lederer, E., 1959. Sur la constitution chimique de la partie glucidique del'asiaticoside. *Bulletin de la Société Chimique de France*, 13:880–887.

Rahajanirina, V., Raoseta, S.O.R., Roger, E., Razafindrazaka, H., Pirotais, S., Boucher, M., Danthu, P., 2012. The infuence of certain taxonomic and environmental parameters on biomass production and triterpenoid content in the leaves of *Centella asiatica* (L.) Urb. from Madagascar. *Chemistry and Biodiversity*, 9:298–308. (<cirad-00826718>).

Rahandraha, T., Chanez, M., Boiteau, P., 1963a. Dosage à l'anthrone de l'asiaticoside de *Centella asiatica*. *Annales Pharmaceutiques Françaises*, 21:313–320.

Rahandraha, T., Chanez, M., Boiteau, P., Jaquard, S., 1963b. Dosage à l'anthrone de l'asiaticoside isolé de *Centella asiatica* par chromatographie quantitative sur poudre de verre en couche mince. *Annales Pharmaceutiques Françaises*, 21:561–567.

Ramiaramanana, E.R., 1984. *Contribution à l'étude du Centella asiatica de Madagascar "Talapetraka"*, Mémoire de Fin d'Etudes d'Ingéniorat en Agronomie, Université d'Antananarivo.

Ratsimamanga, A.R., 1939. *Recherches sur le rôle de l'acide ascorbique, en particulier au cours du travail*. Thèses présentées à la Faculté des Sciences de l'Université de Paris pour obtenir le grade de docteur ès sciences naturelles.

Ratsimamanga, A.R., and Boiteau, P., 1964. Propriétés thérapeutiques des extraits de *Centella asiatica* et de leurs constituants triterpéniques isolés. *Annales de l'université de Madagascar*, 2:101–107.

Reddy, A.S., and Zhang, S., 2013. Polypharmacology: Drug discovery for the future. *Expert Review in Clinical Pharmacology*, 6:41–47.

Rouillard-Guellec, F., Robin, J.R., Ratsimamanga, A.R., Ratsimamanga, S., Rasoanaivo P., 1997. Comparative study of *Centella asiatica* of Madagascar origin and Indian origin. *Acta Botanica Gallica*, 144:489–493.

Shaival, R.P., and Shaival, K.R., 2012. Review on *Centella asiatica*: A wonder drug. *International Journal of Pharmaceutical and Chemical Sciences*, 1(3):1369–1375.

Seevaratnam, B.A., Banumathi, P., Premalatha, M.R., Sundaram, S.P., Arumugam, T., 2012. Functional properties of *Centella asiatica* (L.): A review. *International Journal of Pharmacy and Pharmaceutical Sciences*, 4(Suppl 5):8–14.

Shukla, S.R.Y.N., and Kumar, S., 1997. Chemistry and pharmacology of *Centella asiatica*: A review. *Journal of Medicinal and Aromatic Plants Society*, 19(4):1049–1056.

Singh, S., Gautam, A., Sharma, A., Batra, A., 2010. *Centella asiatica* (L.): A plant with immense medicinal potential but threatened. *International Journal of Pharmaceutical Sciences Review and Research*, 4(2):9–17.

# CHAPTER 6

# Neem, *Azadirachta indica*

**Sunita Facknath**

## CONTENTS

## 6.1 INTRODUCTION

Neem, *Azadirachta indica* (family: Meliaceae), is also known as margosa tree or Indian lilac. Neem is native to India and Southeast Asia. Currently, neem is now spread in the warm lowland tropics as well as in arid and semi-arid areas of the world. Indian immigrants introduced neem to East Africa and Asia during the nineteenth century due to its medicinal properties. The neem tree is now found in Mauritius, Fiji, Malaysia, Indonesia, Thailand, and Cambodia. Neem is also widely cultivated in Mauritania, Senegal, Gambia, Guinea, Ivory Coast, Ghana, Burkina Faso, Mali, Benin, Niger, Nigeria, Togo, Cameroon, Chad, Ethiopia, Sudan, Somalia, Kenya, Tanzania, and Mozambique (Infonet-biovision). In addition, neem has been planted in the United States, Australia, China, Mexico, and several other countries in Latin America.

Neem has been known in India for centuries as a wonder plant, and has been variously described as the "Divine Tree," "Heal All," "Nature's Drugstore," "Village Pharmacy," and "Panacea for all diseases." The word *neem* is derived from Sanskrit "Nimba," which means "bestower of good health." Neem is also referred to as Arishtha, which means "reliever of sickness," and Kalpavriksha, which means "wish fulfilling tree" (Pandey, 1993). In Kenya, it is known as "Muarubaini," which means "the tree of the forty cures." All parts of the tree—the roots, bark, gum, leaves, fruit, seed kernels, and seed oil—are used in therapeutic preparations for both internal and topical uses. Neem is a major ingredient in many Ayurvedic and Unani medicines. Unani medicine lists its pharmacological effects as follows: anti-inflammatory, anti-leprosy, strong blood purifying, antivitiligo, antimicrobial, antipyretic, antiflatulent, antibilephlegm, antiseptic, anti-arthritic, antipurulent, anthelminthic, and wound healing (Rahman and Jairajpuri, 1993).

Neem is nature's systemic purifier, helping to clear toxins and supporting the natural inflammatory response. Neem enhances the body's ability to heal wounds, maintain healthy blood sugar levels, and promotes the natural cleansing mechanisms of the skin and internal organs. Consequently, neem is a powerful blood purifier, detoxifier, and general health promoter. It accelerates wound healing and promotes healthy skin. Neem is used in many different forms—as a powder, decoction, fresh or fermented tea, paste, medicated oil, tablets, pills, and so on.

The tree is evergreen and can grow up to 30 m. It starts to produce fruits from the age of 5 years and can live for over 100 years. The tree can grow in marginal and nutrient-poor soils, and can help in reforestation and in preventing soil erosion and landslides. Being termite resistant, neem wood is useful as building timber, and the leaves, being alkaline, help to neutralize acidic soils. Neem oil and leaves protect crops and stored grain from insects and other pests. The medicinal, cosmetic, pesticidal, and antiparasitic, anthelminthic, antifungal, antidiabetic, antibacterial, antiviral, antifertility, and sedative properties of neem are undisputed and highly impressive, so much so that the National Research Council (NRC), Washington, DC, published a report entitled "Neem: Tree for Solving Global Problems" and has described neem as "one of the most promising of all plants and it may eventually benefit every person on this planet. Probably no other plant yields as many strange and varied products or has as many exploitable by-products." The United Nations has declared neem as the tree of the twenty-first century.

In the early 1990s, some American companies tried to patent neem, but following a court battle, the patents were revoked. Without the possibility of patents, the interest of megacorporations in neem research and development dwindled, and neem has since then remained essentially a home remedy or a traditional medicine.

## 6.2 HISTORY OF NEEM TREE

In ancient India, neem was an integral part of life. Some of the traditional uses of different parts of neem include the following:

- Improvement of quality of life
- Detoxifier and blood purifier
- Preventive as well as curative medicine for a range of internal and external diseases and disorders
- Dental health
- Cosmetic, for hair and skin care
- Contraceptive
- Immuno-fortifier
- Control of pests, parasites, and diseases in crops, livestock, and people
- Protector of food and stored grains
- Improvement of soil health and fertility

Furthermore, the ripe fruits and the tender young leaves were eaten. Its multitude of uses and benefits far surpasses that of any other tree. In fact, the neem tree was considered to be the solution to practically every health- and environment-related problem, and was worshipped as a divine gift from God.

With respect to medicines, neem is a key component of many Ayurvedic and Unani preparations. Consequently, different neem preparations are used at home for the management of various remedies. Unani physicians claim that neem can remove toxic gases from the air and prevent health problems. Furthermore, it was believed that sleeping under a neem tree could cure fever (Rahman and Jairajpuri, 1993). Perhaps the best studied aspect of the immense potential value of the neem tree is the insecticidal effects of this wonder tree (Saxena, 1989). Neem has shown itself to be a potent but safe insecticide for the control of agricultural insect pests, as well as those that act as human disease vectors (e.g., malaria, chikungunya, dengue fever, yellow fever, Chagas disease, etc.). Neem is also useful in the treatment of head and body lice, bedbugs, fleas, and other parasitic insects of humans and pet animals.

The range of diseases that has been traditionally treated with neem includes cancer, malaria, diabetes, hepatitis, duodenal ulcers, kidney disorders, fungal infections, yeast infections, sexually transmitted diseases, all kinds of skin disorders, periodontal disease, mononucleosis, blood disorders, heart diseases, nerve disorders, and allergies. It is particularly popular as a malaria treatment and for diabetes in many traditional pharmacopeia. All of these properties have today been validated by modern science, either in laboratory animals and/or in human subjects in clinical trials, as described in the next section.

## 6.3 GENERAL HEALTH

Taken regularly in one form or another, neem stimulates and strengthens the immune system, improves liver function, and removes blood toxins. It has a generally positive effect on the circulatory, respiratory, and digestive systems, probably due to its immunostimulant property (Dhawan and Patnaik, 1993). Its antiviral properties protect against colds, inflammations, and other viral diseases. The resin produced by the neem tree, powdered and taken orally, is considered a good tonic, blood purifier, and body stimulant. Koley and Lal (1994) have reported that alcoholic extract of neem leaves can substantially decrease blood pressure in a dose-dependent manner.

## 6.4 ANTIFUNGAL ACTIVITY

According to Khan and Wassilew (1987), extracts of neem leaf, neem oil, and neem seed kernels were effective against certain human fungi, including *Trichophyton* spp., *Epidermophyton* spp., *Microsporum* spp., *Trichosporon* spp., *Geotricum* spp., and *Candida* spp.

## 6.5 ANTIBACTERIAL ACTIVITY

Baswa et al. (2001) reported the *in vitro* antibacterial activity of neem seed oil on 14 strains of pathogenic bacteria, while Satyavati et al. (1976) showed that *Vibrio cholerae, Klebsiella pneumoniae, Mycobacterium tuberculosis,* and *Streptococcus pyogenes* were inhibited by neem oil, as were *Streptococcus mutans* and *Streptococcus faecalis* (Almas, 1999).

## 6.6 ANTIVIRAL ACTIVITY

Aqueous leaf extract is virucidal to group-B Coxsackie viruses, while solvent extracts are virucidal to Coxsackie virus B-4 (Badam et al., 1999). *In vitro* studies have demonstrated the antiviral activity against *Vaccinia* spp. virus (Rao et al., 1969), chikungunya, and measles virus (Gogati and Marathe, 1989). Galhardi et al. (2012) reported the *in vitro* antiviral property of neem polysaccharides against poliovirus.

## 6.7 IMMUNOSTIMULANT ACTIVITY

Neem oil, bark, and leaf extracts exhibited strong immunostimulant activity (Upadhyay et al., 1992). Neem tree leaf extracts (100 mg/kg per oral for 3 weeks) significantly increased the immunoglobulin M (IgM), immunoglobulin G (IgG), and anti-ovalbumin antibody levels (Ray et al., 1996).

## 6.8 ANTI-INFLAMMATORY, ANTIPYRETIC, AND ANALGESIC ACTIVITIES

Neem bark extract has been shown to cure inflammatory stomatitis in children (Lorenz, 1976). Neem oil demonstrated an antipyretic effect (Murthy and Sirsi, 1958). Furthermore, the methanolic leaf extract induced an analgesic effect in laboratory animals, which might have been mediated through opioid receptors (Vohra and Dandiya, 1992).

## 6.9 HYPOGLYCEMIC ACTIVITY

Oral administration of aqueous extracts of neem leaves has been shown to significantly decrease blood sugar levels and prevent adrenaline and glucose-induced hyperglycemia (Murty et al., 1978), in normal and experimentally induced diabetic rats (El-Hawary and Kholief, 1990) and rabbits (Khosla et al., 2000).

In non-insulin-dependent diabetics, Neem has a synergistic effect on oral anti-diabetic drugs, and also helps in minimizing diabetic-related complications in the retina and fundus (Riar, 1993).

## 6.10 ANTIMALARIAL ACTIVITY

Neem seed and leaf extracts are effective against malarial parasites (Khalid et al., 1986, 1989). Alcoholic extracts of leaves and seeds are effective against both chloroquine-resistant and sensitive strains of *Plasmodium* spp. (Badani et al., 1987). Dhar et al. (1998) reported that the growth and development of asexual and sexual stages of drug-sensitive and drug-resistant strains of *P. falciparum* were inhibited by neem seed extracts. Furthermore, Luong et al. (2012) reported the effective control of anopheline larvae by neem leaf slurry in West Africa. Neem is not only effective in killing aquatic larvae of mosquitoes and repelling the blood-sucking adult females, which are the vectors of the malarial pathogen, *Plasmodium* spp., but it has also been shown to have some schizonticidal activity (Sharma, 1993). However, this has not been sufficiently investigated. Nonetheless, aqueous neem leaf extracts are used as a remedy for malaria in Thailand and Nigeria (Okpanyi and Ezenkwu, 1981).

## 6.11 ANTIULCER EFFECT

Neem leaf aqueous extract has an antiulcer effect in rats by preventing mucus depletion and mast cell degranulation (Garg et al., 1993) and acting as a strong ant-acid stimulator (Bandyopadhyay et al., 1998). A hot fomentation of neem leaves applied to inflamed joints provides relief from arthritic pains, while tender leaves are very useful in treating diabetes mellitus (Rahman and Jairajpuri, 1993).

## 6.12 ANTICARCINOGENIC ACTIVITY

The anticarcinogenic properties of aqueous neem leaf extracts have been demonstrated on induced oral squamous cell carcinoma, by acting on glutathione and its metabolizing enzymes (Balasenthil et al., 1999). Treatment with neem extracts induced high levels of antioxidants and detoxifying enzymes in the stomach, liver, and blood, and low levels of lipid peroxides, attesting to its anticancer property (Arivazhagan et al., 2000a,b). Furthermore, Neem has been shown to be a potent inducer of apoptosis of cervical cancer cells. Srivastava et al. (2012) reported p53-independent apoptosis and autophagy induced by neem oil limonoids.

## 6.13 HEPATOPROTECTIVE ACTIVITY

Bhanwra et al. (2000) showed that liver necrosis in laboratory rats following high dosages of paracetamol could be prevented by oral administration of aqueous neem leaf extracts, as evidenced by reduced levels of serum aspartate aminotransferase (AST), alanine aminotransferase (ALT), and gamma glutamyl transpeptidase (GGT).

## 6.14 EFFECT ON DIGESTIVE SYSTEM

Infusion of neem leaves mixed with honey is used to treat colic pain. Hot leaves dropped in water and consumed are effective in curing flatulence. Peptic and duodenal ulcers can be treated with neem seed kernels Sudhir et al (2010). A decoction of leaves as well as crushed neem seeds are useful in treating hemorrhoids. Neem flowers can treat diarrhea. Unripe neem fruits are digestive and help in increasing appetite.

## 6.15 CONTRACEPTIVE EFFECT

Neem oil is a strong contraceptive when taken orally, applied topically, or applied subcutaneously. Neem oil can be used as a vaginal spermicide in humans. Apart from killing spermatozoa on direct contact, neem has also been shown to be absorbed through the vaginal mucosa into the circulatory system and exerted reversible antifertility effects for a variable number of days in laboratory rats (Riar,

1993). Talwar et al. (1993) reported that a single administration of 0.1 mL of neem seed extract in rats blocked fertility for up to 180 days without disturbing ovulation or sex steroid hormone production. The same workers observed the same effects in monkeys given 1 mL of neem oil. This effect has been explained as an induction by neem of cell-mediated immunity, which is then triggered by the sperm leading to production of cytokines that kill the sperm (Talwar et al., 1993). A cream based on neem seed extract was shown to be effective in treating leukorrhea caused due to *Chlamydia trachomatis*. This cream is also recommended for use as a herbal vaginal cream contraceptive (Talwar et al., 1993).

## 6.16 DENTAL CARE

In earlier times in India, and even today in villages, people chewed neem twigs or tender branches as an alternative to morning brushing of teeth. The antiseptic, antigingivitis, antiplaque properties of neem provide good oral and dental care and prevent periodontal diseases and foul breath. Burnt neem bark used as a tooth powder is effective in pyorrhea. Gargling with neem leaves or flowers strengthens gums and teeth. One study reported that rinsing with neem mouthwash twice a day was as effective at reducing gingival bleeding, periodontitis, and plaque indices as the commercial chlorhexidine (Balappanavar et al., 2013).

## 6.17 SKIN CARE

Neem is a great skin care product, the leaves and the seed oil being particularly effective. It purifies and clears the skin by removing excess oil and blemishes. It cools and soothes dry, irritated, or itchy skin. It is a powerful antiseptic and antibacterial agent and helps in clearing acne, eczema, psoriasis, ulcers, and boils. Studies have shown that it did not result in bacterial resistance and was not harsh on the skin. Furthermore, an alcoholic extract of neem was shown to be superior to nixoderm, salicylic acid, and benzoic acid preparations in the treatment of ringworm, and to benzyl benzoate and sulfa drugs in the treatment of scabies. It has also been used in the treatment of leprosy, vitiligo, syphilis, and pityriasis (Rahman and Jairajpuri, 1993). The application of a paste made from gently heated leaves promotes liquefaction and drainage of pus and healing of abscesses. A paste of neem leaves and unslaked lime has been used to treat malignant skin ulcers and nonhealing wounds (Rahman and Jairajpuri, 1993). There are reports of neem lightening freckles, blemishes, and even scars, and making them less visible (Rao et al., 1986).

## 6.18 HAIR AND NAIL CARE

Neem oil is an excellent hair oil, promoting shiny, healthy, quick growing hair, preventing dryness, hair loss, and grayness. An extract of neem flowers is also used to prevent hair loss and premature graying. Applied to nails, the antifungal properties of neem oil prevent and cure nail fungus, and keep the nails supple and healthy.

## 6.19 TREATMENT FOR EXTERNAL AND INTERNAL PARASITES

Intestinal worms can be killed by taking the juice of neem leaves or stalks, neem seed oil, or a decoction of the bark or flowers, or eating unripe neem fruits. Its strong pesticidal properties help in clearing scabies and head and body lice. Neem oil spray can also be used as a natural mosquito repellant. Neem keeps mosquitoes away, and unlike the commercial synthetic repellents, it is not toxic to humans. Burning neem leaves and twigs to repel mosquitoes is a common practice even today in many parts of India.

## 6.20 TRADITIONAL NEEM EXTRACTS, PREPARATIONS, AND METHODS OF ADMINISTRATION

Ancient and traditional literature describe a number of different methods of preparation of neem. Some examples are as indicated in the following sections.

### 6.20.1 Aqueous Extracts

• Fresh neem leaves are crushed and applied as a paste to the face affected by acne, freckles, blemishes, or any other skin area affected by psoriasis, ulcers, boils, or eczema. The paste is left until it starts drying and is then rinsed off.
• Fresh neem leaves are soaked in hot water until they soften and then are crushed into a paste and applied as above.
• Neem leaves are boiled in water for a few minutes, then strained and cooled. The water is used for a full body bath or splashed on the face several times a day.
• Dried neem leaf powder is used to make tea or a paste.
• The skin/soft bark of the neem tree is rubbed on a rough surface with some water until a brown paste is obtained.
• The fruits are depulped and the seed separated. The seeds are broken open to remove the kernels. To obtain neem seed kernel oil, the kernels are ground with water and left overnight. The oil floats on top and is skimmed off. To obtain aqueous neem seed kernel extract, the kernels are crushed and placed in a cloth bag. The bag is steeped overnight in a tub of water and then removed the next morning. The water-soluble compounds in the kernels are extracted using water.

### 6.20.2 Alcoholic Extracts

Azadirachtin and the other limonoids are highly soluble in alcohol. Neem extracts using alcohol as a solvent are much more concentrated, and therefore are more active, as compared to aqueous extracts. Neem extracts, using alcohol as a solvent, are much more concentrated, and therefore are more active, as compared to aqueous extracts.

Crushed neem seed kernels are soaked in alcohol (ethanol) overnight, and the extract is then filtered through a cloth. This is meant for external use only.

## 6.21 CHEMISTRY OF NEEM

The principal reason for this extraordinary range of bioactivity is the huge number of compounds present in the neem tree. Over 140 bioactive compounds have been identified so far, and more are being analyzed (Subapriya and Nagini, 2005). The bioactive compounds fall mainly into two groups: isoprenoids and nonisoprenoids. The isoprenoids comprise 31 nortriterpenoids, including 28 limonoids and 3 degraded limonoids, and one diterpenoid. These include protomeliacins, azadiradione, azadirone, limonoids, and derivatives such as vilasinin, nimbin, azadirachtin. nimbinin, nimbolins, nimbolide, margolone, margolonone, isomargolonone, meliantriol, melianone, melianol, and salanin. The nonisoprenoids consist of carbohydrates, proteins, sulfurous compounds, and polyphenolics including flavonoids, dihydrochalcone, coumarin, and aliphatic compounds (Kumar et al., 2010).

It is believed that the numerous uses of the neem tree are directly related to its bioactive compounds. Examples include immunomodulatory, anti-inflammatory, antihyperglycemic, antiulcer, antimalarial, antifungal, antibacterial, antiviral, antioxidant, antimutagenic, and anticarcinogenic properties. Ironically, this versatility of beneficial chemicals has prevented this remarkable gift of nature from being commercially exploited by man to the extent it deserves. The legal requirement for registration, and the need for homogeneity of commercial preparations for obtaining registration, makes it difficult to obtain consistent and pure products from this rich mixture of chemicals in a cost-effective manner. Furthermore, the chemical complexity of the azadirachtins has so far not been matched by human efforts to develop synthetic analogues. Nonetheless, there are a large number of neem-based commercial skin, hair and dental care products, tonics, face creams, face powders, contraceptive vaginal creams, antiseptic creams, soaps, shampoos, pesticides, and fertilizers available in the global market.

Like many other plant-based preparations, the compounds in neem are highly unstable and decompose rapidly, especially in the presence of light. Hence, crude neem extracts need to be prepared and applied fresh. Commercial formulations are stabilized with appropriate additives to increase their shelf life and/or efficacy.

## REFERENCES

Almas, K., 1999. The antimicrobial effects of extracts of *Azadirachta indica* (Neem) and *Salvadora persica* (Arak) chewing sticks. *Indian Journal of Dental Research*, 10:23–26.

Arivazhagan, S., Balasenthil, S., Nagini, S., 2000a. Modulatory effect of garlic and neem leaf extracts on N-methyl-N′-Nitro N-nitrosoguanidine (MNNG) induced oxidative stress in Wistar rats. *Cell Biochemistry and Function*, 18:17–21.

Arivazhagan, S., Balasenthil, S., Nagini, S., 2000b. Garlic and neem leaf extracts enhance hepatic glutathione and glutathione dependent enzymes during N-methyl-N′-nitro-N-nitrosoguanidine (MNNG)-induced gastric carcinogenesis in rats. *Phytotherapy Research*, 14:291–293.

Badam, L., Joshi, S.P., Bedekar, S.S., 1999. 'In vitro' antiviral activity of neem (Azadirachta indica. A. Juss) leaf extract against group B coxsackieviruses. *Journal of Communicable Diseases*, 31:79–90.

Badani, L., Deolankar, R.P., Kulkarni, M.M., Nagsampgi, B.A., Wagh, U.V., 1987. In vitro antimalarial activity of neem (Azadirachta indica A. Juss) leaf and seed extracts. *Indian Journal of Malariology*, 24:111–117.

Balappanavar, A.Y., Sardana, V., Singh, M. 2013. Comparison of the effectiveness of 0.5% tea, 2% neem and 0.2% chlorhexidine mouthwashes on oral health: a randomized control trial. *Indian Journal of Dental Research*, 24:24–34.

Balasenthil, S., Arivazhagan, S., Ramachandran, C.R., Nagini, S., 1999. Chemopreventive potential of neem (*Azadirachta indica*) on 7,12-dimethylbenz[a]anthracene (DMBA) induced hamster buccal pouch carcinogenesis. *Journal of Ethnopharmacology*, 67:189–195.

Bandyopadhyay, U., Chatterjee, R., Bandyopadhyay, R., 1998. US Patent 5,730,986; corresponding to Indian Patent 1100/Del/95.

Baswa, M., Rath, C.C., Dash, S.K., Mishra, R.K., 2001. Antibacterial activity of karanj (*Pongamia pinnata*) and neem (*Azadirachta indica*) seed oil: A preliminary report. *Microbios*, 105:183–189.

Bhanwra, S., Singh, J., Khosla, P., 2000. Effect of *Azadirachta indica* (Neem) leaf aqueous extract on paracetamol-induced liver damage in rats. *Indian Journal of Physiology and Pharmacology*, 44:64–68.

Dhar, R., Zhang, K., Talwar, G.P., Garg, S., Kumar, N., 1998. Inhibition of the growth and development of asexual and sexual stages of drug-sensitive and resistant strains of the human malaria parasite Plasmodium falciparum by Neem (*Azadirachta indica*) fractions. *Journal of Ethnopharmacology*, 61:31–39.

Dhawan, B.N., Patnaik, G.K., 1993. Pharmacological studies for therapeutic potential. In: N.S. Randhawa and B.S. Parmar (Eds.), *Neem Research and Development*. SPS Publication, IARI, India, pp. 242–249.

El-Hawary, Z.M., Kholief, T.S., 1990. Biochemical studies on hypoglycemic agents (I) effect of *Azadirachta indica* leaf extract. *Archives of Pharmacological Research*, 13:108–112.

Galhardi, L.C., Yamamoto, K.A., Ray, S., Ray, B., Linhares, R.E., Nozawa, C., 2012. The in vitro antiviral property of *Azadirachta indica* polysaccharides for poliovirus. *Journal of Ethnopharmacology*, 142(1):86–90.

Garg, G.P., Nigam, S.K., Ogle, C.W., 1993. The gastric antiulcer effects of the leaves of the neem tree. *Planta Medica*, 59:215–217.

Gogati, S.S., Marathe, A.D., 1989. Anti-viral effect of neem leaf (*Azadirachta indica*) extracts on Chinkugunga and measles viruses. *Journal of Research and Education in Indian Medicine*, 8:1–5.

Khalid, S.A., Duddect, H., Gonzalez-Sierra, M.J. 1989. Isolation and characterization of an antimalarial agent of the neem tree *Azadirachta indica*. *Journal of Natural Products*, 52:922–927.

Khalid, S.A., Farouk, A., Geary, T.G., Jensen, J.B., 1986. Potential antimalarial candidates from African plants: An in-vitro approach using *Plasmodium falciparum*. *Journal of Ethnopharmacology*, 15:201–209.

Khan, M., Wassilew, S.W., 1987. The effect of raw material from neem tree, neem oil, and neem extracts on fungi pathogenic to humans. In: H. Schmutterer and K.R.S. Asher (Eds.), *Natural Pesticides from the Neem Tree and Other Tropical Plants*. GTZ, Eschborn, Germany, pp. 645–650.

Khosla, P., Bhanwra, S., Singh, J., Seth, S., Srivastava, R.K., 2000. A study of hypoglycaemic effects of *Azadirachta indica* (Neem) in normal and alloxan diabetic rabbits. *Indian Journal of Physiology and Pharmacology*, 44:69–74.

Koley, K.M. and Lal, J. 1994. Pharmacological effects of *Azadirachta indica* (neem) leaf extract on the ECG and blood pressure of rats. *Indian Journal of Physiology and Pharmacology*, 38:223–225.

Kumar, S.P., Mishra, D., Ghosh, G., Panda, C.S., 2010. Biological action and medicinal properties of various constituents of *Azadirachta indica* (Meliaceae): An overview. *Annals of Biological Research*, 1(3):24–34.

Lorenz, H.K.P., 1976. Neem tree bark extract in the treatment of inflammatory stomatitis. *J. Praxis*, 8:231–233.

Luong, K., Dunkel, F.V., Coulibaly, K., Beckage, N.E., 2012. Potential use of neem leaf slurry as a sustainable dry season management strategy to control the malaria vector *Anopheles gambiae* (Diptera: Culicidae) in West African villages. *Journal of Medical Entomology*, 49(6):1361–1369.

Murthy, S.P., Sirsi, M., 1958. Pharmacological studies on *Melia azadirachta*. Part II. Estrogen and antipyretic activity of neem oil and its fractions. *Indian Journal of Physiology and Pharmacology*, 2:456–460.

Murty, K.S., Rao, D.N., Rao, D.K., Murty, L.B.G., 1978. Effect of *Azadirachta indica* leaf extract on serum lipid profile. *Indian Journal of Pharmacology*, 10:247–250.

Okpanyi, S.N., Ezenkwu, Jr. C., 1981. Anti-inflammatory and antipyretic activities of *Azadirachta indica*. *Planta Medica*, 41:34–39.

Pandey, V.N., 1993. Ancient human medicine. In: N.S. Randhawa and B.S. Parmar (Eds.), *Neem Research and Development*. SPS Publication, IARI, India, pp. 199–207.

Rahman, S.Z., Jairajpuri, M.S., 1993. Neem in Unani medicine. In: N.S. Randhawa and B.S. Parmar (Eds.), *Neem Research and Development*. SPS Publication, IARI, India, pp. 208–219.

Rao, A.R., Kumar, S., Paramsivam, T.B., Kamalakshi, S., Parashuram, A.R., Shantha, M., 1969. Study of antiviral activities of leaves of margosa tree on vaccinia and variola virus: A preliminary report. *Indian Journal of Medical Research*, 57:495–502.

Rao, D.V.K., Singh, L., Chopra, P.C., Ramanujala, G., 1986. In vitro anti-bacterial activity of neem oil. *Indian Journal of Medical Research*, 84:314–316.

Ray, A., Banerjee, B.D., Sen, P., 1996. Modulation of humoral and cell mediated immune responses by *Azardirachta indica* (neem) in mice. *Indian Journal of Experimental Biology*, 34:698–701.

Riar, S.S., 1993. Antifertility and other medical applications. In: N.S. Randhawa and B.S. Parmar (Eds.), *Neem Research and Development*. SPS Publication, IARI, India, pp. 220–226.

Satyavati, G.V., Raina, M.K., Sharma, M. (Eds.), 1976. *Medicinal Plants of India*. Vol. I. Indian Council of Medical Research, New Delhi.

Saxena, R.C. 1989. Insecticides from Neem. In: J.T. Arnason, B.J.R. Philogene, P. Morand (Eds.), *Insecticies of Plant Origin*. Symposium Series 387. American Chemical Society, Washington, DC, pp. 110–135.

Sharma, V.P., 1993. Malaria control. In: N.S. Randhawa and B.S. Parmar (Eds.), *Neem Research and Development*. SPS Publication, IARI, India, pp. 235–241.

Srivastava, P., Yadav, N., Lella, R., Schneider, A., Jones, A., Marlowe, T., Lovett, G., O'Loughlin, K., Minderman, H., Gogada, R., Chandra, D., 2012. Neem oil limonoids induces p53-independent apoptosis and autophagy. *Carcinogenesis*, 33(11):2199–2207.

Subapriya, R. and Nagini, S., 2005. Medicinal properties of neem leaves: A review. *Current Medicinal Chemistry Anticancer Agents*, 5(2):149–160.

Sudhir, P.K., Mishra, D., Ghosh, P. 2010. Biological action and medicinal properties of various constituent of Azadirachta indica. *Annals of Biological Research*, 1(3), 24–34.

Talwar, G.P., Upadhyay, S., Garg, S., Kaushic, C., Kaur, R., Dhawan, S., 1993. Induction of cell mediated immunity in genital tract. In: N.S. Randhawa and B.S. Parmar (Eds.), *Neem Research and Development*. SPS Publication, IARI, India, pp. 227–234.

Upadhyay, S.N., Dhawan, S., Garg, S., Talwar, G.P., 1992. Immunomodulatory effects of neem (*Azadirachta indica*) oil. *International Journal of Immunopharmacology*, 14:1187–1193.

Vohra, S.B., Dandiya, P.C., 1992. Herbal analgesic drugs. *Fitoterapia*, 63:195–207.

# CHAPTER 7

# Commercialization of Plant-Based Medicines in South Africa
## Case Study of Aloe ferox

David R. Katerere

## CONTENTS

## 7.1 INTRODUCTION

South Africa is a culturally and botanically diverse country (Van Wyk and Viljoen, 2011). It is a country with a long history of movement of peoples starting with the first people (Khoi and San) who were nomadic hunter-gatherers (Ives, 2014). After them came the pastoralists and cultivators during the migration of the Bantu people from East Central Africa (Vansina, 1994; Sadr, 2003). Europeans started settling in South Africa, with the Dutch being the first, in the 1650s. As their population grew, they began to move further into the hinterland (Abdi, 1999). The interactions between the newcomers and the locals led to conflict but also cross-pollination of cultures and languages leading to a Eurocentric culture and language with major African influences. The use of indigenous resources and wildcrafting of medicines by the early European settlers was unavoidable, and this contributed to the spreading of knowledge on useful plants beyond precolonial margins. Early examples of this development are evident in the spread and subsequent burgeoning trade of herbal teas such as those from *Aspalathis linearis* (commercially known as rooibos or red bush), bitter tonics such as aloe (*Aloe ferox*), buchu (*Agathosma* spp.), devil's claw (*Harpagophytum procumbens*), and *Pelargonium sidiodes* (umckaloabo) (Grahame and Robinson, 1981; Joubert et al., 2008; Moolla and Viljoen, 2008; Van Wyk, 2011).

Due to South Africa's coastal position as a commercial gateway to the world, colonial-era migrant labor practices, and its cosmopolitan population, the country has a veritable collection of medicinal plant heritage with strong influences from neighboring countries. For example, *Harpagophytum procumbens* was used ethnomedically in present-day Botswana and Namibia and became popular among the German populace in Namibia. Its "modern" use then found itself into South Africa although its geographical footprint is confined to the arid Great Karoo areas bordering Namibia and Botswana. However, devil's claw is still largely exported from Namibia (Wynberg, 2004). Umckaloabo, on the other hand, while it occurs widely in South Africa, the medicinal use of which has made it one of the biggest selling herbs of African origin in Europe, came from a healer in Lesotho (then the protectorate of Basutholand) via an Englishman who observed its use for chest complaints among the locals and then started marketing it for tuberculosis (TB) (so-called consumption) (Brendler and van Wyk, 2008).

There is thus a long history of commercializing indigenous resources in South Africa (whether from within the country's borders or from neighboring countries). This chapter discusses aloe species in general and specifically *Aloe ferox* whose modern commercial trade dates back to the arrival of Dutch settlers in the Cape in the seventeenth century.

## 7.2 ALOE—BOTANICAL DESCRIPTION AND DISTRIBUTION

Members of the *Aloe* genus are cactus-like in appearance (Shane-McWhorter, 2001). They belong to the Xanthorrhoeaceae family (previously Liliaceae/Asphodelaceae) (Shane-McWhorter, 2001; Chen et al., 2012). Members of the genus can be found in Africa (about 405 species), the Arabian Peninsula (45 species), Socotra (Oman and Yemen) (4 species), Madagascar (145 species), and the Mascarene and other Western Indian Ocean islands (7 species) (Klopper and Smith, 2010). Aloe species are mainly concentrated in the southern and eastern regions of the African continent. In the Southern African subcontinent, it is mainly found from the Eastern Cape through southern Lesotho down to the eastern part of the Western Cape in rocky Montane slopes and semi-arid terrain (Van Wyk and Viljoen, 2011). The various species are commonly known by the same name—that is, aloe (English); aalwyn (Afrikaans); hlaba, lekhala (Southern Sotho); icena (Ndebele); imboma (Zulu); and gawakawa (Shona). All of the species excluding *A. vera* (which is now largely cultivated) are listed by Convention on the International Trade in Endangered Species of Wild Fauna and Flora (CITES) in both Appendixes I and II (Klopper and Smith, 2010). The 21 species listed in Appendix I are permitted to be traded only in exceptional circumstances, while the rest of the species in Appendix II can be traded with requisite permits (Klopper and Smith, 2010).

## 7.3  HISTORY OF USE

*Aloe* species have a history of use stretching back to biblical times and are referred to as a spice and part of perfumes in the books of Proverbs and Song of Songs (Dugmore, 2013). There is evidence of their use in ancient civilizations as recorded on Egyptian temple fresco and a Sumerian clay tablet (Sung, 2006), as well as Khoisan rock art (Chen, Van Wyk et al., 2012). Aloes were used by sailors to treat skin abrasions and as sun protectants (van Jaarsveld, 1996). African slaves took aloe across the Atlantic to the Americas and West Indies from the fifteenth to the nineteenth centuries. This shows its significance to Africans at that point in time.

From an ethnobotanical perspective, all aloe species are generally used in the same way—that is, as multipurpose medicines (Mahomoodally, 2013). They have been used for treating wounds, as purgatives or laxatives in constipation and customary "detoxification" or "blood-purifying" treatments, and as a general bitter tonic (Neuwinger, 2000). They are also used as tick repellants in cattle (van Jaarsveld, 1996) and to improve digestibility and growth performance in chickens (Kamba, 2014).

## 7.4  MODERN COMMERCIAL TRADE AND USE

The global aloe trade is anticipated to grow with a compound annual growth rate (CAGR) of over 7% from US\$1.5 million in 2015 to over US\$2.3 million by 2021 (Sunderland et al., 2017). The growth will be mostly due to demand for *Aloe vera*–derived products that range from beverages to topical wound healing and cosmetic products. *Aloe vera* is largely grown in South East Asia, China, and the United States but is not as versatile as *Aloe ferox*. Unlike the other *Aloe* species (including *A. vera*) that possess small leaves, *A. ferox* is more amenable to separation and filleting because of its big leaves. *Aloe ferox* has the longest history of commercial use in South Africa, and it is used in cosmetics, food additives, hygiene products, and complementary medicines (Department of Environmental Affairs, 2014). The commercialization of *Aloe ferox* (more commonly known as Cape aloes) can be traced back to the mid-1700s when the species started being cultivated and exported by Dutch settlers in what is now Cape Town (van Jaarsveld, 1996; Mahomoodally, 2013). The settlers had come to know of its medicinal uses from the local people who tapped the bitters.

Cape aloes, a bitter crude drug prepared from the leaf exudate of *Aloe ferox*, was first exported from South Africa in 1761 and was soon listed in the British Pharmacopoea. It is the main ingredient in "Schweden bitters" used for medicinal, culinary, and beverage purposes (Sung, 2006). *A. ferox* is permitted as a direct food additive for human consumption as a natural flavoring substance by the U.S. Food and Drug Administration (FDA, 2002). The exudate and the drug prepared from Cape aloes are potent laxatives and purgatives rich in anthraquinones, of which the main compound is aloin. The aloin content determines the price of the bitters. The varieties known as the Mossel Bay Aloe contain a high aloin content (18%–25%) compared to the Eastern Cape aloe bitters (also known as Port Elizabeth or Cape aloe variety), which have aloin content under 18%. Thus, the former commands higher prices, particularly in Germany where the minimum aloin requirement is 18% (Melin, 2009; Zapata et al., 2013). As previously alluded to, *A. ferox* results in several by-products, making its potential for commercial exploitation and value addition high. The leaves consist of the outer green skin (rind), the non-bitter containing colorless and tasteless inner leaf fillet (mesophyll), and the yellow bitter sap (exudate) (Reynolds and Dweck, 1999). Each of these components has a modern application in product development, marking distinct progress from when only the bitter sap was commercially marketed. Whole-leaf products are formulated into health supplements; inner-leaf gel may be used in health supplements as fillers in juice blends, yogurts, and cosmetic products; while the bitters are used in laxative products, or increasingly in topical formulations and skin lighteners (Kleinschmidt, 2004).

Apart from the commercialization of processed products from the species, horticultural interest in *Aloe ferox* has also increased. Aloes in general are considered decorative and highly collectable (Grace, 2011). *Aloe ferox* is grown in cactus and rock gardens in tropical and subtropical climates, and is particularly popular in southern California (Christman, 2003). It forms part of living collections in public and private botanic gardens around the world in Switzerland, the United Kingdom, and the United States. While the value of horticultural trade is not available, studies estimated the value of the *Aloe ferox* industry in South Africa in 2006 at about US$90 million per annum, and this was then projected to grow beyond US$2.4 billion by 2010, driven mainly by exports to China (Shackleton and Gambiza, 2007). Whether this was achieved could not be verified, but the trade in bitters was put at R45/kg to R75/kg in 2014 (Department of Environmental Affairs, 2014) and on average 400 tonnes are produced annually. This would approximate the trade in bitters alone to be valued at R18–30 million (about US$2–3 million). The total retail trade has been more recently estimated at between R150 million per annum (US$20 million) and R675 million per annum (US$90 million) (Shackleton and Gambiza, 2007; Grace, 2011). This is because of increased diversity of *A. ferox* products traded over the years. Records show that in 1994, exports were mainly bitters (about 85%) and plant pieces (live or dried) (15%), and this has diversified to include plant pieces, powder, bitters, and derivatives (probably formulated products) in more recent years (Department of Environmental Affairs, 2014).

The *A. ferox* industry, however, goes beyond just benefiting the formal traders and exporters, and also benefits the rural harvesters where the resource grows. In 2014, harvesters and tappers could earn up to R65 (US$13)/kg for bitters. The potential for sustaining rural livelihood has peeked government's interest in setting up cooperatives for the tappers as local enterprises to create local employment and profitability. However, the success of these entities has not been well documented, and anecdotal evidence suggests that the cooperative model has not worked.

## 7.5 SCIENTIFIC RATIONALE FOR THE ETHNOMEDICAL USES OF *ALOE FEROX*

There are many studies that provide scientific rationale for the ethnobotanical use of *Aloe*. It must be noted that most studies on *Aloe* extracts have been done on *A. vera* (as opposed to *A. ferox* which only grows in Southern Africa, and *Aloe chinensis*, native to India and Vietnam and widely found in most of South East Asia). Furthermore, these studies appear to be scanty *vis-à-vis* distinguishing the effects of the three distinct parts of *Aloe*—that is, the outer green ring, the exudate (bitters), and the inner clear pulp (gel). The exudate, which originates from the inner layer of the leaf, contains several phenolics, among them anthraquinones, chromones, anthrones, flavonoids, and cinnamates (Reynolds and Dweck, 1999). But, *A. ferox* gel has been shown to possess arabinogalactans and rhamnogalacturonans (Mabusela et al., 1990), whereas glucomannans are more common in the other species, such as *A. vera*. Polypeptides and glycoproteins have been found in *A. saponaria*, *A. vera*, and *A. arborescens*.

*Aloe vera* gel extract has demonstrated a protective effect comparable to glibenclamide against hepatotoxicity in diabetic rats (Tanaka et al., 2006). There is some evidence that *Aloe* gel extracts may stimulate insulin synthesis, interfere with gluconeogenesis, and ameliorate hyperlipidemia (Bunyapraphatsara et al., 1996). It has also been shown to facilitate faster wound healing in diabetic rodents by increasing collagen formation (Reynolds and Dweck, 1999). Wound healing occurred regardless of whether the administration was oral or topical. Toxicity of aloes has been attributed to anthraquinones, which may induce hyperglycemia (Reynolds and Dweck, 1999). High doses of *Aloe* extracts may reduce central nervous system function, and chronic use has been shown to lead to anemia and sperm damage. Aloe products may also cause contact dermatitis and photo-dermatitis (Vogler and Ernst, 1999). Due to its cathartic effect, *Aloe* intake may result in hypokalemia (Shane-McWhorter, 2001).

## 7.6 CONCLUSION

*Aloe ferox* has been on the market for over 250 years during which time the main product has been the bitters. It is generally acknowledged that the aloe industry in South Africa is operating from a low base with a few producers and manufacturers, and little benefits have flowed to the communities where the resource grows (Department of Environmental Affairs, 2014). The industry has become more formalized in recent years with the inception of the Aloe Council of South Africa whose vision is to develop a globally competitive and sustainable industry through various means, including environmental protection of the natural habitat of aloes, investing in and uplifting rural tapper communities, and promoting research and development in the sector (Aloe Council, 2015). The council will have to work with government and take cognizance of the recent developments in accessing benefit-sharing legislation.

National Environmental Management Biodiversity Act 2004 (Act no. 10 of 2004) (NEMBA) tried to link biodiversity management with economic or socioeconomic benefits to the communities where the resources are exploited. Central to the act is the management and sustainable use of indigenous biological resources and the fair and equitable sharing of benefits arising from the resources. The act is supported by other regulations including the Convention on International Trade in Endangered Species of Wild Fauna and Flora (CITES); Threatened or Protected Species (TOPS); and Bioprospecting, Access and Benefit Sharing regulations (BABS) (Department of Environmental Affairs, 2014). It has, however, led to a waning in business interest in the bioresource industry, because it is seen as onerous and punitive to entrepreneurs. In addition, if the industry follows the trajectory of the global *Aloe vera* industry innovating multiple-use applications for *Aloe ferox* in food and wellness supplements, cosmetics, and pharmaceuticals (Vierhile, 2014), then the growth prospects of the Cape aloe in the future will be even brighter. From government and industry perspectives, there needs to be a concerted effort to support small and medium enterprises (SMEs) to enter the industry. Such enterprises can drive innovation. Furthermore, the documentation of the trade metrics of aloe products needs to be more closely done in order to understand its performance over time, and to make strategic evidence-based interventions.

The lessons that have been learned in the commercial trade of the Cape aloe can and should be applied in the product development and commercialization of other resources used in African indigenous knowledge to the benefit of African communities.

## ACKNOWLEDGMENTS

Dr Oluwaseyi Aboyade is thanked for reviewing and proofreading the draft chapter and her useful suggestions.

## REFERENCES

Abdi, A.A., 1999. Identity formations and deformations in South Africa—A historical and contemporary overview. *Journal of Black Studies*, 30(2):147–163.

Aloe Council, 2015. Aloe Council of South Africa. http://aloesa.co.za/about.html (accessed March 22, 2017).

Brendler, T., and van Wyk, B.E., 2008. A historical, scientific and commercial perspective on the medicinal use of *Pelargonium sidoides* (Geraniaceae). *Journal of Ethnopharmacology*, 119(3):420–433.

Bunyapraphatsara, N., Yongchaiyudha, S., Rungpitarangsi, V., Chokechaijaroenporn, O., 1996. Antidiabetic activity of aloe vera L. juice II. Clinical trial in diabetes mellitus patients in combination with glibenclamide. *Phytomedicine*, 3:245–248.

Chen, W., Van Wyk, B.E., Vermaak, I., Viljoen, A.M., 2012. Cape aloes—A review of the phytochemistry, pharmacology and commercialisation of *Aloe ferox*. *Phytochemistry Letters*, 5(1):1–12.

Christman, S., 2003. 894 *Aloe ferox. Floridata Plant Encyclopedia*. https://floridata.com/Plants/Liliaceae/Aloe%20ferox/894 (accessed November 10, 2017).

Department of Environmental Affairs, 2014. Resource assessment for *Aloe ferox* in South Africa. Republic of South Africa. https://www.environment.gov.za/sites/default/files/docs/aloeferox_report7.pdf (accessed March 22, 2017).

Dugmore, H., 2013. One of the world's greatest plants. Available at: http://heatherdugmore.co.za/one-of-the-worlds-greatest-plants/.

Food and Drug Administration (FDA), 2002. Status of certain additional over-the-counter drug category II and III active ingredients. Final rule, Federal Register 67, 31125–31127.

Grace, O.M., 2011. Current perspectives on the economic botany of the genus Aloe L. (Xanthorrhoeaceae). *South African Journal of Botany*, 77:980–987.

Grahame, R., and Robinson, B.V., 1981. Devils's claw (*Harpagophytum procumbens*): Pharmacological and clinical studies. *Annals of the Rheumatic Diseases*, 40(6):632.

Ives, S., 2014. Farming the South African "Bush": Ecologies of belonging and exclusion in rooibos tea. *American Ethnologist*, 41(4):698–713.

Joubert, E., Gelderblom, W.C.A., Louw. A., de Beer, D., 2008. South African herbal teas: *Aspalathus linearis*, *Cyclopia* spp. and *Athrixia phylicoides*—A review. *Journal of Ethnopharmacology*, 119(3):376–412.

Kamba, E.T., 2014. Effects of *Aloe ferox* in drinking water, on growth performance, blood parameters, meat quality, fatty acid profile and oxidative stability of broiler meat. MSc thesis. University of Fort Hare, South Africa.

Kleinschmidt, B., 2004. South African wild aloe juice enters international market. *Fruit Process*, 14:194–198.

Klopper, R., and Smith, G., 2010. Aloe L. Available at: https://www.plantzafrica.com/plantab/aloe.htm.

Mabusela, W.T., Stephen, A.M., Botha, M.C., 1990. Carbohydrate polymers from *Aloe ferox* leaves. *Phytochemistry*, 29:3555–3558.

Mahomoodally, M.F., 2013. Traditional medicines in Africa: An appraisal of ten potent African medicinal plants. *Evidence-Based Complementary and Alternative Medicine*, 2013:14.

Melin, A., 2009. A bitter pill to swallow: A case study of the trade & harvest of Aloe ferox in the Eastern Cape, South Africa. MSc thesis. Imperial College, London.

Moolla, A., and Viljoen, A.M., 2008. "Buchu"—*Agathosma betulina* and *Agathosma crenulata* (Rutaceae): A review. *Journal of Ethnopharmacology*, 119(3):413–419.

Neuwinger, H.D., 2000. *African Traditional Medicine. A Dictionary of Plant Use and Applications*. Medpharm Scientific Publishers, Stuttgart, Germany.

Reynolds, T., and Dweck, A.C., 1999. *Aloe vera* leaf gel: A review update. *Journal of Ethnopharmacology*, 68:3–37.

Sadr, K., 2003. The neolithic of Southern Africa. *Journal of African History*, 44:195–209.

Shackleton, C.M., and Gambiza, J., 2007. Growth of *Aloe ferox* Mill. at selected sites in the Makana region of the Eastern Cape. *South African Journal of Botany*, 73(2):266–269.

Shane-McWhorter, L., 2001. Biological complementary therapies: A focus on botanical products in diabetes. *Diabetes Spectrum*, 14(4):199.

Sunderland, T., and Ndoye, O., 2017. Indonesia, Center for International Forest Research. 2—Africa. Web references. Available at: http://www.businesswire.com/news/home/20160711005680/en/Global-Aloe-vera-Extract-Market-Worth-USD-2344.2 (Accessed on March 20, 2017).

Sung, C., 2006. History of aloe. In: Y. Park and S. Lee (Eds.), *New Perspectives on Aloe*. Springer, New York, pp. 7–17.

Tanaka, M., Misawo, E., Ito, Y., Habara, N., Nomaguchi, K. et al. 2006. Identification of five phytosterols from *Aloe vera* gel as anti-diabetic compounds. *Biological and Pharmaceutical Bulletin*, 29(7):1418–1422.

van Jaarsveld, E., 1996. The cape aloe—*Aloe ferox* and its uses. *Veld & Flora* 82(2):57.

Vansina, J., 1994. A slow revolution: Farming in subequatorial Africa. *Azania: Archaeological Research in Africa*, 29–30(1):15–26.

Van Wyk, B.E., 2011. The potential of South African plants in the development of new medicinal products. *South African Journal of Botany*, 77(4):812–829.

Van Wyk, B.-E., Viljoen, A., 2011. Special issue on economic botany. *South African Journal of Botany*, 77(4):809–811.

Vierhile, T. 2014. Aloe vera: The next superstar of the plant world. https://www.naturalproductsinsider.com/articles/2014/01/aloe-vera-the-next-superstar-of-the-plant-world.aspx (accessed February 9, 2017).

Vogler, B.K., Ernst, E., 1999. Aloe vera: A systematic review of its clinical effectiveness. *British Journal of Medical Practice*, 49:823–828.

Wynberg, R., 2004. Achieving a fair and sustainable trade in devil's claw (*Harpagophytum procumbens*). In: T. Sunderland and O. Ndoye (Eds.), *Forest Products, Livelihoods and Conservation: Case Studies of Non-Timber Forest Product Systems. Volume 2—Africa.* Centre for International Forestry Research, Indonesia, pp. 53–72.

Zapata, P.J., Navarro, D., Guillén, F., Castillo, S., Martínez-Romero, D., Valero, D., and Serrano, M., 2013. Characterisation of gels from different *Aloe* spp. as antifungal treatment: Potential crops for industrial applications. *Industrial Crops and Products*, 42(Supplement C):223–230.

# CHAPTER 8

# The Story of Niprisan
## *A Clinically Effective Phytomedicine for the Management of Sickle Cell Disorder*

**Charles Wambebe**

## CONTENTS

## 8.1 INTRODUCTION

Sickle cell disorder (SCD) is a genetic disorder that shows its clinical manifestations essentially in the Black race. Indeed about 75% of the global burden of SCD is in sub-Saharan Africa (SSA). Due to lack of early diagnosis and treatment, about 92% of patients with SCD die within the first few years of life from SCD-related complications (Grosse et al., 2011). In most SSA countries, prenatal diagnosis, antibiotic (oral penicillin) prophylaxis, and new screening programs are not institutionalized. SCD emanates from the presence of an abnormal gene leading to production of an abnormal hemoglobin of the sickle or "s" type. Although it is not known how and when the mutation occurred, it is prevalent in malaria endemic regions of the world, especially tropical Africa. The defect causes red blood cells to adopt an abnormal, rigid, sickle shape. In addition to the anemia caused by the reduction in the amount of oxygen that can be transported around the body, sickled cells can cause blockages in blood vessels, restricting blood flow to organs, culminating in SCD-related complications. Subjects with hemoglobin SS genotype (HbSS) manifest recurrent episodes of red blood cell (RBC) sickling, resulting in vaso-occlusive, thrombotic, hemolytic, and sometimes aplastic phenomena. This sequence of events is referred to as sickle cell crisis (SSC). One prominent feature of SSC is the cycle of excruciating pain that the subjects have to endure. However, painful episodes are by far the most common complications of SCD. SCD can be regarded as one of the most neglected diseases in the world. For example, most countries in SSA where about 75%, which may increase to 85% by 2050 (Piel et al., 2013), of the global burden of cases of SCD exist, have no clear policy, government structure, and funding for SCD. Yet, when the governments, relevant organizations, and religious bodies commit themselves to strong awareness campaigns, including mandatory genotype tests before marriage, SCD can be eliminated completely.

## 8.2 PREVALENCE

According to Lesi (1999), SCD is a major public health issue in SSA. For example, in Nigeria, HbSS genotype is found in 2% of live births, while AS/AC genotype carriers account for 25% of the general population (Lesi, 1999). Fleming and his colleagues (1979) as well as Fleming (1989) reported a mortality rate of 95% among children below 5 years of age diagnosed with SCD, who lived in rural areas (Garki, Nigeria). Unfortunately, there are no current reliable data on early childhood mortality among SCD subjects.

## 8.3 GAP IN THE MANAGEMENT OF SCD

Currently, bone marrow transplantation is the most viable option for the cure of SCD. However, the procedure is more successful among children below 10 years of age, while the inclusion criteria are difficult to satisfy. In addition, the procedure is very expensive and unavailable in SSA. Globally, hydroxyurea is used to treat SCD. However, it has some serious side effects (e.g., leukemia, cytopenia, hair loss, infertility, etc.), while only about 50% of those with SCD respond well to hydroxyurea. Furthermore, during treatment with hydroxyurea, close clinical laboratory monitoring is mandatory, which may not be feasible in most medical facilities in SSA.

In view of the above, there is a serious gap in the treatment of SCD in SSA. Evidently, there is no effective, safe, affordable, and accessible medicine for treating SCD in SSA. The response I adopted was to research and develop effective, safe, affordable, and accessible medicine for management of SCD from African indigenous medical knowledge (AIMK).

## 8.4 CLINICAL OBSERVATIONAL STUDY

In rural communities in Africa, traditional medicine is popular, accessible, affordable, and acceptable to the culture of the people. Subsequently, herbal medicines are routinely used to manage SCD in such communities. The most effective way to evaluate such herbal recipes is through a reverse pharmacology approach. This involves clinical observation of patients with SCD who voluntarily visit the traditional health practitioner (THP) with confirmed SCD diagnosis from a hospital. Thereafter, the patient is observed for any positive clinical and laboratory changes, comparing the baseline values to those after administration of the herbal medicine for a specified period of time. In such a situation, ethnomedical survey might not be necessary if credible evidence was provided.

## 8.5 RESEARCH AND DEVELOPMENT OF NIPRISAN

### 8.5.1 Memorandum of Understanding with Traditional Health Practitioner

Research and development of Niprisan began at the National Institute for Pharmaceutical Research and Development (NIPRD) in 1993, when preliminary information was received regarding the apparent effectiveness of a crude herbal product in the management of SCD. At that period, I was the pioneer director-general/chief executive officer of NIPRD. After receiving information regarding an herbal medicine being used by the THP (Late Rev. P.O. Ogunyale), I invited him to NIPRD. After discussion with Rev. Ogunyale, he agreed to release the recipe to me for research and development. Subsequently, a Memorandum of Understanding (MoU) was developed between NIPRD and Rev P.O. Ogunyale. Thereafter, NIPRD started the scientific evaluation of various extracts obtained from the medicinal plants used to prepare the herbal product. Niprisan was extracted and standardized from *Pterocarpus osun* stem bark, *Sorghum bicolor* leaves, *Piper guineensis* seeds, and *Eugenia caryophyllum* fruit.

### 8.5.2 *In Vitro* Effect of Niprisan

Initial scientific studies at the NIPRD laboratory demonstrated that Niprisan protected red blood cells (RBCs) obtained from patients with SCD from being sickled when such cells were exposed to low oxygen tension. The protection was about 91%, and it lasted for 48 hours (Gamaniel et al., 1998). Furthermore, Niprisan reversed already sickled RBCs in a concentration-dependent pattern. The reversal was 100% (Gamaniel et al., 1998). These preliminary data provided scientific insights into the possible beneficial effects of Niprisan in patients with SCD. Figure 8.1 shows the antisickling effect of Niprisan using blood from volunteers diagnosed with SCD. These data are indicative of the potential usefulness of Niprisan as a prophylactic agent in the management of SCD.

Analysis of the effect of Niprisan on HbS oxygen affinity indicated that it slightly shifted the oxygen-dissociation curve of HbSS to the left without any apparent change in the Hill coefficient. These results suggest that the antisickling property of Niprisan may involve direct interaction with Hb molecules. Furthermore, incubation of RBC suspensions with Niprisan did not dehydrate RBCs, cause hemolysis, increase the amount of denatured hemoglobin (Hb), or form met-Hb (Iyamu et al., 2002). It was determined that 0.05 mg/mL induced 50% inhibition of erythrocyte sickling. As for the kinetics of polymerization, addition of 0.05 microg/mL caused a sixfold prolongation of the delay time prior to deoxy-HbS polymerization when

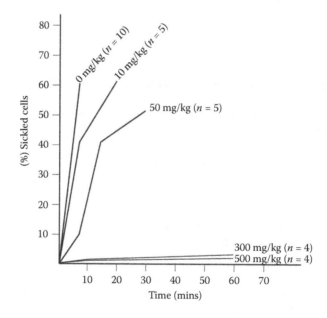

**Figure 8.1**  Concentration-dependent anti-sickling effect of Niprisan using blood from SCD volunteers. Evidently, the higher concentrations of Niprisan completely blocked sickling of Niprisan-pretreated RBCs when exposed to low oxygen tension.

compared with that of untreated HbS samples. The solubility of deoxy-HbS was significantly increased by Niprisan (Iyamu et al., 2002).

The extent of sickling of red blood cells from transgenic mice (Tg sickle mice) which carry human sickle cell genes over time when the mice were exposed to low oxygen environment. Five groups of Tg sickle mice were treated with 0 (n1/410), 10 (n1/45), 50 (n1/45), 300 (n1/44), or 500 (n1/45) mg/kg/day Nix-0699 for 7 days. Thereafter, the mice were exposed to hypoxia for 60 minutes. During hypoxic exposure, aliquots of blood were collected from the tail vein under venous oxygen pressure, and the cells were fixed in 2% glutaraldehyde solution without exposure to air. The percentage of sickled cells was determined by the computer-assisted image analysis system.

### 8.5.3 Chemistry

Bio-guided fractionation of the Niprisan was undertaken. The most bioactive fraction was subjected to nuclear magnetic resonance-mass spectrometry (NMR-MS) leading to the isolation and characterization of vanillin and 5-hydroxyl furfural as the bioactive compounds in the extract.

Subsequently, the total standardized extract and the bioactive compounds were subjected to safety assessment. The extract manifested a better safety profile than the bioactive compounds (either singly or when they were combined). Furthermore, efficacy studies were done. Interestingly, the extract was more effective as an anti-sickling agent than the bioactive compounds (either singly or when they were combined). Apparently, synergy between the components of the extract might have contributed to the efficacy and safety profiles, which were superior to the isolated pure compounds. Furthermore, some components of the extract might be precursors that became active after they were converted to bioactive agents *in vivo*. In view of these results, the standardized ethanol/water extract was used for the clinical trials after formulation into capsule dosage form.

### 8.5.4 *In Vivo* Effect of Niprisan

Figure 8.2 shows that Niprisan improved oxygenation of animals and protected them from death in a dose-dependent manner when they were exposed to low oxygen tension. Figure 8.3 illustrates the protection of the lungs of Niprisan-treated mice compared to the control mice, which had a lot of sickled cells in the alveolar capillary walls. Since patients with SCD can die from acute chest syndrome without warning, it is significant that Niprisan prevents such sudden deaths in animals, thereby providing a scientific basis for the use of Niprisan as a prophylactic medicine in the management of SCD.

Kaplan-Meier survival curves during 60 minutes of hypoxic exposure of transgenic sickle mice showed that niprisan prolonged the lives of the mice dose-dependently. Five groups of Tg sickle mice were treated with 0 (group 1, n1/4 10), 10 (group 2, n1/4 5), 50 (group 3, n1/45), 300 (group 4, n1/44), or 500 (group 5, n1/45) mg/kg/day of Nix-0699 for 7 days. Thereafter, the mice were exposed to hypoxia for 60 minutes, and the survival time of these mice was then determined.

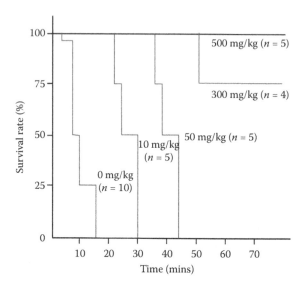

**Figure 8.2** Dose-dependent protection of transgenic mice from death when exposed to low oxygen environment.

The survival time of the drug-treated groups was significantly longer than that of the Tg sickle control mice: group 5 ($P < 0\text{\AE}0001$), group 4 ($P < 0\text{\AE}0001$), group 3 ($P < 0\text{\AE}001$), and group 2 ($P < 0\text{\AE}01$) (Iyamu et al., 2003).

Histopathological analysis of the lungs of control and Nix-0699-treated Tg sickle mice was undertaken. Control and Nix-0699-treated Tg sickle mice were exposed to hypoxia (Figure 8.3). After death, or after the full experimental period of 60 minutes, the mice were sacrificed, and the organs were immediately collected. The alveolar capillary walls of control mice (a) were heavily engorged with sickled cells, resulting in greatly reduced alveolar space. In contrast, the lungs of Tg sickle mice that had

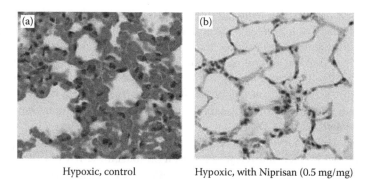

Hypoxic, control                   Hypoxic, with Niprisan (0.5 mg/mg)

**Figure 8.3** Effect of Niprisan on trapping of sickle cells in mouse lung. (Adapted from Iyamu, E.W. et al., 2003. *British Journal of Haematology*, 122(6):1001–1008.)

been pretreated with 500 mg/kg Nix-0699 (b) were remarkably normal compared with the control (alveolar surface area; $P < 0\text{Æ}001$) (hematoxylin and eosin, original magnification 100).

Evidently, the data from both *in vivo* tests in laboratory animals and *in vitro* tests using blood from patients with SCD showed that Niprisan is effective against the sickle cell phenomenon and is devoid of adverse side effects.

### 8.5.5 Safety Assessment of Niprisan

The $LD_{50}$ values in mice and rats were 900 mg/kg (i.p.) and 5 g/kg (per oral), respectively. Furthermore, the subchronic studies indicated that the main tissues and organs were devoid of any defect. Toxicological data including carcinogenicity and mutagenicity assessments indicated that Niprisan was devoid of these adverse effects (Awodogan et al., 1996).

Furthermore, the highest dose used in the animal studies that failed to elicit toxic symptoms is about 500 times higher than the effective clinical dose. This wide gap between the clinically effective dose and the toxic dose (high therapeutic index) provides a strong ethical basis to evaluate Niprisan in human volunteers without compromising on the safety and well-being of the trial participants. Although most herbal recipes are relatively safe due to their long history of clinical use without reported adverse effects, safety evaluation is mandatory. The reasons include the fact that in traditional medicine there is no systematic way of reporting adverse effects of herbal recipes administered to patients. Second, usually, different recipes are prepared for a particular disease because of the holistic nature of traditional medicine practice. Thus, even if an adverse effect is observed, it is difficult to ascribe it to a particular recipe in a typical traditional medicine practice. However, in a research setting, it can be undertaken through evaluation of individual recipes. Other complications include dosage, stability, storage, and hygiene. In traditional medicine practice, dosage cannot be ascertained from batch to batch since quality assurance is not usually instituted. Thus, in my opinion, it is important to undertake a safety evaluation of herbal recipes while developing them as standardized phytomedicines.

### 8.5.6 Standardization of Niprisan

In order to enhance consistency in the quality of Niprisan using different batches of plant samples, a quality assurance system was established. This is particularly relevant while conducting clinical trials with traditional herbal medicines, because there are various factors that can impact on the quality of the product and consequently on the quality of the data and health of the trial subjects. Examples of such factors include method and timing of plant collection, location of plants, harvesting and postharvesting processing, product preparation procedures, storage, natural additives, preservatives, and packaging. Thus, a planned method for standardizing the raw materials, the finished products, and the processes involved right from collection of the raw materials to the manufacturing of the product were articulated and adhered to. A realistic monitoring system was also developed and implemented.

Extensive pharmacological studies were also carried out on various preparations as well as whole animal studies. Based on the favorable outcomes of the safety pharmacology and *in vitro* efficacy tests, Niprisan was evaluated clinically.

## 8.6 CLINICAL TRIAL PHASE I

In view of the robust preclinical data as indicated above, clinical trial phase I was undertaken using Niprisan (500 mg and 250 mg per capsule for adult and children, respectively). The clinical trial phase I was conducted using 20 NIPRD staff who had AA genotype. The purpose of the study was to assess the safety of Niprisan in healthy volunteers. The trial was conducted between March and July 1994. The outcome of the study indicated that the volunteers did not experience any adverse effect.

## 8.7 CLINICAL TRIAL PHASE IIA

Subsequently, clinical trial phase IIA commenced in August 1994 and ended on February 28, 1997. Initially, the staff of NIPRD visited the patients in their homes fortnightly to make vital observations regarding the patients' responses to the new phytomedicine. The subjects experienced improved appetite with appreciable weight gain, significant reduction in hospital admission, while attendance at school profoundly increased. Furthermore, there was no evidence of kidney/liver damage. Due to the encouraging results obtained, the visits were later reduced to once per month. After one and a half years, the clinics were held once every 2 months. The clinical status of the patients was assessed by the medical doctors at the NIPRD clinic during the visits. Laboratory tests were carried out to evaluate the functional status of the liver and the kidney as well as hematological parameters. The data indicated that Niprisan had no detectable adverse effects on the kidney and liver. The values recorded for the parameters monitored were within normal ranges. The pilot study indicated that all the patients benefited from the phytomedicine. There was a lower incidence of anemia and jaundice, probably due to a reduced rate of destruction of the RBCs. Some patients who were hospitalized due to bacterial infection or malaria surprisingly did not experience crisis. Prior to the Niprisan trial, such patients used to experience SCD-related crises during malaria or bacterial infections. Furthermore, there was significant reduction in the frequency and severity of painful crises in about 80% of the volunteers. In addition, the remaining 20% of the volunteers experienced less frequent and less severe crises.

In view of the significance of the data and the public health implications, the pilot clinical trial was repeated at another hospital. The selected study site was Army Base Hospital, Yaba, Lagos. The study in Lagos involved consultant pediatricians, hematologists, and internists. The selection criteria were the same as those used for the site at NIPRD, Abuja. The results were generally similar to those obtained at

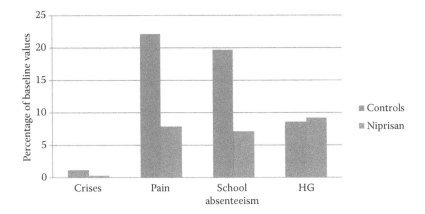

**Figure 8.4** Major clinical outcomes of Niprisan in SCD subjects (Phase II Randomized Placebo-Controlled Clinical Trial).

Abuja. Furthermore, about 73% of the subjects did not experience any crisis during the study period (1 year), while about 63% gained appreciable weight.

The pilot clinical data from Lagos Center confirmed the data at NIPRD, Abuja. Consequently, a phase IIB study was undertaken. The gold standard is a double-blind, placebo-controlled, randomized clinical trial. The study design went beyond the gold standard. Due to the fact that SCD manifestations are unpredictable and vary from patient to patient, a crossover design was used so that each patient served as his or her own control. Furthermore, a health diary was introduced for each patient, and nurses were engaged as monitors to visit each patient every week throughout the duration of the study. A 3-month pretrial period enabled us to identify those who could complete the health diaries correctly and daily. The major outcomes of the clinical trial phase IIB (pivot study) are shown in Figure 8.4.

## 8.8 CLINICAL TRIAL PHASE IIB

The protocol for clinical trial phase IIB was developed by me. The objective of the study was to assess the tolerability and efficacy of Niprisan in patients with SCD. Thereafter, ethical approval was secured while regulatory clearance was obtained. The study site was NIPRD clinic, Abuja, Nigeria. The protocol, among others, included the efficacy criteria, quality assurance systems, and selection criteria. In view of the wide variability of SCD crises, only subjects with at least three episodes of painful or vaso-occlusive crises per year were accepted into the study. The volunteers accepted into the study based on the selection criteria were then randomized to group A or group B. As per the protocol, group A took Niprisan for 6 months before crossing over to placebo for another 6 months. A 1-month washout period was allowed before commencing the administration of the placebo. Group B took placebo for 6 months and then crossed over to Niprisan for 6 months. Efficacy and safety criteria were defined in the clinical protocol. At the beginning of the phase IIB clinical study, 100 patients with SCD satisfied the selection criteria and were registered to undertake the study. However, 84 SCD volunteers completed the study. Some of them were dropped from the study due to noncompliance from the provisions of the study, while others relocated from the study site (Abuja). Based on the protocol for the trial, the main outcome measures were the incidence of crises; the occurrence of painful episodes; certain clinical, hematological, and biochemical measures; patients' daily self-assessment of health; hospitalization; blood transfusion; and absenteeism from school. The criteria used in the evaluation of the clinical effects of the product included changes in

1. Frequency of crisis
2. Severity of crisis
3. Anemia
4. Frequency and duration of hospitalization

The analysis of health diaries showed that severe pains were reported 7.9 and 21 times, respectively, for 6 months on Niprisan and placebo ($P$ <0.01, Wilcoxon Signed Rank test). Furthermore, Niprisan reduced the frequency of crisis from 0.195 to 0.045 per patient per month. Absenteeism reduced from 19.6 (placebo) to 7.1 (Niprisan) in 6 months. Frequency of hospital admission reduced from 0.22 (placebo) to 0.15 (Niprisan) per month (Figure 8.4). In addition, there were no changes in nutritional and metabolic analytes—total protein, albumin, total calcium, fasting total cholesterol, fasting triglyceride, fasting blood glucose, and uric acid. Similarly, AST and ALT levels remained normal indicating no acute liver toxicity. Alkaline phosphatase and gamma glutamyl transpeptidase (GGT) were unchanged indicating that there was no cholestatic and chronic toxicity. Interestingly, creatinine and blood urea nitrogen (BUN) levels remained the same as found in the placebo group, suggesting that there was no kidney toxicity. The data of this study have been published (Wambebe et al., 2001a,b). The major clinical outcomes of the study are depicted in Figure 8.4. The summary of this study as well as previous pilot clinical trials is that Niprisan is safe and efficacious for the management of SCD.

The results of the study indicated that one oral dose of 12 mg/kg Niprisan daily significantly reduced the frequency of sickle cell crises, bone pain, and hospital admission ($P$ <0.05). The mean number of crises per person per month was 0.05 in patients who received Niprisan initially, compared with 0.11 per person per month after the crossover to placebo. Patients generally rated their health as better and reported less sickness and school absenteeism with Niprisan than with placebo. Furthermore, no adverse effect was reported. The results of the phase IIB clinical trial undertaken at the NIPRD clinic, Abuja, were similar to earlier phase IIA studies done at the NIPRD clinic and Army base hospital. For example, about 80% of the study participants did not experience any crisis during the 12 months of trial compared to three major crises experienced by them per year prior to enrollment in the study. Even the remaining participants (about 20%) experienced less frequent and mild episodes of crises. The data from the three clinical trials showed that Niprisan was efficacious in the prophylactic management of patients with SCD (Wambebe et al., 2001a,b).

## 8.9  MULTIPURPOSE EXTRACTION AND MANUFACTURING FACILITIES

Subsequently, through a grant from the UN Development Programme (UNDP), with technical partnership of the UN Industrial Development Organization (UNIDO), a multipurpose pilot-scale extraction facility was established at NIPRD. In addition, NIPCO Pharmaceutical Industry was established to manufacture essential medicines as well as new medicines developed by NIPRD. NIPCO was inspected and approved by the Pharmacists Council of Nigeria (site). Furthermore, NIPCO was inspected by the National Agency for Food and Drug Administration and Control (NAFDAC) and approved for Good Manufacturing Practice (GMP) production of essential medicines in accordance with cGMP requirements.

## 8.10  TRANSFER OF TECHNOLOGY AND LAUNCHING OF NIPRISAN

In order to market Niprisan globally, it was decided to grant the license for commercial production and global marketing to a reputable international company. Subsequently, Xechem International Inc. (United States) applied for the license. The negotiations on granting the company the exclusive license for the production and global marketing of Niprisan involved the NIPRD, the Federal Ministry of Health, and Xechem International Inc. (XECHEM). Eventually, the decision was made to grant Xechem the exclusive license for commercial production and global marketing of Niprisan. Based on the license, Xechem established the manufacturing facility at Abuja, Nigeria, for the commercial production of Niprisan for the global market. A ceremony to mark this remarkable event, the first of its kind in Africa involving the transfer of medicine fully developed in Africa, by African scientists, to the Western world, took place on July 18, 2002. President of the Federal Republic of Nigeria Olusegun Obasanjo personally launched Niprisan after it had been registered by NAFDAC. The uniqueness of the Niprisan case is that the project was initiated and executed by African scientists working in Africa at a time when international provisions for benefit sharing regarding commercial products derived from indigenous medical knowledge were unavailable (Wambebe, 2006). Due to internal conflicts within Xechem Inc., the license was withdrawn. The new licensee is May & Baker.

## 8.11  PATENTING OF NIPRISAN

Through a grant from the UNDP, Niprisan was patented in 46 countries in 1998. In 2006, Niprisan was registered by the National Drug Regulatory Agency of Nigeria and the NAFDAC as a nonprescription prophylactic medicine for the management of SCD. Furthermore, Niprisan was accorded orphan drug status by the U.S. Food and Drug Administration (FDA) in 2003. Furthermore, in 2004, the European Medicine Evaluation Agency accorded Niprisan orphan drug status.

## 8.12 CONCLUSION

It is important to highlight issues related to the research and development of new medicines from African medicinal plants based on AIMK. Partnership with genuine THPs who were accorded proper recognition and were involved in the research and development process was a key factor in the success story of Niprisan. The development of a MoU on fair and equitable benefit sharing was crucial for full disclosure of the contents of herbal recipes by the THP. Cooperation of the national drug regulatory authority facilitated the process. The motivation of technical and research personnel with requisite skills and knowledge was a key factor. The establishment of a quality assurance system ensured product consistency from batch to batch. Sourcing of adequate funds from national government, bilateral arrangements, and UN agencies that were judiciously utilized to acquire relevant equipment was the most crucial factor.

Furthermore, the success story of Niprisan can be linked to crucial commercial milestones. For example, the provision of adequate funds enabled the establishment of standard laboratory facilities and clinic. The robust preclinical data provided convincing results on the safety and efficacy profiles of Niprisan. The availability of a pilot plant facility enabled the validation of concepts and assessment of challenges associated with scaling up processes. The patenting of Niprisan in the United States and other countries was a critical factor in the commercialization of Niprisan. The convincing clinical outcomes from the randomized placebo-controlled clinical trial were a major factor. Indeed, the clinical trial went beyond the gold standard by including health diaries. Being accorded orphan drug status by the U.S. FDA and European Medicine Evaluation Agency was indicative of crucial recognition of the research data. Indeed, it was a great motivation for the commercialization of Niprisan, especially since it is the first phytomedicine to be granted orphan drug status by the U.S. FDA. A champion with a vision, tenacity, and commitment to achieving set goals in spite of tangible obstacles was a crucial advantage.

The establishment of a drug manufacturing facility at Abuja by XECHEM created jobs for Nigerians, built capacity, generated wealth for the economy, and promoted the development of other herbal medicines based on indigenous medical knowledge. To my knowledge, Niprisan is the best medicine for the prophylactic management of SCD *vis-à-vis* safety and efficacy assessments. Obviously, there are many other potential therapeutic agents hidden in African biodiversity and AIMK. The success story of Niprisan should motivate scientists, industry, and governments to invest in the research and development of new medicines from African biodiversity. The reverse pharmacology approach utilized in the development of Niprisan is obviously a good model that can facilitate a high success rate of developing new medicines based on AIMK and also shorten the research and development period and significantly reduce the cost of drug development.

## ACKNOWLEDGMENTS

The author acknowledges the UNDP and the governments of Nigeria and Japan for generous funding for R&D studies and WIPO for guidance on IPR and licensing issues. The late Rev P.O. Ogunyale is thanked for entrusting me with the original recipe for Niprisan.

## REFERENCES

Awodogan, A., Wambebe, C., Gamaniel, K., Okogun, J.I., Orisadipe, A., Akah, P.A., 1996. Acute and short term toxicity of NIPRISAN in rats. I: Biochemical study. *Journal of Pharmaceutical Research and Development*, 1:39–45.

Fleming, A.F., 1989. The presentation, management and prevention of crisis in sickle cell disease in Africa. *Blood Review*, 3:18–28.

Fleming, A.F., Storey, J., Molineaux, L., Iroko, E.A., Attai, E.D., 1979. Abnormal haemoglobins in the Sudan savanna of Nigeria. I. Prevalence of haemoglobins and relationships between sickle cell trait, malaria and survival. *Annals of Tropical Medicine and Parasitology*, 73:161–172.

Gamaniel, K., Amos, S., Akah, P.A., Samuel, B.B., Kapu, S., Olusola, A., Abayomi, O., Okogun, J.I., Wambebe, C., 1998. Pharmacological profile of NIPRD 94/002/1–0: A novel herbal antisickling agent. *Journal of Pharmaceutical Research and Development*, 3:89–94.

Grosse, S.D., Odame, I., Atrash, H.K., Amendah, D.D., Piel, F.B., Williams, T.N., 2011. Sickle cell disease in Africa: A neglected cause of early childhood mortality. *American Journal of Preventive Medicine*, 41(6):398–405.

Iyamu, E.W., Turner, E.A., Asakura, T., 2002. *In vitro* effects of NIPRISAN (Nix-0699): A naturally occurring, potent antisickling agent. *British Journal of Haematology*, 118(1):337–343.

Iyamu, E.W., Turner, E.A., Asakura, T., 2003. Niprisan (Nix-0699) improves the survival rates of transgenic sickle cell mice under acute severe hypoxic conditions. *British Journal of Haematology*, 122(6):1001–1008.

Lesi, F.E.A., 1999. *Sickle Cell Disorder: A Handbook for Patients, Parents, Counselors, and Primary Healthcare Practitioners*. Macmillan, Nigeria, pp. 1–10.

Piel, F.B., Hay, S.I., Gupta, S., Weatherall, D.J., Williams, T.N., 2013. Global burden of sickle cell anaemia in children under five, 2010–2050: Modeling based on demographics, excess mortality, and interventions. *PLOS/Medicine*, July 16. https://doi.org/10.1371/journal.pmed.1001484 (Accessed July 16, 2017).

Wambebe, C., 2006. Guest editorial. *Innovation and Discovery*, 18(1):1–4.

Wambebe, C., Bamgboye, E.A., Badru, B.O., Khamofu, H., Njoku, S.O. et al. 2001a. Efficacy of NIRISANR in the prophylactic management of patients with sickle cell disease. *Current Therapeutic Research*, 62(1):26–34.

Wambebe, C., Khamofu, H., Momoh, J.A., Ekpeyong, M., Audu, B.S. et al., 2001b. Double-blind, placebo-controlled, randomized cross-over clinical trial of NIPRISAN in patients with sickle cell disorder. *Phytomedicine*, 8(4):252–261.

# CHAPTER 9

# Moringa
## The Miracle Plant

Charles Wambebe

## CONTENTS

## 9.1 INTRODUCTION

*Moringa* (Family: Moringaceae) has 13 species that grow in tropical and sub-tropical climates found originally in Africa, India, Arabia, South America, Southeast Asia, the Pacific and Caribbean Islands (Iqbal and Bhanger, 2006).

Examples of *Moringa* species that are native to Africa include:

*M. arborea* Verdc (Kenya).

*M. borziana* Mattei, *M. pygmaea* Verdc, *M. stenopetala* (Somalia).

*M. drouhardii* Jum and *M.hildebrandtii* Engl. (Madagascar).

*M. longituba* Engl., *M. ruspoliana* Engl. (Ethiopia).

*M.stenopetala, M.rivae* Chiov (Kenya and Ethiopia).

*M. ovalifolia* Dinter & Berger (Namibia and Angola).

*M. peregrine* Forssk (Horn of Africa and Egypt).

*M. concanensis* and *M. oleifera* are indigenous to India. Thus, out of the 13 species of Moringa, 11 are indigenous to Africa.

The most widely cultivated *Moringa* species globally is *M. oleifera* (drumstick/horseradish tree), which is indigenous to Himalayas, India. It grows easily even in drought regions (best under warm and dry conditions). The seeds can be sown (e.g., in Sudan) while vegetative propagation is common in India, Indonesia, and in some areas of West Africa.

In Nigeria and other countries, young seed pods and leaves are consumed as vegetables. In Ghana, the leaves are widely used for water purification. Generally, *Moringa oleifera* can be cultivated for its leaves, pods, and/or its kernels for oil extraction and water purification. Ancient Egyptians used *Moringa oleifera* oil for its cosmetic value and skin preparation (Coppin et al., 2013). In different parts of Africa, the leaves, seeds, flowers, pods (fruit), bark, and roots are eaten as a vegetable, and each part is uniquely harvested and utilized. For example, fresh leaves are picked, shade dried, ground to a powder, and then stored and used later as a food flavoring or additive. Dried or fresh leaves are also used in foods such as soups and porridges among the Fulani herdsman in Northern Nigeria (Lockett et al., 2000). Farmers added the leaves to animal feed to attain a healthy livestock (Sánchez et al., 2006), while utilizing the manure and vegetable compost for crop growth (Fahey, 2005). According to Fuglie (1999), the many uses for *Moringa* include alley cropping (biomass production), animal forage (leaves and treated seed-cake), biogas (from leaves), domestic cleaning agent (crushed leaves), blue dye (wood), fencing (living trees), fertilizer (seed-cake), foliar nutrient (juice expressed from the leaves), green manure (from leaves), gum (from tree trunks), honey and sugar cane juice-clarifier (powdered seeds), honey (flower nectar), medicine (all plant parts), ornamental plantings, biopesticide (soil incorporation of leaves to prevent seedling damping off), pulp (wood), rope (bark), tannin for tanning hides (bark and gum), and water purification (powdered seeds). *Moringa* seed oil (yield 30%–40% by weight), also known as Ben oil, is a sweet nonsticking, nondrying oil that resists rancidity. It has been used in salads, for fine machine lubrication, and in the manufacture of perfume and hair care products (Tsaknis et al., 1999). In addition, Foidl et al. (2001) elaborated on the potential of *Moringa oleifera* for agricultural and industrial purposes.

Furthermore, Dongmeza et al. (2006) reported that *Moringa* powder can be added to fish ponds to enhance the protein content in fish meal, while the leaves are used as supplements for feeding cows. Lockett et al. (2000) reported that pregnant women and lactating mothers used the powdered leaves to enhance their children's nourishment.

This chapter looks briefly at *Moringa stenopetala*, which is indigenous to Ethiopia and Kenya and second to *Moringa oleifera vis-à-vis* economic significance. Some of the uses of *Moringa oleifera* in Africa will be highlighted using a few country cases. Thereafter, the chapter reviews the various uses and pharmacological effects responsible for them. Some of the bioactive components of *Moringa oleifera* are also presented.

## 9.2 *MORINGA STENOPETALA*: ETHIOPIA AND KENYA

*Moringa stenopetala* (Family: Moringaceae; Genus, Moringa) is known in Ethiopia as Shferaw (Amharinya), Aleko, Aluko, Halaco, Halako (Gamonya), Kallanki (Benninya), Telahu (Tsemay), Haleko, Shelchada (Konsonya), Wuame, and Mawe (Somalinya). It is the most economically important species after *M. oleifera*.

### 9.2.1 Ethnomedical Uses

*Moringa stenopetala* is indigenous to the southern parts of Ethiopia and Kenya (Figures 9.3). Traditionally, *Moringa stenopetala* leaves are usually boiled and the water is taken for the treatment of malaria, hypertension, asthma, diabetes, stomach pain, etc. (Musa et al., 2016). The leaves of *Moringa stenopetala* are used in ethno-medicine for treatment of malaria, hypertension, asthma, diabetes, stomach pain, kidney infection, fertility disorders, asthma, cancer, worm infestation, milk production in lactating mothers, etc. It also has antioxidant effects. Furthermore, *Moringa stenopetala* contains both primary metabolites (e.g., carbohydrates, proteins, fats, vitamins, and minerals) and secondary metabolites (e.g., alkaloids, flavonoids, glycosides, polyphenols, saponins, sugars, steroids, etc.).

### 9.2.2 Nutritional Significance of *Moringa stenopetala*

According to Endeshaw (personal communication as reported by Seifu, 2014), *Moringa stenopetala* is a favorite and main component of the daily meal of the

Konso, Gamo, and Gofa people in southern Ethiopia. Indeed, *Moringa* leaves are consumed almost every day like spinach together with cereal balls by the inhabitants of the Konso area (Steinmüller et al., 2002). Furthermore, it was reported by Endeshaw (2003) that about 50% of the people in the Konso district of southern Ethiopia obtain their food from *Moringa stenopetala*. Similarly, the inhabitants of Gamo and Gofa areas have an established tradition of eating the leaves of *Moringa stenopetala* (locally called Haleko). In the lowland and middle altitudes of the Konso district, most homesteads have a *Moringa stenopetala* tree. The leaves are cooked and eaten as vegetables. Interestingly, *Moringa stenopetala* persist throughout the year, including in the dry season when most of the other green vegetables are no longer available.

### 9.2.3 Proximate Composition of Fresh Leaves of *Moringa stenopetala*

According to Abuye et al. (2003), *Moringa stenopetala* is the richest source of ß-carotene (vitamin A) among other leafy green vegetables. In 2005, Mathur reported the presence of micronutrients in the leaves of *Moringa stenopetala* (e.g., K, Fe, Zn, P, etc.). Furthermore, the average values of iron and calcium were 3.08 mg/100 g and 792.8 mg/100 g, respectively (Abuye et al., 2003). It is believed that the appropriate use of the leaves of *Moringa stenopetala* can reduce child and maternal mortality rates in Ethiopia by 30%–50% (Anon, 2003).

Furthermore, in 2005, Mathur reported that *Moringa stenopetala* leaves contain seven times the vitamin C of oranges, four times the vitamin A of carrots, four times the calcium of milk, three times the potassium of bananas, and two times the protein of yogurt. In addition, *Moringa stenopetala* leaves contain all the essential amino acids (Mathur, 2005). Raw leaves of *M. stenopetala* contain 9% crude protein on a dry matter basis (Abuye et al., 2003) and a higher percentage of carbohydrates, crude fiber, and calcium compared to kale and Swiss chard (Abuye et al., 2003). Vitamins are present at nutritionally significant levels with mean values of 28 mg/100 g of vitamin C and 160 µg/100 g of ß-carotene. However, significant differences were observed in the proximate composition, mineral, and vitamin contents of the leaves of *M. stenopetala* reported by different authors due to different ecotypes and varieties of the plant used for the studies. In 2005, Beyene reported the findings of his study, which assessed the genetic diversity of 19 *Moringa stenopetala* accessions collected from southern Ethiopia. The study revealed the existence of genetic variability within and between populations. Evidently, further studies are indicated using the various ecotypes and varieties of *Moringa stenopetala vis-à-vis* phytochemistry, pharmacology, macronutrients, and micronutrients.

### 9.2.4 Phytochemistry of the Leaves of *Moringa stenopetala*

In 2010, Amsalu used the crude aqueous leaf extracts of *Moringa stenopetala* and reported the presence of alkaloids, saponins, polyphenols, flavonoids, coumarins, terpenoids, anthraquinones, tannins, phytosterols, and cardiac glycosides, and the presence of all the secondary metabolites except saponins in 70% alcohol fractions.

Sileshi et al. (2014) used another solvent system (butanol fractions of solvent-solvent separate and column chromatographic fractions) of *Moringa stenopetala* leaves. They observed the presence of flavonoids, phenolic compounds, and phenolic glycosides (Sileshi et al., 2014).

## 9.2.5 Toxicity Profile of the Leaves of *Moringa stenopetala*

The acute toxic effect of n-butanol fraction of the leaves of *Moringa stenopetala* in experimental mice was evaluated (Musa et al., 2015). The results of their study indicated that no differences were seen in behavior, gross pathology, and body weights of the experimental mice treated with up to 5000 mg/kg doses of the fraction compared to the control group. Furthermore, Ghebreselassie et al. (2011) evaluated the effects of aqueous leaf extract of *Moringa stenopetala* on blood parameters, and the histopathology of liver and kidney in experimental mice. These workers carried out a subchronic toxicity study. They reported that there were no significant changes in the weight and histopathology of liver and kidney detected in the animals treated with aqueous extract of the plant in comparison with the controls. Recently, Geleta et al. (2016a,b) studied the acute toxic effect of the n-butanol fraction of the leaves of *Moringa stenopetala* in mice. Their results indicated that the n-butanol fraction of the leaves of *Moringa stenopetala* did not cause any mortality up to 5000 mg/kg per oral doses of the fraction. Similarly, no body weight reduction, visible signs of toxicity, and gross pathological alteration (color, size, and texture) were observed. Furthermore, the study results showed that the fraction did not produce adverse effects on hematological and biochemical parameters of the blood.

Evidently, clinical studies are needed using standardized extract of the leaves of *Moringa stenopetala* to ascertain its safety in humans.

## 9.2.6 Pharmacological Effects of Extracts of the Leaves of *Moringa stenopetala*

In 2012, Mengistu et al. as well as Mekonnen and Gessesse (1998) reported the antimalarial, antileishmenial, antifertility, antihyperlipidemic, and hypotensive effects of the extracts of *Morinda stenopetala* leaves in rats. They used aqueous crude extract and 70% ethanol fraction and reported significant prevention of blood pressure increments in a dose-dependent manner. Furthermore, the extracts suppressed increments in cholesterol, glucose, and triglycerides levels in the blood. The antihypertensive and vasodilatory effects of extracts of *Moringa stenopetala* leaves were reported by Geleta et al. (2016a,b), Furthermore, the hypoglycemic (Musa et al., 2016) and antidiabetic effects (Mussa et al., 2008; Toma et al., 2015) of extracts of *Moringa stenopetala* leaves have been reported. Geleta et al. (2015a) evaluated the diuretic activity of a hydro-ethanol extract of *Moringa stenopetala* leaves in Swiss albino mice. The hydro-ethanol extract of the plant showed significant urine output at all doses and significantly increased the excretion of $Na^+$ and $Cl^-$ at higher doses (Geleta et al., 2015a). These pharmacological effects might be attributed to the presence of different phytochemical constituents found in the plant extract, especially glycosides and alkaloids (Geleta et al., 2016a,b).

Furthermore, extracts of the leaves of *Moringa stenopetala* manifested hypoglycemic, antihyperglycemic, and anti hyperlipidemic effects with a wide therapeutic index (Mekonnen, 2016). The antihyperglycemic and antihyperlipidemic effects might be related to the inhibition of intestinal and pancreatic enzymes by extracts of *M. stenopetala*.

## 9.3 NONMEDICAL USES OF *MORINGA OLEIFERA*

The edible oil is contained in the seeds, which can be used as a cooking oil for frying and as an oil for salad dressing. The fatty acid compositions of solvent and enzyme-extracted oil from *Moringa oleifera* seeds showed 67.9% oleic acid in the solvent extract and 70% in the enzyme extracts. According to Abdulkarim et al. (2005), *Moringa* oil contains palmitic (7.8% and 6.8%), stearic (7.6% and 6.5%), and behenic (6.2% and 5.8%) acids for the solvent and enzyme-extracted oils. The monounsaturated-to-saturated fatty acid ratio in *Moringa* seed oil is high. Consequently, it could be considered a good substitute for highly monounsaturated oils such as olive oil (Tsaknis et al., 2002).

Due to its content of zeatin, *Moringa* leaves are used as natural plant growth enhancer (Figure 9.4). Thus, leaf extracts stimulate plant growth, thereby increasing crop yield (Ashfaq et al., 2012).

According to Teixeira et al. (2014), *Moringa* seed powder can be used for water purification, replacing dangerous and expensive chemicals such as aluminum sulfate.

Furthermore, Ashfaq et al. (2012) reported that the extracts of seeds and leaves demonstrated activity against larvae and adults of *Trigoderma granarium* and can reduce the incidence of fungi on groundnut seeds.

*Moringa* seeds are used as biomass for the production of biodiesel. It is anticipated that biodiesel will replace petrodiesel. Some of the advantages of biodiesel over petrodiesel include lack of sulfur and lower emission of monoxides and hydrocarbons. Furthermore, biodiesel is renewable, and it is significantly resistant to oxidative degradation (Rashid et al., 2008). In addition, *Moringa* seeds have 30%–40% content of high-quality fatty acid composition. In fact, about 70% of the oil in *Moringa* seeds is oleic acid. Undoubtedly, *Moringa* seeds present an ideal source for production of biodiesel.

## 9.4 USES OF *MORINGA OLEIFERA* IN AFRICA: COUNTRY CASES

### 9.4.1 Nigeria

In a survey conducted by Stevens et al. (2013), in Nigeria, 78.7% of the respondents used *Moringa* for the treatment of typhoid and malaria. The leaves were the most commonly used (about 83%). However, the stem (12%) and roots (5%) are also used to treat typhoid. The survey revealed that 75.4% and 66.9% essentially use extracts of the leaves to treat ear and eye infections, respectively.

The majority (98.9%) of the respondents indicated that they had used or seen people use *Moringa* for food and medicinal purposes. Specifically, the leaves were used as a vegetable in preparing soup, as salad, and for making tea. Medicinal uses of the leaves included the curing of fever (78.7%) and the treatment of ear infections (71.8%), diabetes mellitus (65.2%), and blood pressure (64.7%).

In addition, *Moringa oleifera* leaves are used to treat toothache, catarrh, common cold, cough, fevers, malaria, typhoid, sore throat, indigestion, snake bites, and skin disorders. It is also used as a purgative, while HIV/AIDS patients use it as an immune booster to reduce the viral load and increase their CD4 counts. Furthermore, *Moringa oleifera* leaves are used to treat male impotency (53.7% of respondents). Mothers use it to improve lactation. In addition, it is employed to reverse malnutrition in both children and adults. It is claimed to be effective in controlling diarrhea and managing high blood pressure (Meresa et al., 2017).

This study is in agreement with the outcomes of the reports of Price (2002) and Fahey (2005) that *Moringa* is efficacious for the treatment of diabetes, high blood pressure, fevers, sores, and skin infections. According to Faizi et al. (1994), the hypotensive effect of extracts of *Moringa oleifera* might be due to its content of nitrile as well as mustard oil and thiocarbamate glycosides.

It is noteworthy that the ethnomedicinal uses of *Moringa* in Nigeria as contained in this survey are substantiated by Farooq et al. (2012). In 2012, Eze reported the potential use of the leaf extract for treating Newcastle disease of poultry in Nigeria. Apparently, *Moringa oleifera* is used as a food supplement and for both prophylactic and therapeutic purposes in Nigeria.

### 9.4.2 Uses of *Moringa oleifera* in Zimbabwe

In Zimbabwe, *Moringa oleifera* is used in all the districts as vegetable, medicine, source of oil, and ornamental purposes. It is also used in the construction of traditional huts, ornamentals, coagulates, for firewood, for making rope, and as fodder for livestock. In both rural and urban communities in Zimbabwe, leaves, young stems with or without flowers of *Moringa oleifera* are cooked and eaten as green vegetables. The leaves are still available during the dry season when no other vegetables are available. The varieties of *Moringa oleifera* in Zimbabwe, like others, contain high quantities of protein, minerals (calcium, oxalic acid, phosphorus, copper, iodine, and iron), vitamins (A, B, and C), and essential amino acids. Thus, the leaves are used as a nutritional supplement. In such cases the leaves can be used fresh or dried and crushed into powder and added to rice, porridge, soups, salads, etc. Young children and pregnant women take it to avert malnutrition. In fact, in different parts of Matabeleland of Zimbabwe, the leaves are consumed by children as well as pregnant and lactating women. Furthermore, pregnant women drink the broth of cooked leaves of *Moringa oleifera* at the commencement of uterine contractions to facilitate delivery. The Tonga people of the Binga district use the root powder as an aphrodisiac. The indigenes mix the root powder with milk to treat asthma, gout, rheumatism, and enlarged spleen or liver. It is also used to alleviate earache and toothache. Due to the presence of vitamin A in *Moringa oleifera,* which boosts the immune system, it is used as a supplement in the treatment of tuberculosis patients. It is also used as a diuretic and to treat gonorrhea, anemia, dysentery, and colitis. Nursing mothers use fresh leaves to improve milk production. Paste made from stem bark is used topically to relieve pain caused by snake, scorpion, and insect bites. The oil from *Moringa oleifera* seeds is used for cooking and lighting, while wristwatch repairers find it very valuable as a lubricant. The oil is also used for the manufacturing of soap and perfumes. In Matabeleland, *Moringa oleifera* leaves are used to feed cattle due to an acute shortage of grass. Generally, the leaves are also used to feed sheep, pigs, goats, and rabbits, while chickens and birds eat the seeds. Crushed seeds of *Moringa oleifera* are poured onto water, and the particles including microorganisms coagulate and sink to the bottom leaving clean water that can be used for drinking. About 2 grams can be used to treat 20 liters of dirty water. It is much cheaper and environmentally friendly compared to the conventional water treatment methods. In Matabeleland, *Moringa oleifera* has become an income-generating tree. The indigenes cultivate it for economic purposes as well. Indeed, the demand for the seedlings is higher than the supply.

### 9.4.3 Nutritional Uses of *Moringa oleifera* Leaves in Zambia, Ghana, Rwanda, and Senegal

Coppin (2008) collected leaves of *Moringa oleifera* from Ghana, Rwanda, Senegal, and Zambia and analyzed them. One sample contained 12 flavonoids including quercetin and kaempferol glycosides. Coppin identified $\alpha$- and $\gamma$-tocopherols, $\alpha$- and $\beta$-carotenes, six analogues of chlorogenic acid including four caffeoylquinic acids and two coumaroylquinic acids (structural and/or spatial isomers). The quantity of vitamin C in the dried leaves was low. Furthermore, Coppin (2008) analyzed 25 samples for their contents of chlorogenic acid isomers analogs (0.181–0.414 mg/100 g DW), tocopherols (7.1–116 mg/100 g DW), carotenoids (4.49–45.94 mg/100 g DW), and flavonoids (0.179%–1.643% g DW). She observed that the concentrations of these phytochemicals varied according to the environment, the country of collection, genetics, and variety of *Moringa oleifera*. It was remarkable that samples bought from the Mitengo women of Lusaka, Zambia, were excellent sources for the recommended daily allowances (RDAs) for calcium, phosphorus, iron, magnesium, manganese, copper, aluminum, and sodium for children as well as pregnant and lactating women. For example, 192 and 250 grams of the Lusaka samples met the RDAs for calcium, iron, and magnesium for pregnant and lactating women, respectively, between the ages of 14 and 50 years old (Coppin, 2008).

In addition to the provitamins, *Moringa* leaves contain minerals (Gupta et al., 1989), polyphenols (Bennett et al., 2003), flavonoids (Lako et al., 2007), alkaloids, and proteins (Soliva et al., 2005). Evidently, these essential nutrients have the potential to be developed and standardized to combat nutritional deficit and chronic inflammatory diseases (Coppin, 2008). The leaves of *Moringa* grown and collected from Ghana, Rwanda, Dakar, Senegal, and Zambia are rich sources of vitamins A and E, phosphorus, potassium, calcium, magnesium, and micronutrients (manganese, iron, copper, boron, aluminum, zinc, and sodium), have a high flavonoid content, and are a moderate source of phenols. Comparatively, the *Moringa* samples collected in 2007 from Rwanda and Zambia exhibited higher contents of all nutrients tested. According to Smolin and Grosvenor (2007), macronutrients and micronutrients contained in the leaves of *Moringa oleifera* provide energy, structure, and regulation, which are needed for growth, maintenance, repair, and reproduction.

Interestingly, the *Moringa* samples from Zambia contained relatively high amounts of total minerals. The highest value of minerals was collected from the Mitengo women in Lusaka, with samples that contained calcium (1.61%), potassium (0.52%), magnesium, (0.60%), iron (40.65 mg/100 g) manganese (14.60 mg/100 g), and copper (0.95 mg/100 g). The leaves collected from Dakar, Senegal, were higher in carotenoid concentration than those collected in both Zambia and Ghana. Due to the high concentration of total carotenoids in the leaves of *Moringa oleifera*, it is generally believed that the use of standardized extracts of *Moringa oleifera* leaves can substantially reduce child mortality in vitamin A–deficient countries.

## 9.5 BIOACTIVE CONSTITUENTS OF *MORINGA OLEIFERA* LEAVES

*Moringa* contains vitamins, flavonoids, carotenoids, polyphenol, phenolic acids, alkaloids, glucosinolates, isothiocyanates, tannins, saponins, oxalates, and phytates (Figures 9.1 and 9.2).

### 9.5.1 Vitamins

*Moringa* contains many vitamins (see Table 9.1). Examples include vitamin A, which is crucial for vision, reproduction, immunity, brain function, cell differentiation, etc. Its deficiency may be directly related to some infant and maternal mortalities, especially in developing countries (Alvarez et al., 2014). *Moringa* also contains ß-carotene, which is useful as an antioxidant. According to Gnagnarella et al. (2017), β-carotene content in *Moringa* is higher than that of carrots, pumpkin, and apricots. Vitamin C is also found in *Moringa* in significant quantities. Vitamin C is involved in the synthesis and metabolism of tyrosine, folic acid, and tryptophan and the hydroxylation of glycine, proline, lysine, carnitine, and catecholamine. Furthermore, vitamin C facilitates the conversion of cholesterol into bile acids, consequently lowering the blood cholesterol levels. In addition, vitamin C is a potent antioxidant.

According to Richter et al. (2003), vitamin E content in *Moringa* is similar to nuts. Vitamin E modulates gene expression, inhibits cell proliferation, inhibits monocyte aggregation, and regulates bone mass. Vitamin E is also a liposoluble antioxidant.

### 9.5.2 Flavonoids

Flavonoids are polyphenols contained in *Moringa* in larger quantities than fruits and vegetables. They are synthesized in plants after microbial infection. In humans, they protect against microbial infections and degenerative disorders. According to

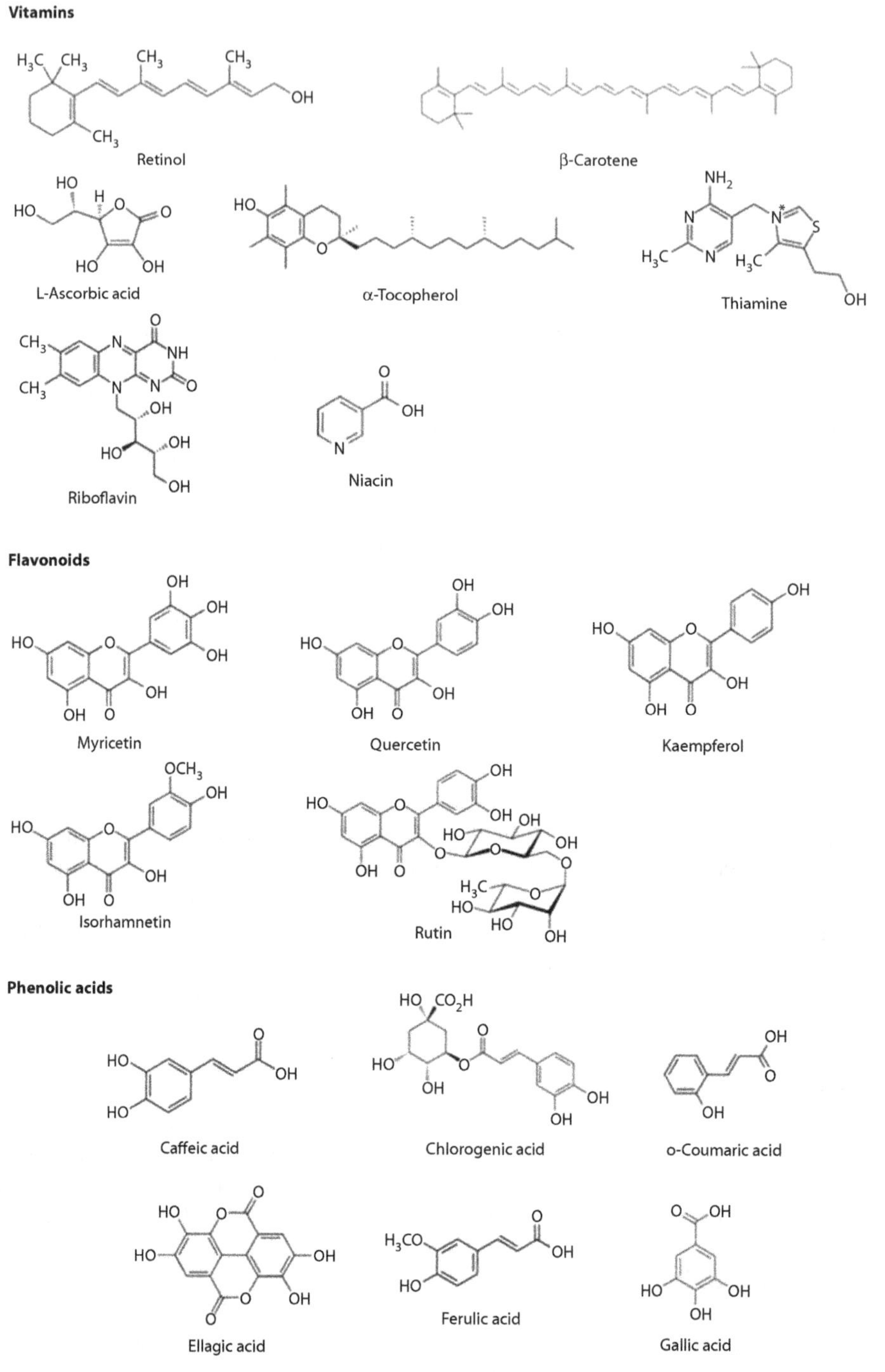

**Vitamins**

Retinol

β-Carotene

L-Ascorbic acid

α-Tocopherol

Thiamine

Riboflavin

Niacin

**Flavonoids**

Myricetin

Quercetin

Kaempferol

Isorhamnetin

Rutin

**Phenolic acids**

Caffeic acid

Chlorogenic acid

o-Coumaric acid

Ellagic acid

Ferulic acid

Gallic acid

**Figure 9.1** Some bioactive compounds in *Moringa oleifera* leaf.

**Alkaloids**

N, α-L-rhamnopyranosyl vincosamide

4-(α-L-rhamnopyranosyloxy)phenylacetonitrile (Niazirin)

Pyrrolemarumine 4″-O-α-L-rhamnopyranoside

methyl 4-(α-L-rhamnopyranosyloxy)-benzylcarbamate

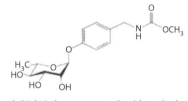

4′-hydroxyphenylethanamide-α-L-rhamnopyranoside (Marumoside A) (R = H)
4′-hydroxyphenylethanamide-α-L-rhamnopyranoside (Marumoside B) (R = D-Glucose)

**Glucosinolates**

4-O-(α-L-rhamnopyranosyloxy)-benzyl glucosinolate (R1, R2, R3 = H)
4-O-(α-L-acetylrhamnopyranosyloxy)-benzyl glucosinolate Isomer 1 (R1, R2 = H; R3 = Ac)
4-O-(α-L-acetylrhamnopyranosyloxy)-benzyl glucosinolate Isomer 2 (R1, R3 = H; R2 = Ac)
4-O-(α-L-acetylrhamnopyranosyloxy)-benzyl glucosinolate Isomer 3 (R2, R3 = H; R1 = Ac)

4-hydroxybenzyl glucosinolate (sinalbin)

**Figure 9.2**  Some bioactive compounds in *Moringa oleifera* leaf.

**Table 9.1  Nutritional Value of 100 Grams (3.5 ounces) of Fresh Leaves of *Moringa oleifera***

**Nutritional Value per 100 g (3.5 oz)**

| | |
|---|---|
| Energy | 64 kcal (270 kJ) |
| Carbohydrates | 8.28 g |
| Dietary fiber | 2.0 g |
| Fat | 1.40 g |
| Protein | 9.40 g |

**Vitamins**

| | |
|---|---|
| Vitamin A equiv. | (47%) 378 µg |
| Thiamine (B1) | (22%) 0.257 mg |
| Riboflavin (B2) | (55%) 0.660 mg |
| Niacin (B3) | (15%) 2.220 mg |
| Pantothenic acid (B5) | (3%) 0.125 mg |
| Vitamin B6 | (92%) 1.200 mg |
| Folate (B9) | (10%) 40 µg |
| Vitamin C | (62%) 51.7 mg |

**Minerals**

| | |
|---|---|
| Calcium | (19%) 185 mg |
| Iron | (31%) 4.00 mg |
| Magnesium | (41%) 147 mg |
| Manganese | (17%) 0.36 mg |
| Phosphorus | (16%) 112 mg |
| Potassium | (7%) 337 mg |
| Sodium | (1%) 9 mg |
| Zinc | (6%) 0.6 mg |

**Other Constituents**

| | |
|---|---|
| Water | 78.66 g |

***M. oleifera* pods, Raw**

| | |
|---|---|
| Energy | 37 kcal (150 kJ) |
| Carbohydrates | 8.53 g |
| Dietary fiber | 3.2 g |
| Fat | 0.20 g |
| Protein | 2.10 g |

**Vitamins**

| | |
|---|---|
| Vitamin A equiv. | (1%) 4 µg |
| Thiamine (B1) | (5%) 0.0530 mg |
| Riboflavin (B2) | (6%) 0.074 mg |
| Niacin (B3) | (4%) 0.620 mg |
| Pantothenic acid (B5) | (16%) 0.794 mg |

*(Continued)*

Table 9.1 *(Continued)*   **Nutritional Value of 100 Grams
(3.5 ounces) of Fresh Leaves of
*Moringa oleifera***

| Nutritional Value per 100 g (3.5 oz) | |
|---|---|
| Vitamin B6 | (9%) 0.120 mg |
| Folate (B9) | (11%) 44 μg |
| Vitamin C | (170%) 141.0 mg |
| **Minerals** | |
| Calcium | (3%) 30 mg |
| Iron | (3%) 0.36 mg |
| Magnesium | (13%) 45 mg |
| Manganese | (12%) 0.259 mg |
| Phosphorus | (7%) 50 mg |
| Potassium | (10%) 461 mg |
| Sodium | (3%) 42 mg |
| Zinc | (5%) 0.45 mg |
| **Other Constituents** | |
| Water | 88.20 g |

*Source:* USDA Nutrient Database.
Note: Percentages are roughly approximated using U.S. recommendations for adults.
Units μg = micrograms; mg = milligrams; IU = International units.

Coppin et al. (2013), myricetin, quercetin, and kaempferol are the main flavonoids identified in *Moringa oleifera* leaves.

### 9.5.3 Phenolic Acids

Phenolic acids are also polyphenols found in *Moringa*. They possess antioxidant, anti-inflammatory, antimutagenic, and anticancer properties (El-Seedi et al., 2012).

### 9.5.4 Alkaloids

Sahakitpichan et al. (2011) reported the presence of $N,\alpha$-L-rhamnopyranosyl vincosamide, 4-($\alpha$-L-rhamnopyranosyloxy) phenylacetonitrile (niazirin), pyrrolemarumine 4''-O-$\alpha$-L-rhamnopyranoside, 4'-hydroxy phenylethanamide-$\alpha$-L-rhamnopyranoside (marumoside A) and its 3-O-$\beta$-D-glucopyranosyl-derivative (marumoside B) and methyl 4-($\alpha$-L-rhamnopyranosyloxy)-benzylcarbamate alkaloids in *Moringa oleifera* leaves.

### 9.5.5 Glucosinolates and Isothiocyanates

Glucosinolates were isolated from *Moringa oleifera* leaves, which are involved in health promotion and prevention of diseases (Dinkova-Kostova and Kostov, 2012).

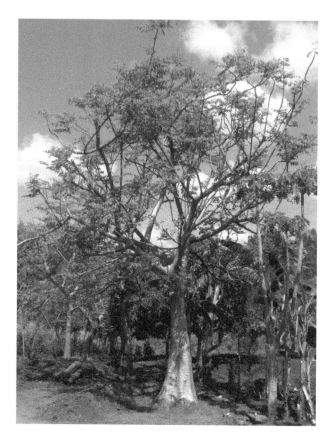

**Figure 9.3**   *Moringa stenopetala* (Ethiopia). Photographed by Trees for the Future, March 28, 2011.

## 9.5.6 Tannins

According to Kancheva and Kasaikina (2013), tannins manifest anticancer, anti-atherosclerotic, anti-inflammatory, antihepatoxic, antibacterial, and anti-HIV replication activity. The tannin content of *Moringa* leaves is greater than that found in nuts.

## 9.5.7 Saponins

Saponins possess anticancer properties. The content of saponins in *Moringa oleifera* leaves is higher than in most plants but lower than what is found in ginseng root (Edeoga et al., 2005).

## 9.5.8 Oxalates and Phytates

Oxalates and phytates are antinutritional compounds that bind to minerals, consequently inhibiting their intestinal absorption. *Moringa oleifera* leaves contain high

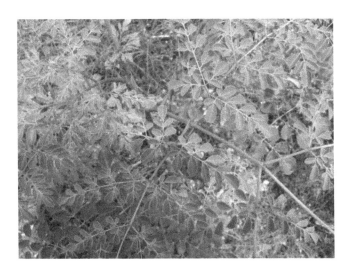

**Figure 9.4**  Photo of *Moringa oleifera* tree.

contents of these compounds. The oxalates content of dried leaves ranges from 430 to 1050 mg/100 g of DW, similar to other plants rich in these compounds, while phytates concentration ranges from 25 to 31 g/kg of DW in dried leaves and from 21 and 23 g/kg of DW in freeze-dried leaves (Richter et al., 2003). These amounts are greater than those found in legumes and cereals but lower than brans (García-Estepa et al., 1999).

## 9.6 PHARMACOLOGICAL EFFECTS OF EXTRACTS OF *MORINGA OLEIFERA* LEAVES

### 9.6.1 Antioxidant Effects

The antioxidant effects of extracts of *Moringa* leaves have been reported by different authors (Siddhuraju and Becker, 2003; Vongsak et al., 2013). The antioxidant effects were concentration dependent with $EC_{50}$ of about 0.08–0.2 mg/mL. The best results were obtained with methanol and ethanol extracts. In addition to the solvent system, significant seasonal variations were observed *vis-à-vis* the antioxidant effects of *Moringa* leaves (Iqbal and Bhanger, 2006; Shih et al., 2011). The results also showed that both environmental temperature and soil properties are crucial in determining the antioxidant effects of extracts of *Moringa* leaves. In 2009, Verma and his colleagues reported their study involving the effects of extracts of *Moringa* leaves on markers of oxidative stress in rats. They observed that administration of *Moringa oleifera* leaves extract in CCl4-intoxicated rats prevented the increment of lipid peroxide oxidation (LPO) levels and decreased glutathione (GSH) concentration and the activities of superoxide dismutase (SOD) and catalase (CAT) antioxidant enzymes in liver and kidney compared to the controls. Furthermore, the effects obtained in the group treated with 100 mg/kg body weight/day of leaves extract were comparable to those obtained in the standard group treated with 50 mg/kg body weight/day of vitamin E. In addition, the antioxidant effects of *Moringa* using goats fed with dried leaves of *Moringa* were reported by Moyo et al. (2012). They found a significant increase in GSH activity in goats supplemented with *Moringa* leaves as compared with the control group. In comparison, the activities of catalase (CAT) and superoxide dismutase (SOD) of diet supplemented with *Moringa oleifera* were increased appreciably compared to the controls given normal feed. Furthermore, MDA generated in the liver homogenate was inhibited by *Moringa oleifera* extracts, which suggests protection against oxidative stress.

In 2008, Chumark and his coworkers reported that *Moringa oleifera* leaves extract dose-dependently suppressed the initiation and propagation of lipid peroxidation using human plasma in *ex vivo* assay. Plants are rich sources for natural antioxidants; the best known are tocopherols, flavonoids, vitamin C, and other phenolic compounds (Laandrault et al., 2001). Other contributors to the antioxidant activity include alkaloids, proteins, minerals, and other vitamins such as the carotenoids and vitamins B6, B12, and K (Smolin and Grosvenor, 2007).

Furthermore, polyphenols scavenge free radicals such as peroxide, hydroperoxide, or lipid peroxyl, and inhibit the oxidative mechanisms that can lead to degenerative diseases. There are a number of clinical studies confirming the powerful anticancerous and anticardiac disease properties of polyphenols (Siddhuraju and Becker, 2003; Bajpai et al., 2005).

### 9.6.2 Anti-Inflammatory and Immunomodulatory Effects

Inflammation is a protective immunovascular response that involves immune cells, blood vessels, and molecular mediators. The goal of treatment of inflammation is to eliminate the initial cause of cell injury, clear necrotic cells and tissues damaged from the original injury and the inflammatory process, and then initiate tissue repair. According to Waterman et al. (2014), *Moringa oleifera* concentrate and isothiocyanates isolated from the leaves significantly decreased gene expression and production of inflammatory markers in RAW macrophages. Thus, both the expression of inducible nitric oxide synthase (iNOS), IL-1β and production of NO and TNFα at 1 and 5 μM were attenuated.

The immunomodulatory effect of methanolic and ethanolic extracts of *Moringa oleifera* leaves using cyclophosphamide-induced immunodeficient mice have been reported, respectively, by Sudha et al. (2010) and Gupta et al. (2010). Their data indicated a significant increase in white blood cells, percentage neutrophils, and serum immunoglobulins. Apparently, both cellular and humoral immune responses were stimulated. In 2015, Waterman et al. reported the molecular basis of the anti-inflammatory effect of extracts of *Moringa oleifera*. In their experiment, obese-induced mice were supplemented with *Moringa oleifera* leaves concentrate. The authors observed a reduction of gene expression of pro-inflammatory markers, TNFα, IL-6, and IL-1β in the liver and ileum tissues in mice treated with *Moringa oleifera* concentrate compared to the control group. Furthermore, gene expression of TNFα was reduced in adipose tissue, while adiponectin had enhanced expression in the treated mice compared to the controls.

Similarly, Das et al. (2013) compared the anti-inflammatory effects of *Moringa oleifera* leaves extract to that of quercetin in mice fed with a high-fat diet. The authors found that both *Moringa oleifera* leaves extract and quercetin inhibited the translocation of the p65 subunit of NF-κB (4.2- and 2.3-fold reduction in the expression level, respectively) when compared with the control group fed only with a high-fat diet. Furthermore, both *Moringa oleifera* leaves extract and quercetin downregulated the expressions of iNOS, interferon gamma (IFN-γ), and C-reactive protein (CRP) compared to the control group fed only with a high-fat diet. The release of serum inflammatory cytokines TNF-a and IL-6 was significantly decreased in the group treated with the extract (30% and 27% reduction for TNF-a and IL-6, respectively) and in the group treated with quercetin (27% and 21% reduction for TNF-a and IL-6, respectively) when compared to the control group.

Evidently, both the anti-inflammatory and immunomodulatory effects of supplementation with *Moringa oleifera* leaves have been validated using *in vitro* and *in vivo* methods. Das et al. (2013) suggested that quercetin (one of the bioactive components of *Moringa oleifera*) may be responsible for inhibiting the activation of NF-kB as well as the subsequent NF-kB–dependent downstream events associated with inflammation. In addition, many other bioactive compounds naturally present in *Moringa oleifera* leaves, such as other flavonoids and phenolic acids, may be involved in the anti-inflammatory effect of *Moringa oleifera* leaves. However, the mechanism of action of other bioactive entities' compounds naturally present in *Moringa oleifera* leaves, which may be involved in its anti-inflammatory effects, requires further research. Data showed that extracts of *Moringa oleifera* leaves activated both the cellular and the humoral immunity processes, which may account for its immunomodulatory effect. However, the mechanism of the activation is not yet known (Gupta et al., 2010). Furthermore, studies involving human subjects are required *vis-à-vis* the anti-inflammatory and immunomodulatory effects of *Moringa oleifera* leaves.

### 9.6.3 Hypoglycemic Effect

In 2007, Ndong et al. reported their investigation on the hypoglycemic effect of extracts of the leaves of *Moringa oleifera* using male spontaneously diabetic Goto-Kakizaka (GK) rats and nondiabetic rats. Their findings suggested that *Moringa oleifera* induced a glucose intolerance ameliorating effect in both GK and Wistar rats. However, the effect was more pronounced in the diabetic than in the normoglycemic rats.

Furthermore, Edoga et al. (2013) observed that the aqueous extract produced a dose-dependent reduction in blood glucose levels of normoglycemic and hyperglycemic rats. For example, in normoglycemic rats, 100, 200, and 300 mg/kg of leave extracts of *Moringa oleifera* resulted in the reduction of 23.14%, 27.05% and 33.18%, respectively, of the blood glucose levels within 6 hours of administration. However, in alloxan-induced diabetic rats, the reduction in blood glucose levels was more pronounced. Thus, 100, 200, and 300 mg/kg, respectively, induced 33.29%, 40.69%, and 44.06% reduction in blood glucose levels. It is significant that the authors reported similar reductions in blood glucose levels using 200 mg/kg of the reference medicine (i.e., tolbutamide).

Yassa and Tohamy (2014) reported the hypoglycemic effect of extracts of *Moringa oleifera* leaves using streptozotocin-induced diabetic rats. These workers also observed that the histopathological damage of islet cells associated with diabetes was profoundly reversed by the extracts of *Moringa oleifera* leaves.

Various workers have reported the diabetic effect of *Moringa oleifera* leaves using human subjects. For example, Kumari (2010) reported the hypoglycemic effect of *Moringa oleifera* leaves in non-insulin-dependent type 2 diabetes mellitus subjects aged 30–60 years old. The volunteers were divided into test and control groups. The subjects in the test group were given 8 grams of dried *Moringa oleifera* leaves for 40 days, while the control group was not given any *Moringa oleifera* leaves. Daily meals were comparable between the two groups in terms of relative food type consumption, nutrients, and calories. Fasting and postprandial blood glucose concentrations were taken at baseline and at the end of the experiment. Fasting and postprandial blood glucose did not differ much from baseline in the control group, while they were significantly reduced in the experimental group (−28% and −26%, respectively).

The hypoglycemic effect of *Moringa oleifera* leaves might be partly due to its content of isothiocyanates. According to Waterman et al. (2015), isothiocyanates decreased phosphoenolpyruvate carboxykinase and glucose-6-phosphatase gene expression, suggesting that they act via blocking these rate-limiting steps in liver gluconeogenesis. Furthermore, isothiocyanates reduced glucose production in liver cells, even at very low concentrations. The same authors suggested that isothiocyanates isolated from leaves of *Moringa oleifera* reduced insulin resistance and hepatic gluconeogenesis. It is also possible that phenolic acids and flavonoids present in *Moringa oleifera* might act on cellular signaling pathways in pancreas, liver, skeletal muscle, and white adipose tissue. Such effects may be related to their antioxidant, enzyme inhibition, receptor agonist, or antagonist activity or through other mechanisms not yet known (Babu et al., 2013; Bahadoran et al., 2013; Oh and Jun, 2014).

Studies have suggested the potential use of *Moringa oleifera* leaves in human patients with diabetes. However, randomized controlled clinical trials involving larger numbers of subjects are needed before *Moringa oleifera* leaves can be considered as a supplement in the management of diabetes.

### 9.6.4 Hypolipidemic Effect

In 2008, Chumark et al. (2008) reported the hypolipidemic effect of *Moringa oleifera* leaves using rabbits fed with a high-cholesterol diet. They observed that the test rabbits treated with *Moringa oleifera* leaves manifested significant reductions in total cholesterol (52%), low-density lipoproteins (LDL) (42.7%), high-density lipoproteins (HDL) (44.2%), and triglycerides (75.4%) compared to control rabbits fed only with a high-cholesterol diet. The same authors also reported that they observed similar reductions in the group treated with 5 mg/kg of simvastatin (reference medicine).

Furthermore, the hypolipidemic effect of the extracts of *Moringa oleifera* leaves was reported in hyperlipidemic human subjects (Nambiar et al., 2010). The authors observed a reduction of 1.6% in plasma total cholesterol while HDL was increased (6.3%). However, there were no significant changes in LDL, very low-density lipoproteins (VLDL), and triglycerides compared to the control group. Phenolic compounds, especially flavonoids, present in *Moringa oleifera* might be partly responsible for its hypolipidemic effect (Siasos et al., 2013).

## 9.6.5 Hepatic and Kidney Protective Effects

Fakurazi et al. (2008) reported hepatic and kidney protective effects of the extracts of *Moringa oleifera* leaves against isoniazid, rifampicin, pyrazinamide, acetaminophen, and gentamicin. Serum ALT, AST, ALP, and BUN and creatinine were reduced in animals treated with the extract of *Moringa oleifera* leaves. The mechanism underlying the observed protection of liver and kidney by extracts of *Moringa oleifera* leaves is not yet elucidated.

## 9.6.6 Anticancer Effects

Sikder et al. (2013) as well as Sreelatha and Padma (2011) have reported the protective effect of extracts of *Moringa oleifera* leaves against organisms and cells from oxidative DNA damage associated with cancer and degenerative diseases. Apparently, the antiproliferative effect involved induction of apoptosis, morphological changes, and DNA fragmentation. The apoptosis induction and tumor cell growth inhibitory effects of aqueous extract of *Moringa oleifera* leaves on human lung cancer cells were reported by Jung (2014). Significant inhibition of pancreatic cancer cells was reported by Berkovich et al. (2013). Furthermore, *Moringa oleifera* leaves extracts inhibited the viability of acute myeloid leukemia, acute lymphoblastic leukemia, and hepatocellular carcinoma cells (Parvathy and Umamaheshwari, 2007). However, the extract was devoid of toxic effects against normal mononuclear cells. In addition, Pamok et al. (2011) reported that both aqueous and ethanolic extracts inhibited cell proliferation of three different types of colon cancer cell lines.

Purwal et al. (2010) studied the effects of oral administration of hydro-methanolic and methanolic extracts of *Moringa oleifera* leaves in a murine melanoma tumor model. The authors reported that an oral administration of 500 mg/kg for 15 days of the extracts delayed tumor growth and significantly increased the lifespans of the animals.

Evidently, *in vitro* studies indicate potential anticancer effects of *Moringa oleifera* leaves on various cancer cell lines. Abdull Razis et al. (2014) ascribed the anticancer effects of *Moringa* to the presence of 4-($\alpha$-L-rhamnosyloxy) benzyl isothiocyanate, niazimicin, and $\beta$-sitosterol-3-O-$\beta$-D-glucopyranoside. More studies are needed to confirm these effects that have profound potential application in the management of cancer.

## 9.7 CONCLUSION

The brief review of the multipurpose uses of *Moringa* in this chapter clearly demonstrates its immense potential applications in nutrition, agriculture, animal husbandry, human health, energy, house construction, among others. The review also shows that among the 13 *Moringa* species, only two have been studied. More studies are needed for *Moringa stenopetala* and the other 10 *Moringa* species that are indigenous to Africa. In view of the diverse uses of *Moringa oleifera*, it is one of the most studied plants. Different parts of the plant can be consumed for their nutritional claims. Examples include immature seed pods, young leaves, mature seeds, oil pressed from the seeds, flowers, etc. It is also used for water purification as well as for biopesticides and the production of biodiesel. Its ethnomedical uses (both for treatment and prevention) include different types of cancer, diabetes, infective diseases, cardiovascular disorders, dyslipidemia, among others. It is remarkable that many *in vivo* and *in vitro* data have confirmed the various ethnomedical uses of *Moringa oleifera*. It is therefore not surprising that it is referred to as "The Miracle Plant." Indeed, there is no plant that has such wide applications in agriculture, animal husbandry, medicine, nutrition, and water purification.

Nutrition is a critical area of concern in Africa, since malnutrition leads to both morbidity and mortality. It is indicative that at the level of the African Union and member states of the African Union, strategic plans need to be articulated to harness and utilize the nutritional potentials of the *Moringa* plant. The mechanism should involve appropriate policies and the establishment of structures for coordination and empowerment to ensure that policies are fully implemented.

According to the World Health Organization (WHO, 2017), 3.4 million people, mostly children, die annually from water-related diseases. Furthermore, most of these illnesses and deaths can be prevented through simple, inexpensive measures. In 2017, WHO also reported that about 1 billion people get their water supplies from unhygienic sources. Insects that carry malaria, filaria, and trypanosome parasites need water to breed. For example, about 300 million people suffer from malaria every year, while about 1 million people die from malaria in sub-Saharan Africa annually. Furthermore, lack of good quality, reliable water forces people (mostly women and children) to get water from alternative, unsafe sources, exposing them to diseases such as diarrhea or dysentery, cholera, typhoid, and schistosomiasis. Since *Moringa* species are routinely used for water purification in Africa and elsewhere, member states of the WHO can engage with stakeholders to scale up the processes to ensure clean water is available to the populace, especially in rural settings.

Interestingly, *Moringa oleifera* and other *Moringa* species have abundant bioactive compounds that may be responsible for their diverse ethnomedical uses. Such bioactive components include vitamins, carotenoids, polyphenol, phenolic acids, flavonoids, alkaloids, glucosinolates, isothiocyanates, tannins, and saponins.

*Moringa* has significant quantities of both macronutrients and micronutrients. Genetic variations, climatic conditions, soil characteristics, age of plant at harvesting, postharvesting processes, and so on, affect the quantities of the bioactive components of *Moringa oleifera*. Thus, when extracts of *Moringa oleifera* or any other *Moringa* species are standardized and formulated as nutritional supplements, quality assurance systems must be instituted to ensure consistent quality of different batches of the product. Another challenge is the high content of oxalates and phytates in *Moringa oleifera* leaves, which is known to limit the intestinal adsorption of minerals. Furthermore, randomized controlled clinical trials are very few using standardized extracts of *Moringa oleifera* leaves. In view of the potential therapeutic applications of *Moringa* species for both preventive and curative purposes as well as improvement in quality of life, more randomized clinical trials should be undertaken. Such clinical studies should also include chronic aspects to ascertain the safety profiles in human subjects when it is used as a supplement, especially for purposes of improving quality of life and preventing some chronic disorders.

According to Leone et al. (2015), the diversifications and high morphological variability exhibited by *Moringa* species may be utilized for the conservation and selection of *Moringa oleifera* germplasm. The same authors advocated for the collection and characterization of world accessions (both cultivated and natural) and for the setting of a collaborative network among institutions conducting research on *Moringa oleifera*. This will help scientists and farmers to have reliable access to information and materials, which will consequently enhance the quality of *Moringa* products in the market. Furthermore, researchers interested in the association between phenotypical and molecular data and genetic maps (both association map and physical map) in order to identify genes for breeding will be facilitated by the existing collaborative network. Next-generation sequencing (NGS) can be used to discover genome-wide genetic markers and to build saturated genetic maps in a timely fashion and economically.

Based on the case studies of the uses of *Moringa* in some African countries, it also has potential in food security. African governments, scientists, and the private sector need to collaborate to develop strategic plans for *Moringa* yield improvement, cultivation, and standardization as well as marketing of *Moringa* products for various nutritional conditions. It is significant that both *Moringa oleifera* and *Moringa senopetala* are drought resistant and grow very well even in dry seasons when other green leafy vegetables are not available. Farmers in Africa should be guided and trained to know the nutritional values inherent in *Moringa* species and take advantage. Subsequently, they should be empowered to cultivate them. The economic potentials of *Moringa* business in Africa and globally are immense. It is interesting that in Africa, most of the people involved in the processing, production, and marketing of *Moringa* are women. Consequently, empowering the women involved in *Moringa* business in Africa will support their families and elevate their socioeconomic status.

The potential uses of *Moringa* in agriculture are crucial. The private sector should take advantage of the plant hormones in *Moringa* to cultivate, process, and market the plant hormone. Positive effects on the health and growth of animals fed with *Moringa* supplement should also be explored and widely applied. Awareness by all the relevant sectors of the potentials of *Moringa* should be appropriately articulated and spearheaded by member states of the WHO so that the private sector can become interested. The use of *Moringa oleifera* seeds as a source of producing biodiesel is remarkable. The economic implications and the environmental benefits of such a venture are obvious. Member states of the WHO should endeavor to create the enabling environment so that the private sector can partner with local communities to launch such ventures.

## REFERENCES

Abdulkarim, S.M., Long, K., Lai, O.M., Muhammad, S.K.S., Ghazali, H.M., 2005. Some physico-chemical properties of *Moringa oleifera* seed oil extracted using solvent and aqueous enzymatic methods. *Food Chemistry*, 93(20):253–263.

Abdull Razis, A.F., Ibrahim, M.D., Kntayya, S.B., 2014. Health benefits of *Moringa oleifera*. *Asian Pacific Journal of Cancer Prevention*, 15:8571–8576.

Abuye, C., Urga, K., Knapp, H., Selmar, D., Omwega, A.M., Imungi, J.K., 2003. A compositional study of *Moringa stenopetala* leaves. *East African Medical Journal*, 80(5):247–252.

Alvarez, R., Vaz, B., Gronemeyer, H., de Lera, A.R., 2014. Functions, therapeutic applications, and synthesis of retinoids and carotenoids. *Chemistry Review*, 114:1–125.

Amsalu, N., 2010. An ethinobotanical study of medicinal plants in Farta Woreda, South Gondar Zone of Amhara Region, Ethiopia. MSc Thesis. Published by Addis Ababa University 127.

Anon, 2003. Ethiopia forms Moringa tree promotion committee. Available at: http://www.pan-apress.com/newslat.aspcode=eng00444&dte=16/07/2003 (Accessed on July 8, 2017).

Ashfaq, M., Basra, S.M., Ashfaq, U., 2012. Moringa: A miracle plant for agro-forestry. *Journal of Agriculture and Social Sciences*, 8:115–122.

Babu, P.V., Liu, D., Gilbert, E.R., 2013. Recent advances in understanding the anti-diabetic actions of dietary flavonoids. *Journal of Nutrition and Biochemistry*, 24:1777–1789.

Bahadoran, Z., Mirmiran, P., Azizi, F., 2013. Dietary polyphenols as potential nutraceuticals in management of diabetes: A review. *Journal of Diabetes and Metabolic Disorder*, 12:43. doi:10.1186/2251-6581-12-43.

Bajpai, M., Pande, A., Tewari, S.K., Prakash, D., 2005. Phenolic contents and antioxidant activity of some food and medicinal plants. *International Journal of Food Science and Nutrition*, 56:287–291.

Bennett, R.N., Mellon, F.A., Foidl, N., Pratt, J.H., Dupoint, S.M., Perkins, L., Kroon, P.A., 2003. Profiling glucosinolates and phenolics in vegetative and reproductive tissues of the multi-purpose trees *Moringa oleifera* L. (Horseradish Tree) and *Moringa stenopetala* L. *Journal of Agriculture and Food Chemistry*, 51:3546–3553.

Berkovich, L., Earon, G., Ron, I., Rimmon, A., Vexler, A., Lev-Ari, S., 2013. *Moringa oleifera* aqueous leaf extract down-regulates nuclear factor-kappa B and increases cytotoxic effect of chemotherapy in pancreatic cancer cells. *BMC Complementary Alternative Medicine*, 13:12, doi:10.1186/1472-6882-13-212.

Beyene, D., 2005. Genetic variation in *Moringa stenopetala* germplasm of Ethiopia by using RAPD as genetic marker. MSc Thesis. Addis Ababa University, Ethiopia.

Chumark, P., Khunawat, P., Sanvarinda, Y., Phornchirasilp, S., Morales, N.P., Phivthong-Ngam, L., Ratanachamnong, P., Srisawat, S., Pongrapeeporn, K.U., 2008. The *in vitro and ex vivo* antioxidant properties, hypolipidaemic and antiatherosclerotic activities of water extract of *Moringa oleifera* Lam. leaves. *Journal of Ethnopharmacology*, 116:439–446.

Coppin, J., 2008. A study of the nutritional and medicinal values of Moringa oleifera leaves from sub-Saharan Africa: Ghana, Rwanda, Senegal and Zambia. M.Sc. thesis, Rutgers University-Graduate School-New Brunswick, New Brunswick.

Coppin, J.P., Xu, Y., Chen, H., Pan, M.H., Ho, C.T., Juliani, R., Simon, J.E., Wu, Q., 2013. Determination of flavonoids by LC/MS and anti-inflammatory activity in *Moringa oleifera*. *Journal of Functional Foods*, 5:1892–1899.

Das, N., Sikder, K., Bhattacharjee, S., Majumdar, S.B., Ghosh, S., Majumdar, S., Dey, S., 2013. Quercetin alleviates inflammation after short-term treatment in high-fat-fed mice. *Food Functions*, 4:889–898.

Dinkova-Kostova, A.T., Kostov, R.V., 2012. Glucosinolates and isothiocyanates in health and disease. *Trends in Molecular Medicine*, 18:337–347.

Dongmeza, E., Siddhuraju, P., Francis, G., Becker, K., 2006. Effects of dehydrated methanol extracts of Moringa (Moringa oleifera Lam.) leaves and three of its fractions on growth performance and feed nutrient assimilation in Nile tilapia (Oreochromis niloticus (L.)). *Aquaculture*, 261(1): 407–422.

Edeoga, H.O., Okwu, D.E., Mbaebie, B.O., 2005. Phytochemical constituents of some Nigerian medicinal plants. *African Journal of Biotechnology*, 4:685–688.

Edoga, C.O., Njoku, O.O., Amadi, E.N., Afomezie, P.I., 2013. Effect of aqueous extract of *Moringa oleifera* on serum protein of *Trypanosoma brucei* infected rats. *International Journal of Science and Technology*, 3(1):85–87.

El-Seedi, H.R., El-Said, A.M., Khalifa, S.A., Göransson, U., Bohlin, L., Borg-Karlson, A.K., Verpoorte, R., 2012. Biosynthesis, natural sources, dietary intake, pharmacokinetic properties, and biological activities of hydroxycinnamic acids. *Journal of Agriculture and Food Chemistry*, November 7;60(44):10877–10895. doi:10.1021/jf301807g. Epub 2012 October 30.

Endeshaw, H.G., 2003. Promoting the miracle tree of hope. Ethiopian Herald, Addis Ababa University, Ethiopia.

Eze, D.C., Okwor, E.C., Okoye, J.O.A., Onah, D.N., Shoyinka, S.V.O., 2012. Effects of *Moringa oleifera* methanolic leaf extract on the morbidity and mortality of chickens experimentally infected with Newcastle disease virus (Kudu 113) strain. *Journal of Medicinal Plant Research*, 6(27):4443–4449.

Fahey, J.W., 2005. *Moringa oleifera*: A review of the medical evidence for its nutritional, therapeutic, and prophylactic properties. Part 1. *Trees for Life Journal*, 1:5.

Faizi, S., Siddiqui, B., Saleem, R., Saddiqui, S., Aftab, K., 1994. Isolation and structure elucidation of new nitrile and mustard oil glycosides from *Moringa oleifera* and their effect on blood pressure. *Journal of Natural Products*, 57:1256–1261.

Fakurazi, S., Hairuszah, I., Nanthini, U., 2008. *Moringa oleifera* Lam prevents acetaminophen induced liver injury through restoration of glutathione level. *Food Chemistry and Toxicology*, 46:2611–2615.

Farooq, F., Rai, M., Tiwari, A., Khan, A.A., Farooq, S., 2012. Medicinal properties of *Moringa oleifera*: An overview of promising healer. *Journal of Medicinal Plant Research*, 6(27):4368–4374.

Foidl, N., Makkar, H.P.S., Becker, K., 2001. The potential of *Moringa oleifera* for agricultural and industrial uses. *What Development Potential for Moringa Products*? Dar Es Salaam, Ethiopia. *Workshop Proceedings*, pp. 10–30.

Fuglie, L.J., 1999. *The Miracle Tree: Moringa oleifera: Natural Nutrition for the Tropics.* Church World Service, Dakar, p. 68.

García-Estepa, R.M., Guerra-Hernández, E., García-Villanova, B., 1999. Phytic acid content in milled cereal products and breads. *Food Research International*, 32:217–221.

Geleta, B., Makonnen, E., Debella, A., Abebe, A., Fekadu, N., 2016a. *In vitro* vasodilatory activity of the crude extracts and fractions of *Moringa stenopetala* (Baker f.) Cufod. leaves in isolated thoracic aorta of guinea pigs. *Journal of Experimental Pharmacology*, 8:35–42.

Geleta, B., Makonnen, E., Debella, A., Tadele, A., 2016b. *In vivo* antihypertensive and antihyperlipidemic effects of the crude extracts and fractions of *Moringa stenopetala* (Baker f.) Cufod. leaves in 29 rats. *Frontiers in Pharmacology B*, 7:97.

Ghebreselassie, D., Mekonnen, Y., Gebru, G., Ergete, W., Huruy, K., 2011. The effects of *Moringa stenopetala* on blood parameters and histopathology of liver and kidney in mice. *Ethiopian Journal of Health Development*, 25(1): 51–57.

Gnagnarella, P., Salvini, S., Parpinel, M., 2017. Food Composition Database for Epidemiological Studies in Italy. Available at: http://www.bda-ieo.it/ (Accessed on July 16, 2017).

Gupta, A., Gautam, M.K., Singh, R.K., Kumar, M.V., Rao, C.H.V., Goel, R.K., Anupurba, S., 2010. Immunomodulatory effect of *Moringa oleifera* Lam. extract on cyclophosphamide induced toxicity in mice. *Indian Journal of Experimental Biology*, 48:1157–1160.

Gupta, K., Barat, G.K., Wagle, D.S., Chawla, H.K.L., 1989. Nutrient contents and antinutritional factors in conventional and non-conventional leafy vegetables. *Food Chemistry*, 31(2):105–116.

Iqbal, S., and Bhanger, M.I., 2006. Effect of season and production location on antioxidant activity of *Moringa oleifera* leaves grown in Pakistan. *Journal of Food Composition and Analysis*, 19:544–551.

Jung, I.L., 2014. Soluble extract from *Moringa oleifera* leaves with a new anticancer activity. *PLoS ONE*, 9:e95492.

Kancheva, V.D., and Kasaikina, O.T., 2013. Bio-antioxidants—A chemical base of their antioxidant activity and beneficial effect on human health. *Current Medicinal Chemistry*, 20:4784–4805.

Kumari, D.J., 2010. Hypoglycemic effect of *Moringa oleifera* and *Azadirachta indica* in type-2 diabetes. *Bioscan*, 5:211–214.

Laandrault, N., Pouchert, P., Ravel, P., Gase, F., Cros, G., Teissedro, P.L., 2001. Antioxidant activities and phenolic level of French wines from different varieties and vintages. *Journal of Agriculture and Food Chemistry*, 49:3341–3343.

Lako, J., Trenerry, V.C., Wahlqvist, M., Wattanapenpaiboon, N., Southeeswaran, S., Premier, R., 2007. Phytochemical flavonols, carotenoids and the antioxidant properties of a wide selection of Fijian fruit, vegetables and other readily available foods. *Food Chemistry*, 101(4):1727–1741.

Leone, A., Alberto Spada, A., Battezzati, A., Schiraldi, A., Aristil, J., Bertoli, S., 2015. Cultivation, genetic, ethnopharmacology, phytochemistry and pharmacology of *Moringa oleifera* leaves: An overview. *International Journal of Molecular Science*, 16:12791–12835.

Lockett, C.T., Calvert, C.C., Grivetti, L.E., 2000. Energy and micronutrient composition of dietary and medicinal wild plants consumed during drought. Study of rural Fulani, northeastern Nigeria. *International Journal of Food Science Nutrition*, 51:195–208.

Mathur, B.S., 2005. *Moringa Book*. Trees for Life International, St. Louis, MO.

Mekonnen, D., 2016. Miracle tree: A review on multi-purposes of *Moringa oleifera* and its implication for climate change mitigation. *Journal of Earth Sciences and Climate Change*, 7:366.

Mekonnen, Y., and Gessesse, A., 1998. Documentation on the uses of *Moringa stenopetala* and its possible antileishmanial and anti-fertility effects. *SINET: Ethiopian Journal of Science*, 21:287–295.

Mengistu, M., Abebe, Y., Mekonnen, Y., Tolessa, T., 2012. In vivo and in vitro hypotensive effect of aqueous extract of Moringa stenopetala. *African Health Sciences*, 12(4): 545–551.

Meresa, A., Fekadu, N., Degu, S., Tadele, A., Geleta, B., 2017. An ethnobotanical review on medicinal plants used for the management of hypertension. *Clinical and Experimental Pharmacology*, 7:228. doi:10.4172/2161-1459.1000228.

Moyo, B., Oyedemi, S., Masika, P.J., Muchenje, V., 2012. Polyphenolic content and antioxidant properties of *Moringa oleifera* leaf extracts and enzymatic activity of liver from goats supplemented with *Moringa oleifera* leaves/sunflower seed cake. *Meat Science*, 91:441–447.

Musa, A.H., Vata, P.K., Debella, A., 2015. Acute toxicity studies of butanol fraction of leaves of *Moringa stenopetala* in rats. *Asian Pacific Journal of Health Sciences*, 2(2):160–164.

Musa, A.H., Vata, P.K., Gebru, G., Mekonnen, Y., Debella, A., 2016. Biochemical and hematological study on butanol fraction of leaves of *Moringa stenopetala* in experimental rats. *IOSR Journal of Pharmacy*, 6:64–68.

Mussa, A., Makonnen, E., Urga, K., 2008. Effects of the crude aqueous. extract and isolated fraction of *Moringa stenopetala* leaves in normal and diabetic mice. *Pharmacology Online*, 3:1049–1055.

Nambiar, V.S., Guin, P., Parnami, S., Daniel, M., 2010. Impact of antioxidants from drumstick leaves on the lipid profile of hyperlipidemics. *Journal of Herbal Medicine and Toxicology*, 4:165–172.

Ndong, M., Uehara, M., Katsumata, S.I., Suzuki, K., 2007. Effects of oral administration of *Moringa oleifera* Lam on glucose tolerance in Goto-kakizaki and Wistar rats. *Journal of Clinical Biochemistry and Nutrition*, 40:229–233.

Oh, Y.S., and Jun, H.S., 2014. Role of bioactive food components in diabetes prevention: Effects on beta-cell function and preservation. *Nutrition and Metabolic Insights*, 7:51–59.

Pamok, S., Saenphet, S., Vinitketkumnuen, V., Saenphet, K., 2011. Antiproliferative effect of *Moringa oleifera* Lam. and *Pseuderanthemum palatiferum* (Nees) Radlk extracts on the colon cancer cells. *Journal of Medicinal Plant Research*, 6:139–145.

Parvathy, M.V.S., and Umamaheshwari, A., 2007. Cytotoxic effect of *Moringa oleifera* leaf extracts on human multiple myeloma cell lines. *Trends in Medical Research*, 2:44–50.

Price, M.L., 2002. *The Moringa Tree*. ACHO Staff, Florida, USA.

Purwal, L., Pathak, A.K., Jain, U.K., 2010. *In vivo* anticancer activity of the leaves and fruits of *Moringa oleifera* on mouse melanoma. *Pharmacology Online*, 1:655–665.

Rashid, U., Anwar, F., Moser, B.R., Knothe, G., 2008. *Moringa oleifera* oil: A possible source of biodiesel. *Bioresource Technology*, 99:8175–8179.

Richter, N., Siddhuraju, P., Becker, K., 2003. Evaluation of nutritional quality of Moringa (*Moringa oleifera* Lam.) leaves as an alternative protein source for Nile tilapia (*Oreochromis niloticus* L.). *Aquaculture*, 217:599–611.

Sahakitpichan, P., Mahidol, C., Disadee, W., Ruchirawat, S., Kanchanapoom, T., 2011. Unusual glycosides of pyrrole alkaloid and 4′-hydroxyphenylethanamide from leaves of *Moringa oleifera*. *Phytochemistry*, 72:791–795.

Sánchez, N.R., Spörndly, E., Ledin, I., 2006. Effect of feeding different levels of foliage of *Moringa oleifera* to Creole dairy cows on intake, digestibility, milk production and composition. *Livestock Science*, 101(1–3):24–31.

Seifu, E., 2014. Actual and potential applications of *Moringa stenopetala*, underutilized indigenous vegetable of Southern Ethiopia. A review. *International Journal of Agricultural and Food Research*, 3(4):8–19.

Shih, M.C., Chang, C.M., Kang, S.M., Tsai, M.L., 2011. Effect of different parts (leaf, stem and stalk) and seasons (summer and winter) on the chemical compositions and antioxidant activity of *Moringa oleifera*. *International Journal of Molecular Science*, 12:6077–6088.

Siasos, G., Tousoulis, D., Tsigkou, V., Kokkou, E., Oikonomou, E., Vavuranakis, M., Basdra, E.K., Papavassiliou, A.G., Stefanadis, C., 2013. Flavonoids in atherosclerosis: An overview of their mechanisms of action. *Current Medicinal Chemistry*, 20:2641–2660.

Siddhuraju, P., and Becker, K., 2003. Antioxidant properties of various solvent extracts of total phenolic constituents from three different agroclimatic origins of drumstick tree (*Moringa oleifera* Lam.) leaves. *Journal of Agriculture Food Chemistry*, 51:2144–2155.

Sikder, K., Sinha, M., Das, N., Das, D.K., Datta, S., Dey, S., 2013. *Moringa oleifera* leaf extract prevents *in vitro* oxidative DNA damage. *Asian Journal Pharmacology and Clinical Research*, 6:159–163.

Sileshi, T., Makonnen, E., Debella, A., Tesfaye, B., 2014. Antihyperglycemic and subchronic toxicity study of *Moringa stenopetala* leaves in mice. *Journal of Coastal Life Medicine*, 2:214–221.

Smolin, L.A., and Grosvenor, M.B., 2007. *Nutrition: Science and Application*. 3rd edition, Wiley, ISBN:978-1-118-54960-5.

Soliva, C.R., Kreuzer, M., Foidl, N., Foidl G., Machmüller, A., Hess, H.D., 2005. Feeding value of whole and extracted *Moringa oleifera* leaves for ruminants: Their effects on ruminal fermentation *in vitro*. *Animal Feed Science Technology*, 118:47–62.

Sreelatha, S., and Padma, P.R., 2011. Modulatory effects of *Moringa oleifera* extracts against hydrogen peroxide-induced cytotoxicity and oxidative damage. *Human and Experimental Toxicology*, 30:1359–1368.

Steinmüller, N., Sonder, K., Kroschel, J., 2002. Fodder tree research with *Moringa stenopetala*—A daily leafy vegetable of Konso people, Ethiopia. Available at: http://www.tropentag.de/2002/proceedings/node62.html (Accessed on July 15, 2017).

Stevens, G.C., Baiyeri, K.P., Akinnagbe, O., 2013. Ethnomedicinal and culinary uses of *Moringa oleifera* Lam. Nigeria. *Journal of Medicinal Plants Research*, 7(13):799–804.

Sudha, P., Asdaq, S.M., Dhamingi, S.S., Chandrakala, G.K., 2010. Immunomodulatory activity of methanolic leaf extract of *Moringa oleifera* in animals. *Indian Journal of Physiology and Pharmacology*, 54:133–140.

Teixeira, E.M.B., Carvalho, M.R.B., Neves, V.A., Silva, M.A., Arantes-Pereira, L., 2014. Chemical characteristics and fractionation of proteins from *Moringa oleifera* Lam. leaves. *Food Chemistry*, 147:51–54.

Toma, A., Makonnen, E., Mekonnen, Y., Debella, A., Adis Akwattana, S., 2015. Antidiabetic activities of aqueous ethanol and n-butanol fraction of *Moringa stenopetala* leaves in streptozotocin-induced diabetic rats. *BMC Complementary and Alternative Medicine*. Available at: http://www.bmc.complementaryalternmed.biomedcentral.com. (Accessed on July 16, 2017).

Tsaknis, J., and Lalas, S. 2002. Stability during frying of *Moringa oleifera* seed oil variety "Periyakulam 1". *Journal of Food Composition and Analysis*, 15(1):79–101.

Tsaknis, J., Lalas, S., Gergis, V., Douroglou, V., Spiliotis, V., 1999. Characterization of *Moringa oleifera* variety Mbololo seed oil of Kenya. *Journal of Agriculture and Food Chemistry*, 47:4495–4499.

Verma, A.R., Vijayakumar, M., Mathela, C.S., Rao, C.V., 2009. In vitro and in vivo antioxidant properties of different fractions of *Moringa oleifera* leaves. *Food Chemistry and Toxicology*, 47:2196–2201.

Vongsak, B., Sithisarn, P., Mangmool, S., Thongpraditchote, S., Wongkrajang, Y., Gritsanapan, W., 2013. Maximizing total phenolics, total flavonoids contents and antioxidant activity of *Moringa oleifera* leaf extract by the appropriate extraction method. *Indian Crop Production*, 44:566–571.

Waterman, C., Cheng, D.M., Rojas-Silva, P., Poulev, A., Dreifus, J., Lila, M.A., Raskin, I., 2014. Stable, water extractable isothiocyanates from *Moringa oleifera* leaves attenuate inflammation *in vitro*. *Phytochemistry*, 103:114–122.

Waterman, C., Rojas-Silva, P., Tumer, T., Kuhn, P., Richard, A.J., Wicks, S., Stephens, J.M., Wang, Z., Mynatt, R., Cefalu, W., 2015. Isothiocyanate-rich *Moringa oleifera* extract reduces weight gain, insulin resistance and hepatic gluconeogenesis in mice. *Molecular Nutrition Food Research*, 59(6): 1013–1024.

World Health Organization, 2017. Available at: http://www.who.int/water_sanitation_health/ (Accessed on July 17 and 18, 2017).

Yassa, H.D., and Tohamy, A.F., 2014. Extract of *Moringa oleifera* leaves ameliorates streptozotocin-induced diabetes mellitus in adult rats. *Acta Histochemistry*, 116:844–854.

# CHAPTER 10

# African Traditional Medicine
## *The Way Forward*

**Kofi Busia**

### CONTENTS

## 10.1 INTRODUCTION

Traditional medicine involves health practices, approaches, knowledge, and beliefs incorporating plant-, animal-, and mineral-based medicines, spiritual therapies, and manual techniques and exercises, applied singularly or in combination, to treat, diagnose, and prevent illnesses or maintain well-being. By the broad definition of the World Health Organization (WHO), traditional medicine is "the sum total of the knowledge, skills and practices based on the theories, beliefs and experiences indigenous to different cultures, whether explicable or not, used in the maintenance of health, as well as in the prevention, diagnosis, improvement or treatment of physical and mental illnesses" (WHO, 1978).

African traditional medicine is the oldest, and perhaps the most diverse of all the world's indigenous medical systems. This is based on the premise that Africa is the cradle of human civilization with a rich biological and cultural diversity marked by regional differences in healing practices (Gurib-Fakim, 2006).

Several types of African traditional medicine are practiced in the region, although not all of them are recognized by communities and governments. Examples of African traditional medicine practices that are recognized by almost all communities in the African region include general traditional health services, traditional midwifery, bone setting and mental health care, while those that are not often recognized by all communities and governments include divination and circumcision (Mhame et al., 2010).

African traditional practitioners include herbalists, traditional birth attendants, bone setters, diviners, traditional surgeons, and spiritualists (Trease and Evans, 2002), who are variously described as *Babalawo*, *Adahunse*, or *Oniseegun* among the Yoruba-speaking people of Nigeria; Marabou in Senegal, and many parts of French-speaking West Africa and Odunseni among the Akans of Ghana. Among the Igbos of Nigeria they are known as the *Dibia*; the Hausas call them *Boka*, while in South Africa *Sangoma* or *Nyanga* are the terms used (Cook, 2009). They are highly respected in their communities, and are therefore consulted for the treatment of a wide variety of diseases ranging from simple bruises to chronic conditions such as cancer, diabetes, and hypertension.

African traditional medicine is characteristically holistic with the body and spirit considered as an integral unit, and disease, good health, success or failure are believed to be the products of the actions of individuals and ancestral spirits (Helwig, 2010). It is generally believed that displeasure of the gods or God due to a breach of a universal moral code by a person, family, or village has the potential to trigger an illness (Onwuanibe, 1979). In administering treatment, the healers attempt to reconnect the social and emotional equilibrium of patients based on community rules and relationships (Hillenbrand, 2006). The healing practices involve considerable mysticism and secrecy (Twumasi, 1975). The practitioners use a range of treatment approaches including "magic," fasting, dieting, bathing, massaging, herbs, and certain surgical procedures (Conserve Africa Foundation, 2010). This approach to medical care has its roots in Egyptian medicine (Porter, 1997). Before prescribing medicines, African traditional healers typically make their diagnosis through incantations, which are believed to help establish mystical and cosmic connections. However, in cases where the illness cannot be identified, the patient may be advised to consult a diviner who can make the diagnosis by establishing contact with the spirit world through a process whereby objects are thrown and the patterns in which they fall are given metaphysical interpretations. The process of divination often requires not only medication, but also sacrifices (Onwuanibe, 1979). Diagnosis may also involve confessions with the aim of extracting vital information, as it is done in some religions (Heinrich et al., 2004). Treatment will be prescribed according to the seriousness of the condition and often involves a combination of herbal therapy, incantations, rituals, and sacrifices (Heinrich et al., 2004). As part of the treatment regimen, healers will typically address possible psychological causes such as effects of breakdown in relationships with friends and family, or neighbors, or work colleagues, the guilt of immorality, as well as violation of religious codes and cultural taboos. In some cases, the method of "bleed-cupping" was used to treat conditions such as migraines, coughs, abscesses, and pleurisy, followed by application of an herbal ointment and oral intake of herbal medicines. In some cultures, headaches are treated by rubbing hot herbal ointment across a patient's eyelids, while malaria is treated with both oral intake of herbal mixtures and steam inhalations, and vomiting is induced with herbal emetics. In the Bight of Benin, gout and rheumatism are treated with the fat of a boa constrictor (Onwuanibe, 1979; Gurib-Fakim, 2006; Gurib-Fakim et al., 2010; Gurib-Fakim and Mahomoodally, 2013). Thus, in many African communities, traditional healers often act, in part, as intermediaries between the visible and invisible worlds, between the living and the dead with a view to establishing harmony between the sick person and the ancestors.

## 10.2 HISTORY OF AFRICAN TRADITIONAL MEDICINE

The history of traditional medicine in Africa dates back to about 3200 BC, when King Menes became the first Pharaoh of ancient Egypt. During this period, medical knowledge was recorded in the form of wall paintings in tombs and on papyrus. The Ebers Papyrus, which dates back to around 1500 BC, was the most notable of these documents, and is reputed to be the oldest surviving medical document. It contained information on diagnosis and treatment methods as well as medicinal plants including aloe, cannabis, cassia, castor oil, frankincense, fennel, henna, juniper, linseed, myrrh, opium, senna, and thyme. Ancient Egyptians were known to be voracious consumers of garlic and onions, as they believed the two herbs had the ability to promote survival (Patrick et al., 2009). Imhotep, who lived about 2980 BC during the reign of Pharaoh Zosar of the Third Dynasty, and is credited with the title of first African physician in a scientific sense (Porter, 1997; Mungwini, 2009), treated his patients by making them sleep overnight in the inner precincts of the temples so they would be cured through dream experiences with a god, or an emissary such as a snake (Porter, 1997).

In ancient Egypt, good health was linked with proper diet and lifestyle as well as the maintenance of peaceful relationships with the gods, spirits, and the dead, while illness was believed to be the result of imbalance, which could be restored to equilibrium by supplication, spells, and rituals (Porter, 1997). The Egyptians believed that humans were born healthy, and that both earthly and supernatural forces, particularly evil spirits, could invade the body through the orifices to consume vital tissues and organs and cause disorders (Porter, 1997). However, Egyptian medicine was not entirely superstitious or magical. Indeed, Egyptians were advanced medical practitioners and had great expertise in human anatomy and many other medical disciplines due to their skills in mummification (Aboelsoud, 2010) and also through their interaction with the Greeks and other cultures.

Ancient Egyptians also practiced massage and manipulation, but also made extensive use of medicinal plants and foods (Aboelsoud, 2010). Records show that there was a high degree of specialization among Egyptian physicians (Halioua et al., 2005; Aboelsoud, 2010). For example, surgery was well advanced, although it was limited to repairing injuries and bone fractures. In terms of workings of the human body, the Egyptians believed that human life was contained in breath, and a speculative vascular network that was likened to the Nile and its canals. Good health could only be achieved if this vascular network was kept free of obstructions, which may be undigested food and feces. For this reason, the Egyptians were reputed to set aside 3 days each month for purging (Porter, 1997) with remedies such as senna, colocynth, and castor oil.

Ancient Egyptians were also skilled in pharmacy. Medications were administered while reciting certain incantations. Herbs such as aloe, caraway, castor, cumin, glue, fennel, linseed oil, pomegranates, and safflower were all used. Remedies were also made from mineral substances including copper salts, plain salt, and lead as well as eggs, liver, hairs, milk, animal horns and fat, honey, and wax (Rosen, 1979; Aboelsoud, 2010). The Egyptians also used honey and grease in many wound treatments, while breast milk was sometimes given as an antiviral against the common cold (Sauneron, 1958; Aboelsoud, 2010).

Contrary to the widespread belief that African traditional medicine is mystic, superstitious, and demonic rather than scientific, some evidence suggests that the practitioners were probably aware of the natural causes of illness (Oke, 1995; Erinosho, 1998, 2005, 2006). For example, in sub-Saharan Africa, the ancient kingdoms and empires of Asante, Benin, Borno, Ethiopia, Jukun, Monomotapa and Mali, Nubia, Nri, Nupe, Oyo, and Songhai had remarkably codified healing recipes (Mungwini, 2009), which prominently featured medicinal plants as key components. Indeed, the folkloric claims of a number of these plants have been scientifically validated, possible evidence that they were used not only for their spiritual and symbolic significance, but also for their perceived "pharmacological" effects. Notable among these plants include *Acacia senega* (Gum Arabic), *Agathosma betulina* (Buchu), *Aloe ferox* (Cape Aloes), *Aloe vera* (North African Aloes), *Artemisia afra* (African wormwood), *Boswellia sacra* (Frankincense), *Commiphora myrrha* (Myrrh), *Harpagophytum procumbens* (Devil's Claw), *Hibiscus sabdariffa* (Hibiscus, Roselle), *Hypoxis hemerocallidea* (African potato), *Prunus africana* (African Cherry), and *Catharanthus roseus* (Rosy Periwinkle) (Sofowora 1993; Hostettmann et al., 2000).

As in conventional medicine, herbal medications have different routes of administration, the most common being oral, nasal, rectal, or topical. However, in some cases such medications may be worn as amulets, necklaces, or talismans around the waist or ankles, while others may also be hanged on doors and windows or placed under a mat or pillow or some obscure place in the house to ward off spirits (Heinrich et al., 2004).

Africans have also been known to practice a traditional form of inoculation against diseases such as yaws and smallpox, whereby the disease is transferred "from arm to arm," using a thorn to scratch material from the pustule of a smallpox-infected patient, and rubbing it into the skin of uninfected persons (Herbert, 1975; Schneider, 2009).

Thus, prior to the introduction of modern medicine, traditional medicine was the only source of health care available to the vast majority of Africans (Romero-Daza, 2002). African traditional health knowledge has spread across the world, into many cultures, maintaining a unique and distinctive character. In more recent years, African traditional medicine has been successfully integrated into Western healthcare delivery systems, especially for HIV/AIDS, malaria, tuberculosis, and other infectious and chronic diseases. Unfortunately, the healing practices and materia medica of the time were not documented (WHO, 1978; Harley, 1941).

## 10.3 INFLUENCE OF EUROPEAN COLONIAL RULE

The advent of European colonial rule on the African continent in the nineteenth century marked a significant turning point in the history of African traditional medicine. The Witchcraft Suppression Ordinance of 1896 enacted in Great Britain, which criminalized the "witch-doctor," was also enacted in the British colonies with similar consequences. In some countries, African traditional medicine practices were thought to be associated with "witchcraft," "backwardness," and "superstition," and were therefore outrightly banned. The result was that the practitioners lost much of their authority over communal affairs, although their knowledge survived through informal transmission to trusted members of the family.

Besides the attempts made to suppress African traditional medicine, its decline was also instigated by the influence of "Western" culture, which had conventional medicine as a key component. As the colonial authorities sought to expand "modern" health services with the establishment of medical and nursing schools, hospitals, and other health facilities, the populations gradually rejected their indigenous medicine in favor of this "refined" system of health care. In addition, the introduction of Christianity, which sought to purge Africans of what was considered to be demonic belief systems, contributed to the gradual demise of African traditional medicine. The problem was further compounded by the emergence of a new African elite, which adopted European cultural practices to the neglect of their own (Guthrie, 1951; Okere, 1983; Mungwini, 2009).

The suppression of African traditional medicine continued even after independence, leading to protests and agitations in some countries (Erinosho, 1998, 2006). However, with the realization that African traditional medicine was an integral part of African culture, and had the potential to contribute meaningfully to health-care delivery in many countries (WHO, 2001), attitudes began to change, especially after the Alma Ata Declaration (WHO, 1978) that called on WHO member states to incorporate traditional medicine in their national health systems.

In spite of the negative attitudes shown toward traditional medicine in Africa that have contributed largely to its neglect (Feierman, 2002), it still enjoys a high degree of patronage. Indeed, in certain African countries, up to 90% of the population still relies exclusively on plants for their health-care needs (Okigbo and Mmeka, 2006). For example, in Ghana, Mali, Nigeria, and Zambia, herbal medicines are routinely used as the first line of treatment for 60% of children with malaria-induced high fever (WHO, 2002a, b; Busia and Kasilo, 2010; Kasilo et al., 2010a, b). In Burkina Faso, there is an increasing demand for traditional medicine for the treatment of rheumatic and neurological complaints (Carpentier et al., 1995), and in Ghana, about 70% of the population depends primarily on traditional medicine (Roberts, 2001). In rural Tanzania, traditional medicine is used to treat convulsion, which is locally referred to as "*degedege*" (Makundi et al., 2006). There are also reports that the vast majority of South Africans use traditional medicine to treat a variety of ailments (Mander et al.,

2007; Lekotjolo, 2009). In some instances, patients use traditional medicine simultaneously with modern medicine, especially in the management of chronic disorders, such as hypertension (Amira and Okubadejo, 2007).

## 10.4 REASONS FOR THE UPSURGE OF INTEREST IN TRADITIONAL MEDICINE

Globally, there is now a general recognition that traditional medicines, the medicines once described as primitive, could be mankind's saving grace—and, therefore, within the past three decades, the changing view of herbs in particular, as medicines moved from that of "witches brew" to major medicine (Busia, 2005).

Several factors have contributed to the growing recognition of traditional medicine worldwide. It has been shown that traditional medicines, especially herbal medicines, have promising therapeutic potential, which can be exploited for the management of a wide range of diseases, which may not respond well to conventional treatments. For example, some herbal medicines are known to be effective for the treatment of diseases such as malaria and/or HIV/AIDS, which disproportionately affect Africans more than other races (Mander et al., 2007). Plants have also been found to be sources of some useful compounds that can be used therapeutically or as leads for the synthesis of essential medicines. Table 10.1 provides examples of some phytomedicines of African origin that are available on the international market (Lai and Roy, 2004; Falodun et al., 2005; Falodun and Usifoh, 2006; Tapsell et al., 2006).

Traditional medicine holds enormous economic potential, which can be harnessed to alleviate poverty, especially in developing countries such as Africa. The global market for herbal medicines, which currently stands at over US$60 billion annually, is growing steadily. In South Africa, traditional medicine (TM) is reported to have contributed as much as R2.9 billion to the economy (Mander et al., 2007). In China, traditional herbal preparations account for 30%–50% of the total medicines consumption, with sales revenue from traditional Chinese medicines in 2005 totaling $14 billion, a 23.8% increase over the previous year. Annual revenues in Western Europe reached US$5 billion in 2003–2004, while the sales of products totaled US$160 million in Brazil in 2007. According to a report published in HerbalGram, sales of herbal dietary supplements in the United States in 2008 reached $4.8 billion. In the United Kingdom, annual expenditure on alternative medicine is US$230 million. A South Australian study showed that in 2000, Australians spent $2.3 billion on alternative therapies, a 62% increase since 1993 (MacLennan et al., 1996, 2002; Bensoussan, 1999). In 1996, about 2.8 million traditional Chinese medicine consultations were reported in Australia. This represented an annual turnover of about 84 million Australian dollars (WHO, 2000). In addition, various reports indicate that in San Francisco, London, and South Africa, 75% of people living with HIV/AIDS seek alternative forms of medicines for treatment. In Germany, 90% of people take a natural remedy at some point in their life (Boon, 2002; Stange et al., 2008; Chinsembu and Hedimbi, 2010; Mbeh et al., 2010; Shim et al., 2011). In China, traditional preparations from plants represent 30%–50% of total medicine consumption (WIPO,

Table 10.1   Examples of Phytomedicines on the International Market

| Plant Species | Action | Constituents | Countries |
|---|---|---|---|
| Ancistrocladus abbreviatus | Anti-HIV | Michellamine B | Cameroon and Ghana |
| Corynanthe pachyceras | Male stimulant | Corynanthidine, corynanthine, yohimbine | Ghana |
| Tamarindus indica | Insecticides | Pectins | Egypt |
| Rauvolfia vomitoria | Tranquilizer and antihypertensive | Reserpine, yohimbine | Nigeria, Zaire, Rwanda, Mozambique |
| Cinchona succirubra | Antimalarial | Quinine | West African countries |
| Syzigium aromaticum | Dental remedy | Eugenol, terpenoids | East African countries, Madagascar |
| Agava sisalana | Oral contraceptives | Corticosteroids Hecogenin | Tanzania |
| Physostigma venenosum | Opthalmia | Physostigimine (eserine) | Calabar (Nigeria), Ghana, Cote d'Ivoire |
| Prunus africana | Prostate gland hypertrophy | Sterols, triterpenes, n-docosanol | Cameroon, Kenya, Madagascar |
| Catharanthus roseus | Antileukemia and Hodgkin's disease | Triterpenoids, tannins, and alkaloids | Madagascar |
| Zingiber officinale | Anti-inflammatory, circulatory stimulant, carminative | Gingerol, zingibrene | Nigeria |
| Chrysanthemum cinerariifolium | Insecticides | Pyrethrins | Ghana, Kenya, Rwanda, Tanzania, South Africa |

Source: Adapted from Okigbo, R.N., and Mmeka, E.C. 2006. *KMITL Science and Technology Journal*, 6(2):83–94. Abiodun et al. (2007), Falodun (2010), Hostettmann and Marston (2002), Olaniyi (2005), Sofowora (1992), WHO (1977).

2001), and in Australia, government surveys show that 42% of the people report using complementary and alternative medicine (CAM) treatments (Bensoussan, 1999). It has also been reported that between 1959 and 1980, of all the medical prescriptions dispensed from community pharmacies in the United States, 25% contained plant extracts or active ingredients derived from higher plants. Moreover, about 119 chemical substances derived from 90 plant species often through plant-based bioactivity-guided fractionation studies, are important medicines currently in use in one or more countries (Farnsworth et al., 1985).

Furthermore, limited access to modern medicines and drugs to treat and manage diseases in middle- and low-income countries, especially in Africa, may have contributed to the widespread use of TM in these regions, especially in poor households. In a recent study by the WHO and Health Action International (HAI) in 36 low- and middle-income countries, drugs were reportedly way beyond the reach of large sections of the populations (Cameron et al., 2008).

Other important factors that have influenced the growing popularity of TM are the lack of effective treatments for many diseases (e.g., age-related disorders, such as coronary heart disease, strokes, parkinsonism, and cancers), side effects associated with many conventional medicines, limited modern health-care facilities, and shortage of health professionals in some countries. For example, in Ghana, the ratio of traditional medicine practitioners (TMPs) to the population is estimated at 1:200, whereas that of medical doctors to the population is 1:20,000. In Nigeria the ratio of TMPs to the population is estimated at 1:110 in Benin City and that of medical doctors at 1:16,400 (WHO, 2003, 2006) (Figure 10.1).

Indeed, the majority of medical doctors available in Africa are concentrated in urban areas and cities at the expense of rural areas. Therefore, for millions of people in rural areas, native healers remain the most easily accessible and affordable health resource available to the local community and at times the only therapy that subsists.

Another often-ignored, but important factor for the widespread use of TM in Africa is the belief systems of the people. TM provides an avenue through which the diverse cultural heritages of Africans are preserved and respected (Owumi, 2002). TM is sought when the population's health conditions respond poorly to orthodox treatment, or carry the burden of stigma, or are thought to have resulted from supernatural causes (Izugbara et al., 2005; Okigbo and Mmeka, 2006).

Nevertheless, in developed countries, the resurgence of interest in TM is due to factors other than accessibility, affordability, and cultural compatibility. The WHO (2002a, b) reported that anxiety about the adverse effects of chemical drugs, improved access to health information, changing values, increased cases of chronic diseases, and reduced tolerance of paternalism are some of the factors responsible for the growing demand for CAM in developed countries (Thorne et al., 2002).

In view of the growing demand for African TM, there have been calls for its integration into the national health systems to improve access to quality health care (Obute, 2005; Erinosho, 2006; Okigbo and Mmeka, 2006). It is generally believed that integrating TM into mainstream health care will enhance quality of care and

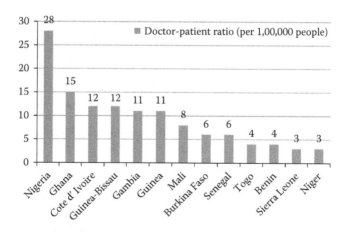

**Figure 10.1**  Doctor-patient ratio (per 1,00,000 people) in ECOWAS. (Adapted from WHO, 2006). Doctor to patient ratio in Africa. Available at: http://hdr.undp.org/hdr2006/statistics/indicators/58.html [Accessed on July 25, 2014].)

also make primary health care readily available and affordable to the populations (Obute, 2005). Nevertheless, the lingering mistrust between practitioners of conventional and traditional medicine in Africa has continuously hampered and thwarted the process of integration and efforts to promote collaboration between the practitioners of traditional and conventional medicine (Nevin, 2001; Ebomoyi, 2009).

## 10.5 CHALLENGES

With about 80% of Africans known to patronize TM, and credible reports indicating that in countries such as Ghana, Mali, and Nigeria, 60% of cases of malaria-induced fever in children are treated with herbal medicines, the importance of TM in primary health care in the subregion cannot be overemphasized. Many African governments recognize the need to promote the sector to improve access to quality health care for the people, but the issue of funding remains a major stumbling block. Having made the provision of modern health-care services a priority, it is a huge challenge for any government to have adequate resources to develop its TM sector. The TM sector is therefore hugely underfunded, resulting in a proliferation of quacks with doubtful abilities and intentions preying on the vulnerabilities of the people.

Efforts to promote African TM are hampered by the absence of national policies and regulatory frameworks; lack of appropriate mechanisms and approaches to control safety, efficacy, and quality of TM products; low-technological methods of preparation and poor manufacturing practices; inadequate support for TM research and development; lack of preservation and protection of indigenous knowledge and biodiversity; poor/absent conservation methods resulting in high rates of deforestation; and lack of training/education programs and licensing practice for qualified TMPs.

In addition, the general belief among orthodox medicine practitioners that TM practices have not or cannot be scientifically validated remains a very serious challenge. While it is true that subjecting the metaphysical aspects of African TM to conventional scientific studies can be a challenge, that the physical aspects of African TM can be scientifically studied and analyzed is not in doubt (Oyelakin, 2009). As mentioned earlier, several scientific studies have validated the ethnomedical uses of many African plants. It has also been argued that given the inherent epistemological and ideological differences between African traditional medicine and conventional medicine, it is difficult to use orthodox scientific methods to determine the efficacy and effectiveness of TM. It is feared that if African TM is integrated into the modern medical system, it would erode its identity and integrity and further justify and promote the "supremacy" or "superiority" of conventional medicine. For this reason, it has been suggested that African TM can be better developed if it is allowed to operate, develop, and flourish independent of conventional medicine (Konadu, 2008; Oyelakin, 2009).

Another fundamental challenge to the development of African TM is the widespread proliferation of quacks, although this is not limited to TM practice. This situation is due in part to the prevailing, weak regulatory regime and also to the perennial mass unemployment characteristic of many African countries. According to Pretorius (1999), "in the current economic climate and amid the concomitant unemployment, there is a marked increase in the ranks of traditional healers, among whom there are, unfortunately, quite a number of charlatans." Moreover, the influence of Western religion, education, urbanization, and globalization (Feierman, 2002) has led to a "passionate ambivalence" toward African TM among some segments of the African population, particularly the educated elite (Kiringe, 2005; Teshome-Bahiru, 2006). These challenges have led to calls for more education and training and stricter regulatory controls to foster consumer confidence.

It is also worthy of note that research and development of herbal medicines is often constrained by the relatively smaller quantities of biologically active ingredients they contain, which makes large-scale production and commercialization extremely difficult. For this reason, the pharmaceutical industry would prefer total synthesis from sources that would provide higher yields or from structural analogues that frequently have more pharmacological activity than the parent compound (Ekong, 1986; Nworgu et al., 2007).

The use of herbal medicines also carries with it the potential for drug-herbal interactions or herbal-herbal interactions, which may arise from concomitant intake of drugs and herbal medicines, the use of herbal medicines for different ailments, and the multicomponent nature of herbal preparations. These interactions could be pharmacological, chemical, or biochemical in nature.

Several biochemical and pharmacological mechanisms are involved in the metabolism of herbal medicines, which elicit body responses. In the metabolism of drugs, the initial elimination route, known as presystemic "first-pass" metabolism, involves the small intestine, the portal vein, and the liver. First-pass metabolic degradation often determines the peak and mean concentrations of an ingested drug, food supplement, or herbal medicine. Drugs such as terfenadine (an antihistamine formerly used for the treatment of allergic conditions), requires 100% presystemic, first-pass metabolism to convert it to its active and less toxic metabolite, terfenadine carboxylate. Like many other drugs and herbs, the metabolism and bioactivation of terfenadine involve oxidation by the cytochrome P450 microsomal enzyme system (Strandell et al., 2004; Chaudhary and Willett, 2006; Guengerich, 2008; Drugs.com, 2012). It has been shown that some natural bioactive compounds from plants and certain drugs could inhibit the enteric cytochrome P450 3A4 isozyme and produce toxic effects. For example, drugs such as erythromycin and ketoconazole, or foods such as grapefruit juice that inhibit or compete with these enzymes, will partially or completely block the metabolism of terfenadine and result in the absorption of unmetabolized terfenadine, with the potential for very serious toxic reactions including cardiac arrest and death (Bailey and Dresser, 2004; Drugs. com, 2012).

Another issue of great concern is the adulteration of some herbal medicines with orthodox medications to enhance their efficacy. Some adulterated herbal preparations have been reported to be the cause of kidney failure in some populations. A study by Lai et al. (2010), showed a dose-dependent association between consumption of aristolochic acid–containing Chinese herbal products and an increased risk of urinary tract cancer. Aristolochic acid is metabolized by the action of cytochrome P450 enzymes (Leoper et al., 1994; Lekechal et al., 1996; Fau et al., 1997). Adulterated products contaminated with potentially harmful ingredients such as heavy metals and toxins are occasionally encountered and withdrawn from the market (Parab et al., 2003; Ang, 2003; Ang et al., 2004; Ostrander et al., 2004).

## 10.6 THE WAY FORWARD

In response to these challenges, *vis-a-vis* the growing recognition of the contribution African TM can make to the attainment of the health-related provisions of the Millennium Development Goals (WHO, 1988), several African governments have taken steps to institutionalize it in their national health systems. Governments have identified certain priority interventions in the sector that have the potential to impact meaningfully on the health of the populations. These include the establishment of subregional associations of TMPs for efficient policy and program implementation; development of guidelines and standards of registration modalities for TMPs; development of an integrated program for training of TMPs and health personnel; protection of intellectual property rights (IPRs) and traditional medical knowledge; promotion of dialogue between TMPs and orthodox health personnel to enhance mutual trust and respect; promotion of research into traditional medicine, particularly herbal medicines; as well as promotion of conservation, local production, and cultivation of medicinal plants (Bannerman, 1983).

WHO established a Regional Expert Committee on traditional medicine in 2001 to put in place a regional mechanism for supporting countries to effectively monitor and evaluate progress made in the implementation of the traditional medicine strategy (Kasilo et al., 2010a, b). WHO also published tools for institutionalizing TM in health systems (WHO, 2005) and guidelines for the clinical evaluation of TMs (WHO, 2004) to facilitate development of national TM policies, regulatory frameworks for the practice of TM, and implementation plans, and to enhance research data on their safety, efficacy, and quality. WHO facilitated the exchange of country experiences and the dissemination and utilization of research results (WHO, 2004a,b,c), and they assessed the Centre for Scientific Research into Plant Medicine in Ghana (2007) and the Department of TM of the National Institute for Research in Public Health in Mali (2008) in view of their proposed designation as WHO Collaborating Centres in TM research. In 2008, the 61st World Health Assembly adopted a global strategy on public health, innovation, and intellectual property, which sets research priorities in TM, and whose effective implementation of this research agenda will go a long way toward improving access to medicines for the people of the African region.

It has become increasingly clear that promotion of rational TM practices and products can only be successful by identifying the safest and most effective therapies. For herbal medicines, this can be achieved through research and development (R&D) to isolate therapeutically active ingredients. R&D on higher medicinal plants have the potential to identify breakthrough chemical entities for treating several diseases for which there are no satisfactory therapies in modern medicine. Several countries are conducting research on TMs used for the treatment of malaria, HIV/ AIDS, diabetes, sickle cell anemia, and hypertension in order to produce evidence on safety, efficacy, and quality, and some have reported promising results. Such R&D activities can contribute meaningfully to health-care delivery on the continent and must be provided with the necessary financial, technical, and human resources to ensure their success (Chaudhury, 1992; Valiathan, 1998).

Collaboration among institutions of higher learning, industry, and government must be promoted in order to ensure that meaningful benefits can be realized from research on traditional knowledge and its application in science and technology.

As part of this R&D effort, the compilation of inventories of herbal medicines of proven efficacy and preparation of monographs on medicinal plants commonly used by the populations are being pursued in earnest. Countries such as Benin, Burkina Faso, Cameroon, Chad, Cote d'Ivoire, Gabon, Guinea, Madagascar, Mali, and Senegal are all engaged in these activities. However, only Ghana has published the second edition of its *National Herbal Pharmacopoeia* (GHP, 1992, 2007), while Nigeria printed a first edition (NHP, 2008). The West African Health Organization (WAHO) in collaboration with the WHO Regional Office for Africa has developed the first volume of a *West African Herbal Pharmacopoeia*. Governments could play a crucial role here by translating these activities into policies to ensure that adequate legal and regulatory mechanisms are established for promoting and maintaining good TM practices and products as well as equitable access and safety, efficacy, and quality. Besides emphasizing the strengths of TM, these policies should also underscore its limitations to highlight the fact that although TM has much to offer, it cannot always substitute for access to highly effective modern drugs and emergency measures that make such a critical difference between life and death for many people (WHO, 1998).

Another important area that deserves closer attention is the need to protect IPRs and traditional knowledge, to safeguard the TM sector from wanton exploitation. The African Union published the African Model Law for the protection of the rights of the local communities, farmers, and breeders and for the regulation of access to biological resources such as plants and animals (OAU Model Law, 1998). The AU also published the African Model Legislation for the Protection of the Rights of Land of Communities, Farmers, and Breeders and for the regulation of access to biological resources, including agricultural genetic resources and knowledge and technologies (Ekpere, 2000). Many African countries have yet to adopt this model legislation, but generally significant progress has been made. Also in the African Science and Technology Consolidated Plan of Action (2006), the importance of protecting and promoting indigenous knowledge and related technological innovations is emphasized. The document notes the disturbing lack of protection and promotion of indigenous knowledge in most African countries due to the weakness of the institutions to safeguard the rights of indigenous knowledge holders and also the lack of coordination between formal research and development institutions and local communities that hold and use traditional knowledge. In order to establish mechanisms to protect cultural rights and IPRs for countries to adapt to their specific situations,

WHO developed guidelines and a regulatory framework for the protection of traditional medical knowledge (Twarog and Kapoor, 2004), which are complementary to
the OAU Model Law (1998). Specialized training in this area is essential in achieving this goal. WHO and other regional institutions must continue to work in close
collaboration with organizations dealing with IPR issues, particularly the African
Union, the African Regional Intellectual Property Organization (ARIPO), and the
African Organization for Intellectual Property Rights (OAPI), to strengthen and provide formal training to traditional herbal practitioners.

Above all, promotion of TM can never succeed without proper training of the
practitioners and other key stakeholders. Unfortunately, to date many countries have
not taken this issue as seriously as they should, although West Africa appears to have
made some progress. The Kwame Nkrumah University of Science and Technology in
Kumasi, Ghana, established a bachelor of science degree in herbal medicine in 2001
to train medical herbalists, and Nigeria is in the process of introducing a similar
course in five of its medical schools. Elsewhere in Africa, Uganda (Traditional and
Modern Health Practitioners Together against AIDS and Other Diseases [THETA])
and the United Republic of Tanzania (Tanga AIDS Working Group [TAWG]) have
reported to have institutionalized training programs for THPs.

## 10.7 CONCLUSION

TM has gained public acceptance because of its accessibility, affordability,
and effectiveness, but the real challenge facing its development is lack of adequate
funding. This situation needs to be addressed if its potential is to be fully harnessed to help the countries meet the enormous health challenges of the twenty-
first century and beyond. Although the sector enjoys political goodwill in many
countries, it would need more than political goodwill to translate the many policy
orientations into tangible products. Overall, there is an urgent need to promote
more empirical research on how traditional medicine can be utilized to complement the modern medicine to improve access to quality health care for the African
people. Africa has immense potential in developing and repositioning itself in the
global knowledge economy. The challenges of repackaging traditional knowledge
can be turned into opportunities that will facilitate the rise of a new information-
driven economy.

The upsurge of herbal medicines in Africa has bright prospects, but the pace of
its development can be accelerated with promotional plans and government funding
for research and development, continuous education of the practitioners, support for
the local production of herbal medicines of proven efficacy, and establishment of an
enforceable regulatory framework.

As we traverse the second decade of the twenty-first century, African governments will have to take total responsibility for the health of their people. Institutions
such as the WHO or WAHO will obviously provide the needed financial and technical assistance, but in the end the key decisions to drive the sector will have to come
from the countries.

## REFERENCES

Abiodun, F., Igwe, A., Osahon, O., 2007. Anti-microbial evaluation of a herbal dental remedy stem bark of *Nauclea latifolia*-family Rubiaceae. *Journal of Applied Sciences*, 7:2696–2700.

Aboelsoud, N.H., 2010. Herbal medicine in ancient Egypt. *Journal of Medicinal Plants Research*, 4(2):082–086.

African Science and Technology Consolidated Plan of Action, 2006. NEPAD Office of Science and Technology, Lynnwood, Pretoria, South Africa. Available at: http://www.nepad.org/system/files/ast_cpa_2007.pdf (Accessed on July 29, 2014).

Amira, O.C., and Okubadejo, N.U., 2007. Frequency of complementary and alternative medicine utilization in hypertensive patients attending an urban tertiary care centre in Nigeria. *BMC Complementary and Alternative Medicine*, 7(30):1–5.

Ang, H.H., 2003. Analysis of lead content in herbal preparations in Malaysia. *Human and Experimental Toxicology*, 22:445–451.

Ang, H.H., Lee, E.L., Cheang, H.S., 2004. Determination of mercury by cold vapor atomic absorption spectrophotometer in Tongkat Ali preparations obtained in Malaysia. *International Journal of Toxicology*, 23:65–71.

Bailey, D.G., and Dresser, G.K., 2004. Interactions between grapefruit juice and cardiovascular drugs. *American Journal of Cardiovascular Drugs*, 4:281–297.

Bannerman, R.H., 1983. The role of traditional medicine in primary health care. In: R.H. Bannerman, J. Burterand, and Wen (Eds.), *Traditional Medicine and Health Care Coverage*. WHO, Geneva, Switzerland, pp. 318–327.

Bensoussan, A., 1999. Complementary medicine—Where lies its appeal? *Medical Journal of Australia*, 170:247–248.

Boon, H., 2002. Regulation of complementary/alternative medicine: A Canadian perspective. *Complementary Therapies in Medicine*, 10(1):14–19.

Busia, K., and Kasilo, O.M.J., 2010. Overview of traditional medicine in ECOWAS. *African Health Monitor, Special Issue*, 14:15–24.

Busia, K., 2005. Medical provision in Africa—Past and present. *Phytotherapy Research*, 19:919–923.

Cameron, A., Ewen, M., Ross-Degnan, D., Ball, D., Laing, R., 2008. *Medicine Prices, Availability, and Affordability in 36 Developing and Middle-Income Countries: A Secondary Analysis*. WHO, Geneva, Switzerland.

Carpentier, L., Prazuck, T., Vincent-Ballereau, F., Ouedraogo, L.T., Lafaix, C., 1995. Choice of traditional or modern treatment in West Burkina Faso. *World Health Forum*, 16:198–210.

Chaudhary, A., and Willett, K.L., 2006. Inhibition of human cytochrome CYP 1 enzymes by flavonoids of St. *John's wort. Toxicology*, 217:194–205.

Chaudhury, R.R., 1992. *Herbal Medicines for Human Health*. WHO-SEARO, New Delhi, India.

Chinsembu, K.C., and Hedimbi, M., 2010. An ethnobotanical survey of plants used to manage HIV/AIDS opportunistic infections in Katima Mulilo, Caprivi region, Namibia. *Journal of Ethnobiology and Ethnomedicine*, 6(25). doi:10.1186/1746-4269-6-25

Conserve Africa Foundation, 2010. *Medicinal Plants and Natural Products*. Conserve Africa Foundation. Available at: http://www.conserveafrica.org.uk/medicinal_plants.pdf (Accessed on May 5, 2014).

Cook, C.T., 2009. Sangomas: Problem or solution for South Africa's health care system. *Journal of the National Medical Association*, 101(3):261–265.

Drugs.com, 2012. Grapefruit juice and medicine may not mix. Available at: http://www.drugs.com/fda-consumer/grapefruit-juice-and-medicine-may-not-mix-208.html    (Accessed on July 25, 2014).

Ebomoyi, E.W., 2009. Genomics in traditional African healing and strategies to integrate traditional healers into western-type health care services—A retrospective study. *Researcher*, 1(6):69–79.

Ekong, D.E., 1986. Medicinal plants research in Nigeria: Retrospect and prospects. In: A. Sofowora (Ed.), *The State of Medicinal Plants Research in Nigeria*. Ibadan University Press, Nigeria, pp. 5–6.

Ekpere, J.A., 2000. *The OAU Model Law: The Protection of the Rights of Local Communities, Farmers, and Breeders, and for the Regulation of Access to Biological Resources—An Explanatory Booklet*. OAU/STRC, Lagos.

Erinosho, O.A., 1998. *Health Sociology for Universities, Colleges and Health Related Institutions*. Sam Bookman, Ibadan.

Erinosho, O.A., 2005. *Sociology for Medical, Nursing, and Allied Professions in Nigeria*. Bulwark Consult, Abuja.

Erinosho, O.A., 2006. *Health Sociology for Universities, Colleges and Health Related Institutions*. Bulwark Consult, Ibadan, Abuja.

Falodun, A., 2010. Herbal medicine in Africa—Distribution, standardization and prospects. *Research Journal of Phytochemistry*, 4:154–161.

Falodun, A., and Usifoh, C.O., 2006. Isolation and characterization of 3-carbomethoxypyridine from the leaves of *Pyrenacantha staudtii* (Hutch and Dalz). *Acta Poloniae Pharmaceutica Drug Research*, 63:235–237.

Falodun, A., Usifoh, C.O., and Nworgu, Z.A.M., 2005. Phytochemical and active column fractions of *Pyrenacantha staudtii* leaf extract on isolated rat uterus. *Pakistan Journal of Pharmaceutical Sciences*, 18:31–35.

Farnsworth, N.R., Akerele, O., Bingel, A.S., Soejarto, D.D., and Guo, Z.-G., 1985. Medicinal plants in therapy. *Bulletin WHO*, 63:965–981.

Fau, D., Lekchal, M., Farrell, G., Moreau, A., Moulis, C. et al., 1997. Diterpenoids from germander, an herbal medicine, induce apoptosis in isolated rat hepatocytes. *Gastroenterology*, 113:1334–1346.

Feierman, S., 2002. Traditional medicine in Africa: Colonial transformations. New York Academy of Medicine, March 13. Reported by Carter, GM, The Foundation for the Integrative AIDS Research.

Ghana Herbal Pharmacopoeia (GHP), 1992. The Advent Press, Accra, Ghana.

Ghana Herbal Pharmacopoeia (GHP), 2007. The Advent Press, Accra, Ghana.

Guengerich, F.P., 2008. Cytochrome p450 and chemical toxicology. *Chemical Research in Toxicology*, 21:70–83.

Gurib-Fakim, A., 2006. Medicinal plants: Traditions of yesterday and drugs of tomorrow. *Molecular Aspects of Medicine*, 27(1):1–93.

Gurib-Fakim, A., Brendler, T., Phillips, L.D., Eloff, L.N., 2010. *Green Gold—Success Stories Using Southern African Plant Species*. AAMPS Publishing, Mauritius.

Gurib-Fakim, A., and Mahomoodally, M.F., 2013. African flora as potential sources of medicinal plants: Towards the chemotherapy of major parasitic and other infectious diseases—A review. *Jordan Journal of Biological Sciences*, 6:77–84.

Guthrie, D., 1951. Observations on primitive medicine, with special reference to native African medicine. *Proceedings of the Royal Society of Medicine, Section of the History of Medicine*, 45.91–94.

Halioua, B., Ziskind, B., and DeBevoise, M.B., 2005. *Medicine in the Days of the Pharaohs.* Harvard University Press, Cambridge, MA.

Harley, G.W., 1941. *Native African Medicine, with Special Reference to Its Practice in the Mano Tribe of Liberia.* The Harvard University Press, Cambridge, MA.

Heinrich, M., Barnes, J., Gibbons, S., Williamson, E.M., 2004. *Fundamentals of Pharmacognosy and Phytotherapy.* Churchill Livingstone, Elsevier Ltd., London.

Helwig, D., 2010. Traditional African Medicine. Encyclopedia of Alternative Medicine. Available at: http://findarticles.com/p/articles/mig2603/is0007/ai2603000708/ (Accessed on May 5, 2014).

Herbert, E.W., 1975. Smallpox inoculation in Africa. *Journal of African History,* 16(4):539–559.

Hillenbrand, E., 2006. Improving traditional-conventional medicine collaboration: Perspectives from Cameroonian traditional practitioners. *Nordic Journal of African Studies,* 15(1):1–15.

Hostettmann, K., and Marston, A., 2002. Twenty years of research into medicinal plants: Results and perspectives. *Phytochemistry Review,* 1:275–285.

Hostettmann, K., Marston, A., Ndjoko, K., Wolfender, J.-L., 2000. The potential of African plants as a source of drugs. *Current Organic Chemistry,* 4:973–1010.

Izugbara, C.O., Etukudoh, I.W., Brown, A.S., 2005. Transethnic itineraries for ethnomedical therapies in Nigeria: Igbo women seeking Ibibio cures. *Health and Place,* 11:1–14.

Kasilo, O.M.J., Mawuli, K.-T., Busia, K., 2010a. Towards sustainable local production of medicines in the African Region. *African Health Monitor, Special Issue,* 14:80–98.

Kasilo, O.M.J., Trapsida, J.-M., Mwikisa, C.N., Lusamba-Dikassa, P.S., 2010b. An overview of the traditional medicine situation in the African Region. *African Health Monitor,* 3:7–15.

Kiringe, J.W., 2005. Ecological and anthropological threats to ethno-medicinal plant resources and their utilization in Maasai communal ranches in the Amboseli region of Kenya. *Ethnobotany Research and Applications,* 3:231–241.

Konadu, K., 2008. Medicine and anthropology in twentieth century Africa: Akan medicine and encounters with (medical) anthropology. *African Studies Quarterly,* 10(2&3). Available at: http://africa.ufl.edu/asq/v10/v10i2a3.htm (Accessed on July 31, 2014).

Lai, M.N., Wang, S.M., Chen, P.C., Chen, Y.Y., Wang, J.D., 2010. Population-based case–control study of Chinese herbal products containing aristolochic acid and urinary tract cancer risk. *Journal of the National Cancer Institute,* 102(3):179–186.

Lai, P.K., and Roy, J. 2004. Antimicrobial and chemopreventive properties of herbs and spices. *Current Medicinal Chemistry,* 11:1451–1460.

Lekechal, M., Pessayre, D., Lereau, J.M., Moulis, C., Fouraste, I., Fau, D., 1996. Hepatotoxicity of the herbal medicine germander: Metabolic activation of its furano diterpenoids by cytochrome P450 3A depletes cytoskeleton-associated protein thiols and forms plasma membrane blebs in rat hepatocytes. *Hepatology,* 24:212–218.

Lekotjolo, N., 2009. Wits starts training of first 100 Sangomas this year. *The Times.*

Leoper, J., Descatoire, V., Letteron, P., Moulis, C., Degott, P. et al., 1994. Hepatotoxicity of germander in mice. *Gastroenterology,* 106:464–472.

MacLennan, A.H., Wilson, D.H., Taylor, A.W., 1996. Prevalence and cost of alternative medicine in Australia. *Lancet,* 347:569–573.

MacLennan, A.H., Wilson, D.H., Taylor, A.W., 2002. The escalating cost and prevalence of alternative medicine. *Preventive Medicine,* 35:166–173.

Makundi, E.A., Malebo, H.M., Mhame, P., Kitua, A.Y., Warsame, M., 2006. Role of traditional healers in the management of severe malaria among children below five years of age: The case of Kilosa and Handeni Districts, Tanzania. *Malaria Journal,* 5(58):1–9.

Mander, M., Ntuli, L., Diederichs, N., Mavundla, K., 2007. Economics of the traditional medicine trade in South Africa. Available at: http://www.hst.org.za/uploads/files/chap13_07 (Accessed on August 21, 2013).

Mbeh, G.N., Edwards, R., Ngufor, G., Assah, F., Fezeu, L. et al., 2010. Traditional healers and diabetes: Results from a pilot project to train traditional healers to provide health education and appropriate health care practices for diabetes patients in Cameroon. *Global Health Promotion*, 17(2):17–26.

Mhame, P.P., Busia, K., Kasilo, O.M.J., 2010. Clinical practices of African traditional medicine. *African Health Monitor*, Issue 13. Available at: http://www.aho.afro.who.int/fr/ahm/issue/13/reports/clinical-practices-african-traditional-medicine (Accessed on July 31, 2014).

Mungwini, P., 2009. Down but not out: Critical insights in traditional Shona metaphysics. *Journal of Pan African Studies*, 2(9):177–196.

Nevin, T., 2001. Day of the Sangoma. *African Business*, 261:16–18.

NHP, 2008. *The Nigeria Herbal Pharmacopoeia*. Federal Ministry of Health, Abuja, Federal Republic of Nigeria.

Nworgu, Z.A.M., Falodun, A., Usifoh, C.O., 2007. Inhibitory activity of 3-carbomethoxypyridine and 3-carbobutoxypyridine on isolated rat uterus. *Acta Poloniae Pharmaceutica–Drug Research*, 64:179–182.

OAU Model Law, 1998. The OAU Model Law for the Protection of the Rights of Local Communities and the Regulations of Access to Biological Resources.

Obute, G.C., 2005. Ethnomedicinal plant resources of South Eastern Nigeria. Available at: http://www.siu.edu/~ebl/leaflets/-obute.htm (Accessed on September 18, 2009).

Oke, E.A., 1995. Traditional health services: An investigation of providers and the level and pattern of utilization among the Yoruba. *Ibadan Sociological Series*, 1:2–5.

Okere, T., 1983. *African Philosophy: A Historico Hemeneutical Investigation of the Conditions of Its Possibility*. University Press of America, New York.

Okigbo, R.N., and Mmeka, E.C., 2006. An appraisal of phytomedicine in Africa. *KMITL Science and Technology Journal*, 6(2):83–94.

Olaniyi, A.A., 2005. *Essential Medicinal Chemistry*. 3rd ed., Ibadan Shaneson CI Ltd., Ibadan, Nigeria, pp. 346–349.

Onwuanibe, R.C., 1979. The philosophy of African medical practice. *A Journal of Opinion (African Studies Association)*, 9(3):25–28.

Ostrander, G.K., Cheng, K.C., Wolf, J.C., Wolfe, M.J., 2004. Shark cartilage, cancer and the growing threat of pseudoscience. *Cancer Research*, 64:8485–8491.

Owumi, B.E., 2002. The political economy of maternal and child health in Africa. In: U.C. Isiugho-Abanihe, A.N. Isamah, and J.O. Adesina (Eds.), *Currents and Perspectives in Sociology*. Malthouse Press Limited, Ibadan, pp. 212–226.

Oyelakin, R.T., 2009. Yoruba traditional medicine and the challenge of integration. *Journal of Pan African Studies*, 3(3):73–90.

Parab, S., Kulkarni, R.A., Thatte, U., 2003. Heavy metals in herbal medicines. *Indian Journal of Gastroenterology*, 22:111–112.

Patrick, E.M., Armen, M., Gretchen, R.H., 2009. Ancient Egyptian herbal wines, PNAS website, quoted in the Article Study: Herbs added to 5,100-year-old Egyptian wine on the LD News website (Accessed on May 31, 2014).

Porter, R., 1997. *The Greatest Benefit to Mankind: A Medical History of Humanity from Antiquity to the Present*. Harper Collins, London, UK.

Pretorius, E., 1999. *South African Health Review*. 5th ed. Health Systems Trust. Traditional Healers, Durban, pp. 249–256.

Roberts, H., 2001. ACCRA: A way forward for mental health care in Ghana? *Lancet*, 357(9271):1859.

Romero-Daza, N., 2002. Traditional medicine in Africa. *Annals of the American Academy of Political and Social Science*, 583:173–176.

Rosen, G., 1979. *Journal of the History of Medicine and Allied Sciences*, Yale University, Department of the History of Medicine, Project Muse. H. Schuman.

Sauneron, S., 1958. Une recette égyptienne de collyre. *BIFAO*, 57:158.

Schneider, W.H., 2009. Smallpox in Africa during colonial rule. *Medical History*, 53(2):193–227.

Shim, J.M., Bodeker, G., Burford, G., 2011. Institutional heterogeneity in globalization: Co-development of western-allopathic medicine and traditional-alternative medicine. *International Sociology*, 26(6):769–788.

Sofowora, A., 1992. *Medicinal Plants and Traditional Medicine in Africa*. 24th edn., John Wiley and Sons, New York, p. 8.

Sofowora, A., 1993. *Medicinal Plants and Traditional Medicine in Africa*. 1st edn., John Wiley and Sons, Somerset, New Jersey, pp. 96–106.

Stange, R., Amhof, R., Moebus, S., 2008. Complementary and alternative medicine: Attitudes and patterns of use by German physicians in a national survey. *Journal of Alternative and Complementary Medicine*, 14(10):1255–1261.

Strandell, J., Neil, A., Carlin, G. 2004. An approach to the in vitro evaluation of potential for cytochrome p450 enzyme inhibition from herbals and other natural remedies. *Phytomedicine*, 11:98–104.

Tapsell, L.C., Hemphill, I., Cobiac, L., Patch C.S., Sullivan, D.R. et al., 2006. Health benefits of herbs and spices: The past, the present, the future. *Medical Journal of Australia*, 185:S4–S24.

Teshome-Bahiru, W., 2006. Impacts of urbanisation on the traditional medicine of Ethiopia. *Anthropologist*, 8(1):43–52.

Thorne, S., Paterson, B., Russell, C., Schultz, A., 2002. Complementary/alternative medicine in chronic illness as informed self-care decision making. *International Journal of Nursing Studies*, 39:671–683.

Trease, G.E., and Evans, W.C., 2002. *Pharmacognosy*. 15th ed. WB Saunders, London, UK.

Twarog, S., and Kapoor, P., 2004. *Protecting and Promoting Traditional Knowledge: Systems, National Experiences and International Dimensions*. United Nations Publications, New York and Geneva.

Twumasi, P.A., 1975. *Medicinal Systems in Ghana: A Study in Medicinal Sociology*. Ghana Publishing Company, Accra, Ghana, pp. 3–6.

Valiathan, M.S., 1998. Healing plants. *Current Sciences*, 75:1122.

WHO, 1977. *Resolution Promotion and Development of Training and Research in Traditional Medicine*. World Health Organization, Rome, Italy, p. 49.

WHO, 1978. Primary Health Care: Report on the International Conference on Primary Health care. Alma Ata, USSR. Available at: http://whqlibdoc.who.int/publications/9241800011.pdf (Accessed on July 31, 2014).

WHO, 1988. *Resolution WHA41.19 Traditional Medicine and Medicinal Plants*. Forty-First World Health Assembly, Geneva, Switzerland.

WHO, 1998. *Regulatory Situation of Herbal Medicines: A World Wide Review*. World Health Organization, Geneva, Switzerland.

WHO, 2000. *Traditional and Modern Medicine: Harmonising the two Approaches Western Pacific Region*. World Health Organization, Geneva, Switzerland.

WHO, 2001. *Legal Status of Traditional Medicine and Complementary/Alternative Medicine: A Worldwide Review*. World Health Organization, Geneva, Switzerland.

WHO, 2002a. *Traditional Medicine—Growing Needs and Potential*. World Health Organization, Geneva, Switzerland.

WHO, 2002b. *WHO Traditional Medicine Strategy 2002–2005*. World Health Organization, Geneva, Switzerland.

WHO, 2003. Traditional medicine: Our culture, our future. *African Health Monitor*, 4:1.

WHO, 2004. *Tools for Institutionalizing Traditional Medicine in Health Systems of Countries in the WHO African Region*. WHO Regional Office for Africa (WHO/AFRO/EDM/ TRM/2004.4).

WHO, 2004a. *Guidelines for Clinical Study of Traditional Medicines in WHO African Region*. WHO Regional Office for Africa, Brazzaville, Republic of the Congo (AFR/ TRM/04.4).

WHO, 2004b. *Final Report of Regional workshop on Research and Development of Traditional Medicine and Intellectual Property Rights held in Johannesburg*, South Africa, November 25–27. WHO Regional Office for Africa, Brazzaville, Republic of the Congo (AFR/TRM/04.2).

WHO, 2004c. *Pre-Clinical Safety Testing of TMs, Johannesburg, South Africa September*. WHO Regional Office for Africa, Brazzaville, Republic of the Congo (unpublished).

WHO, 2005. WHO Regional Expert Committee on Traditional Medicine. *Final Report of the Fourth Meeting*. Brazzaville, Republic of the Congo, November 16–19, 2004. WHO Regional Office for Africa, Brazzaville, Republic of the Congo (Document reference, AFR/ TRM.05.02).

WHO, 2006. Doctor to patient ratio in Africa. Available at: http://hdr.undp.org/hdr2006/ statistics/indicators/58.html (Accessed on July 25, 2014).

WIPO, 2001. Intellectual property needs and expectations of traditional knowledge holders, WIPO, Geneva, Switzerland.

# Index